Current Progress in Endoscopy

Current Progress in Endoscopy

Edited by Christoph Fox

hayle
medical

New York

Hayle Medical,
750 Third Avenue, 9ᵗʰ Floor,
New York, NY 10017, USA

Visit us on the World Wide Web at:
www.haylemedical.com

ISBN: 978-1-63241-581-3

Cataloging-in-Publication Data

Current progress in endoscopy / edited by Christoph Fox.
    p. cm.
Includes bibliographical references and index.
ISBN 978-1-63241-581-3
1. Endoscopy. 2. Diagnosis. 3. Endoscopic surgery. I. Fox, Christoph.
RC78.7.E5 C87 2019
616.075 45--dc23

Table of Contents

Preface

The purpose of the book is to provide a glimpse into the dynamics and to present opinions and studies of some of the scientists engaged in the development of new ideas in the field from very different standpoints. This book will prove useful to students and researchers owing to its high content quality.

An endoscopy is a medical diagnostic technique, which uses an endoscope to examine the interior of a cavity or a hollow organ in the body. A patient is either put under anesthesia or is fully conscious during the procedure. It is performed to investigate the conditions of the digestive system, diagnose conditions such as cancers, inflammation, anemia or bleeding, and also treat a bleeding vessel, a narrow esophagus, a polyp or a foreign object. Endoscopy can be done for the investigation of the gastrointestinal tract (GI tract), the respiratory tract, the female reproductive system, the urinary tract, ears and closed body cavities such as the abdominal or pelvic cavity. It is also performed during pregnancy, orthopedic surgery, plastic surgery, endodontic surgery, etc. This book contains some path-breaking studies in the domain of endoscopy. It outlines the processes and applications of endoscopy in detail. This book includes contributions of experts and scientists, which will provide innovative insights into this field.

At the end, I would like to appreciate all the efforts made by the authors in completing their chapters professionally. I express my deepest gratitude to all of them for contributing to this book by sharing their valuable works. A special thanks to my family and friends for their constant support in this journey.

Editor

Observation of the Pharynx to the Cervical Esophagus Using Transnasal Endoscopy with Blue Laser Imaging

Kenro Kawada, Tatsuyuki Kawano, Taro Sugimoto, Toshihiro Matsui, Masafumi Okuda, Taichi Ogo, Yuuichiro Kume, Yutaka Nakajima, Katsumasa Saito, Naoto Fujiwara, Tairo Ryotokuji, Yutaka Miyawaki, Yutaka Tokairin, Yasuaki Nakajima, Kagami Nagai and Takashi Ito

Abstract

Background In 2014, the new transnasal endoscopy with Blue laser Imaging (BLI) has been developed. Aim We present the usefulness of the observation of from the pharynx to the cervical esophagus using transnasal endoscopy with BLI. Patients and Methods This study was conducted between June 2014 and October 2014. During this period, 70 consecutive patients (60 men, 10 women; mean age 67.9 years old) with esophageal or head and neck cancer underwent endoscopic screening at the oropharynx and hypopharynx by transnasal endoscopy with BLI system We performed this endoscopic observation from oral cavity to pharynx before inserting into the cervical esophagus.The visibility of subsites of the hypopharynx and the orifice of the esophagus was evaluated. The extent of the view of hypopharyngeal opening was classified into 3 categories (excellent, good, poor). Then, the diagnostic accuracy of transnasal endoscopy with BLI system was estimated. Our screening is as follows. First, the patient is asked to bow their head deeply in the left lateral position. We put a hand on the back of the patient's head and push it forward. The patient is then asked to lift the chin as far as possible. In order to inspect the oral cavity, we insert an endoscope without a mouthpiece. After observation of the oral cavity, the endoscope was inserted through the nose. When the tip of the endoscope reached caudal to the uvula, the patient opened his mouth wide, stuck his tongue forward as much as possible and made a vocal sound like "ayyy". The endoscopist caused the endoscope to U-turn and observed the oropharynx, in particular the radix linguae (Intra-oropharyngeal U-turn method). For examination of the hypopharynx and the orifice of the esophagus, the patient is asked to blow hard and puff their cheeks while the mouth remains closed (Trumpet maneuver). Results 8 elderly cases were excluded because they could not perform the adequate ballooning. Finally, 62 cases were investigated. The ballooning the pyriform sinus and posterior wall not only allows accurate assessment of the stretched pharyngeal mucosa but also gives a view of postcricoid subsite and the orifice of the esophagus. The wide endoscopic view of the pharynx was obtained in a series of the procedures (excellent=53/62, 85.4%; good=7/52, 4.5%; and poor=2/62, 7.6%). Among 70 patients, 6 superficial lesions (8.6%) at the oropharynx(n=1) and hypopharynx (n=5) were discovered with BLI system. Mucosal redness, a pale thickened mucosa, white deposits or loss of a normal vascular pattern, well demarcated areas covered with scattered dots are important characteristics to diagnose superficial carcinoma. Conclusion The more progress achieved in transnasal endoscopy rapidly in the last few years, it can improve for observing the blind area using trans-oral endoscopy, therefore the trans-nasal endoscope will be a standard tool for the screening of the upper gastrointestinal tract in the near future.

Keywords: Transnasal endoscopy, Blue laser imaging, Superficial pharyngeal cancer

1. Introduction

According to the "field cancerization" concept [1], head and neck cancer, especially pharyngeal cancer, frequently coexist with esophageal cancer. Recently several reports [2, 3] have indicated the possibility of applying narrow-band imaging (NBI) endoscopy with magnification to improve the detection of superficial pharyngeal cancer. Compared with conventional endoscopy, NBI results in dramatic improvements in the rate detection of superficial lesions and significant enhancement in visualizing the microvascular structure of the mucosal surface [4]. The superiority of NBI was also recently demonstrated in a multicenter randomized controlled trial in Japan [5]. As more progress has been achieved in the field of endoscopy, the number of superficial cancers in the head and neck region has increased.

However, some areas are difficult to observe with transoral endoscopy. In particular, achieving circumferential observation of the hypopharyngeal mucosa is difficult during conventional endoscopy due to the anatomically closed field, effects of the pharyngeal reflex and accumulation of saliva. On conventional endoscopic screening, the physician usually inserts the endoscope from the left pyriform sinus of the hypopharynx to the cervical esophagus, with a blind space in the posterior wall and postcricoid subsite of the hypopharynx as well as radix linguae. Therefore, detecting early signs of cancer in the blind space is difficult for gastrointestinal endoscopists. On the other hand, transnasal endoscopy may be performed comfortably due to attenuation of the gag reflex. In Japan, the transnasal endoscopy is a very popular procedure and can be performed without sedation. It has also been reported that transnasal endoscopy may be performed less invasive with respect to the cardiopulmonary function [6,

7], and the technique is considered to be more comfortable for the patient than conventional endoscopy.

Since we developed the pharyngolaryngeal observation method using transnasal endoscopy in 2009, we have constantly evolved the procedure in order to better detect carcinoma in the head and neck at earlier stages in cases often coexistent with esophageal cancer. In 2014, a new transnasal endoscopy device with Blue laser Imaging (BLI) was developed. The pharynx is the orifice of the gastrointestinal tract. In this article, we present the usefulness of observing the pharynx to the cervical esophagus using transnasal endoscopy with BLI.

2. Simple questionnaire

A complete medical history, including demographic and clinical data, was obtained prior to the endoscopy procedure. Selected patients constituting a high-risk group for pharyngeal carcinoma are beneficial targets of endoscopic surveillance. Epidemiological studies have detected several strong predictors for identifying persons at high risk for pharyngeal and esophageal squamous cell carcinomas. For example, alcohol drinking and tobacco smoking synergistically increase the risk of both cancers [8, 9], as does a reduced intake of greenish-yellow vegetables and fruits [10] and a low body mass index [11]. The presence of distinct esophageal iodine-unstained lesions and melanosis is also associated with a risk of cancer [12, 13], and alcohol consumption combined with inactive aldehyde dehydrogenase-2 (ALDH2) and less active alcohol dehydrogenase (ADH1B) enhances cancer risks in a multiplicative fashion [14, 15]. The detection of an enlarged mean corpuscular volume (MCV) [16], as induced by heavy drinking or smoking, a high level of acetaldehyde exposure, and/or poor nutrition, may be useful for identifying high-risk persons.

The results of a simple flushing questionnaire have been reported to predict the ALDH2 phenotype with a high accuracy [17].

3. Preparation

Transnasal endoscopy was performed without sedation. Prior to commencement of the procedure, each nasal cavity was sprayed with 0.05% naphazoline nitrate to induce vasocon-striction, followed by premedication with 100 mg of dimethylpolysiloxane and 10 000 U of pronase, with sodium bicarbonate to remove mucus and foam in the stomach. Nasal anesthesia was started by spraying a solution of 4% lidocaine into the nostril for three minutes, after which a swab covered with 8 % lidocaine spray was inserted into the deeper nasal cavity for two minutes. The patient was then placed in the lateral decubitus position to receive endoscopy. Antispasmodics such as scopolamine were not used for premedication.

3.1. Equipment

Recently, we applied a new transnasal esophagogastroduodenoscopy (EGD) device [EG-L580NW, Fuji Film, Tokyo, Japan] with the LASEREO system (a video processor (VP-4450:

FUJIFILM Co. Tokyo) including a light source (LL-4450; FUJIFILM Co. Tokyo)) under modification of the endoscopic technique for observing head and neck cancers and obtained excellent results. The endoscope is a transnasal endoscope that can provides high quality endoscopic images to be viewed on a monitor and digitally recorded with a wide field view of 140 degrees. The LASEREO system (FUJIFILM Co. Tokyo) is a novel endoscopic system employing a semiconductor LASER as a light source. This system is equipped with two LASERs with different in a wavelengths, one for white light sources (wavelength: 450 nm), and one for BLI (wavelength: 410 nm). The white light observation mode consists of a 450 nm LASER and fluorescence of white light phosphor, which is excited by a 450 nm LASER. The phosphor exists in the endoscope. BLI observation mode, which consists of a 410 nm LASER and feeble fluorescence light excited by a 450 nm LASER and is useful for acquiring mucosal surface information, including patterns of the surface blood vessels and structures. The endoscope allows for detailed observations in close view, as it has a focal length of 3 mm to achieve good endoscopic images. The endoscope also has a forceps with channel measuring 2.4 mm in diameter, which improves the ability to aspirate saliva and gastric juices and remove gastric mucus adhering to the tip of the endoscope. It has been reported that BLI is useful for making the diagnosis of colorectal tumors [18], or upper gastrointestinal lesions [19]. An abnormal microvascular pattern in brownish areas can be detected in most pharyngeal and esophageal cancers in the near view with white light images and clearly observed on BLI images. The color contrast of pharyngeal and esophageal cancers rises with BLI, resulting in useful screening result.

3.2. Endoscopic examinations-from the oral cavity to the oropharynx

Our screening procedure is as follows. First, the patient is asked to bow their head deeply in the lateral decubitus position. We then place a hand on the back of the patient's head and push it forward. The patient is then asked to lift the chin as far as possible (lateral sniffing position).

In order to avoid overlooking cancers in the floor of the mouth, soft plate and uvula, we first observe the oral cavity (Figure 1). and then insert the endoscope without a mouthpiece and subsequently observe the upper, lateral and posterior wall of the oropharynx while the patient sticks their tongue forward (Figure 2).

After observing the buccal cavity, further oropharyngeal observation is carried out with a retroflexed endoscope inserted via the nose. When the tip of the endoscope reachs the area caudal to the uvula, the patient opens their mouth wide and sticks their tongue forward as much as possible while making a vocal sound similar to "ayyy". The endoscopist causes the endoscope to make a U-turn (intra-oropharyngeal U-turn method) and observes the oropharynx, in particular the radix linguae. A schematic drawing of the procedure is shown in (Figure 3). We previously reported the usefulness of the intra-oropharyngeal U turn method [20]. One hundred and seventy-two patients underwent treatment with this method from April to October 2012. It was possible to observe all areas of the tongue from the radix linguae to the apex linguae, in 160 cases (93%) [21], and a frontal view of the papillae vallatae was obtained in all patients (Figure 4). After completing the intra-oropharyngeal U-turn method, the tip of the endoscope is inserted gently between the epiglottis and the tongue to observe the vallecula and the tonsil side of the epiglottis.

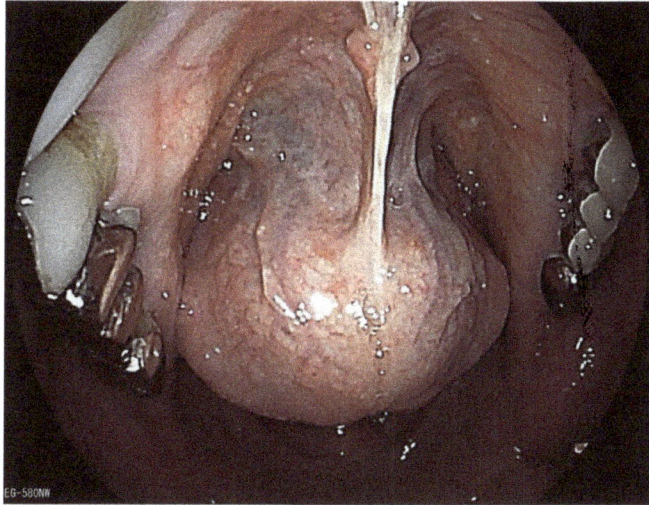

Figure 1. A view of the floor of the mouth through a trans-oral approach.

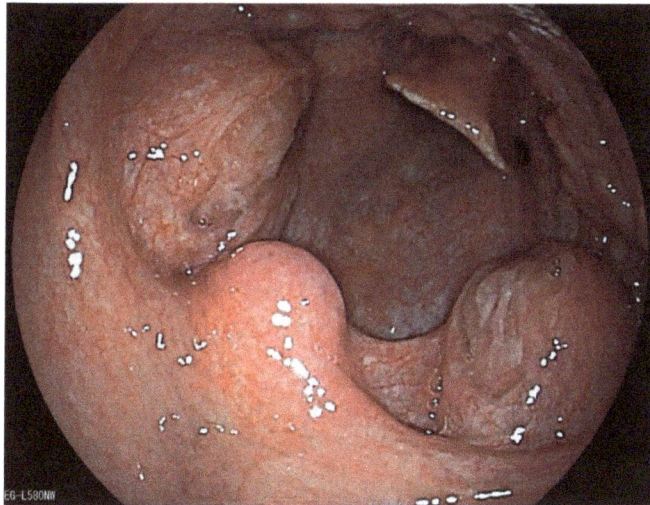

Figure 2. A view of the oropharynx through a trans-oral approach.

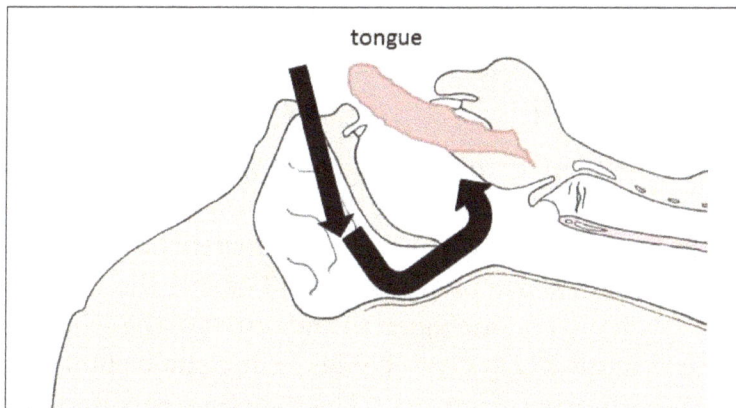

Figure 3. Schema of intra-oropharyngeal U-turn method.

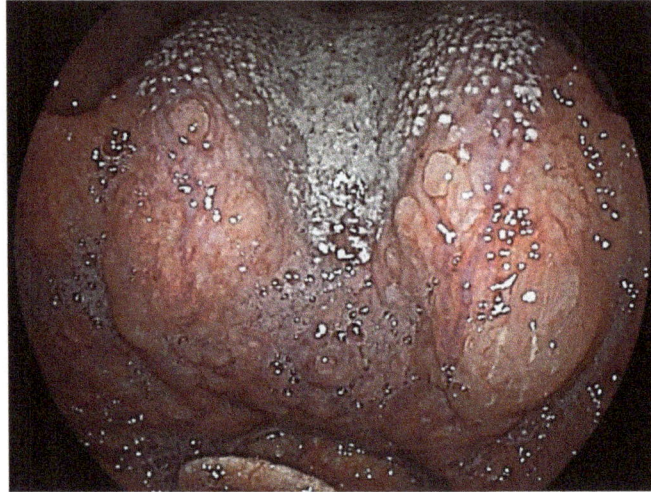

Figure 4. A view of the radix linguae through a trans-nasal approach.

3.3. Endoscopic examination from the hypopharynx to the cervical esophagus

The vocal cords and right and left pyriform sinus should be observed (Figure 5). When the patient vocalizes, the vocal cords move to the anterior region, making observation of the pyriform sinus easier. The technique of esophagogastroduodenoscopy (EGD) has also been improved, although it is not possible to observe otorhinolaryngeal sites in some patients due to the gag reflex. The postcricoid subsite and orifice of the esophagus are especially difficult to visualize using flexible laryngopharyngoscopy. Several reports have suggested techniques for improving the view of the hypopharynx with a flexible fiber optic laryngoscope. Spraggs and Harris described a modified Valsalva technique involving the nose being squeezed shut by the examiner's hand while the patient attempts to blow through the obstructed nose [22, 23]. Other reports have described the trumpet maneuver [24], the anterior neck skin traction maneuver [25] or a combination of the two [26]. However, these maneuvers have not been attempted in conventional EGD due to the effects of the gag reflex.

Since we introduced the modified Valsalva maneuver using transnasal endoscopy in 2009 [27], a total of 94 superficial head and neck cancers were found in 70 patients using transnasal ESD over the last four years [28]. Furthermore, it has been reported the modified Valsalva maneuver using transnasal endoscopy is prospectively useful for detecting superficial pharyngeal cancer [29].

For the examination of the hypopharynx and orifice of the esophagus, the patient is asked to blow hard and puff their cheeks while keeping their mouth closed. The endoscopist pulls the patient's chin forward with the right hand, and the characteristics of the posterior wall of the hypopharynx and postcricoid subsite pharyngeal wall enable the pharyngeal mucosa to be stretched out and the postcricoid region (Figure 6) and orifice of the esophagus to be visualized in an open space. The transnasal BLI system enables clear visualization of the palisade vessels of the pharyngoesophageal junction (Figure 7). The total time required to perform the procedure is approximately two minutes. This technique is easy to perform and feasible in almost all high-risk patients. The endoscope is then passed into the cervical esophagus.

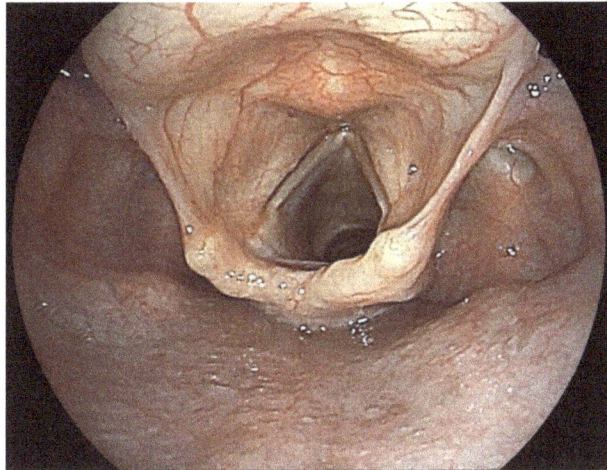

Figure 5. A view of the larynx and the hypopharynx.

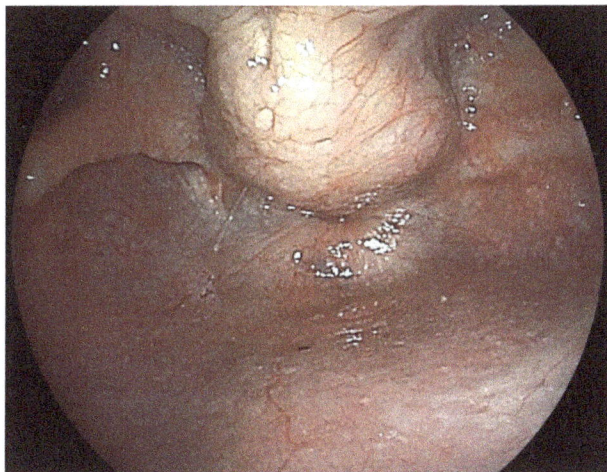

Figure 6. Transnasal endoscopy using trumpet maneuver improves the visualization of the hypopharynx and the pharyngoesophageal junction.

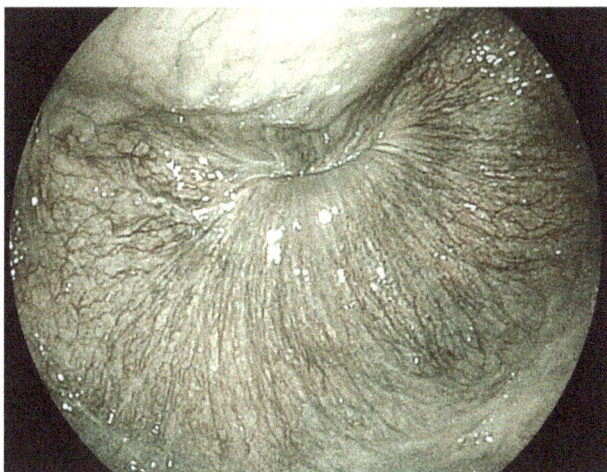

Figure 7. The endoscopic image of the pharyngoesophageal junction using Blue lasar imaging (BLI).

4. Patients and Methods

This study was conducted between June 2014 and October 2014. During this period, 70 consecutive patients (60 males, 10 females; mean age: 67.9 years old) with esophageal or head and neck cancer underwent endoscopic screening of the oropharynx and hypopharynx using transnasal endoscopy with the BLI system at the Department of Esophageal and General Surgery, Tokyo Medical and Dental University. We performed endoscopic observation from the oral cavity to pharynx before inserting the endoscope into the cervical esophagus. BLI images were obtained on a color video monitor by pushing a fingertip control switch. The visibility of subsites of the hypopharynx and the orifice of the esophagus was evaluated, and the extent of view of the hypopharyngeal opening was classified into three categories (excellent, good, poor). The diagnostic accuracy of transnasal endoscopy with the BLI system was subsequently estimated. Two experienced endoscopists (K.K., N.F.) performed all of the examinations, using the same endoscope.

The examinations were recorded onto video cassettes. Written informed consent was obtained from all patients prior to the endoscopic examinations.

5. Results

Eight elderly patients were excluded due toinadequate ballooning. Finally, 62 patients were investigated. Ballooning of the pyriform sinus and posterior wall allows for both an accurate assessment of the stretched pharyngeal mucosa and provides a view of the postcricoid subsite and orifice of the esophagus.

A wide endoscopic view of the pharynx was obtained in a series of the procedures (excellent=53/62, 85.4%; good=7/52, 4.5%; and poor=2/62, 7.6%). Among the 70 patients, six superficial lesions (8.6%) at the oropharynx (n=1) and hypopharynx (n=5) were discovered with the BLI system (Table 1). Three lesions were located at the piriform sinus and two lesions were located on the posterior wall of the pharyngoesophageal junction, which in the blind area on conventional screening. A representative lesion is shown in Figure 8. The hypopharynx was stretched according to the trumpet maneuver, whicn allowed us to detect a slightly depressed area. On BLI observation, a well demarcated brownish area was recognized, with scattered brown dots within the areas on a close view (Figure 9). The lesion was resected via endoscopic laryngopharyngeal surgery (ELPS). The area unstained with iodine was similar to the brownish area observed on BLI (Figure 10).

The histopathological examination revealed a diagnosis of squamous cell carcinoma with microinvasion beneath the epithelium (Figure 11).

In one case, superficial oropharyngeal cancer was located at the radix linguae (Figure 12), and the intra-oropharyngeal U-turn method was very effective for making the diagnosis.

Case	Sex	Age	Esophageal cancer	location	Macroscopic type	Size	Treatment	Tumor thickness
1	Male	72	Synchronous	PW	0-IIa	21mm	ELPS	350μm
2	Female	56	Metachronous	PW	0-IIc	12mm	ELPS	250μm
3	Male	69	Metachronous	rtPS	0-IIb	※10mm	-	
4	Male	63	Synchronous	rtPS	0-IIb	※15mm	-	
5	Male	66	Metachronous	ltPS	0-IIb	※15mm	-	
6	Male	60	Metachronous	Oro	0-IIc	※25mm	TORS	

PW=posterior wall of hypopharynx, rtPS= right piriform sinus
lt PS=left piriform sinus, Oro=oropharynx, TORS=transoral robotic surgery
ELPS=endoscopic laryngopharyngeal surgery ※=endoscopic findings

Table 1. The oropharyngeal and hypopharyngeal cancers detected by transnasal endoscopy with BLI.

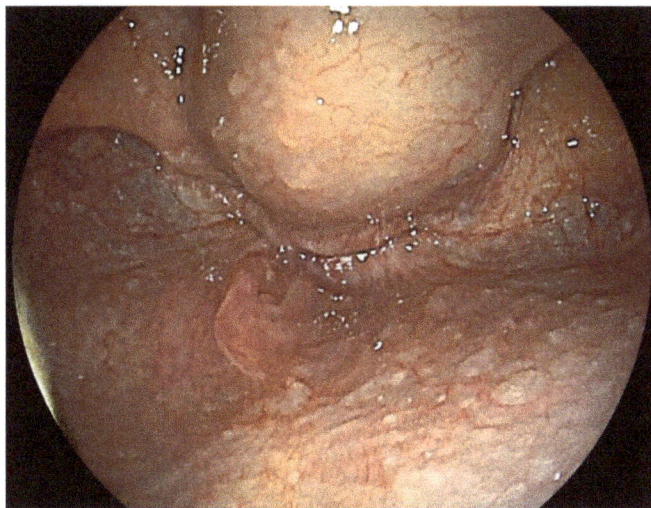

Figure 8. A slightly depressed lesion was observed in the posterior wall of the hypopharynx using the trumpet maneuver.

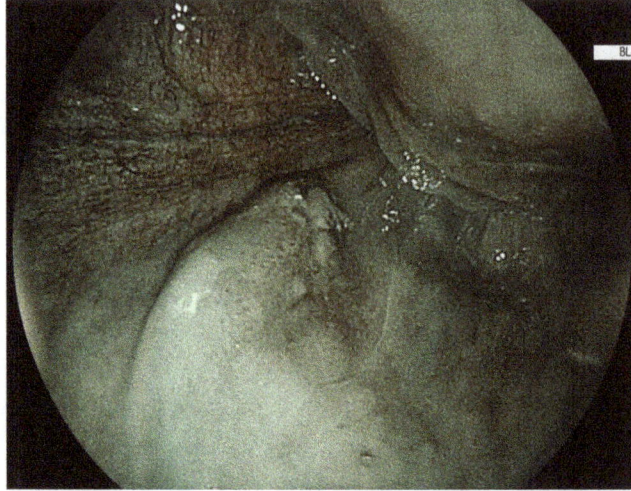

Figure 9. The endoscopic image using the BLI during the trumpet maneuver

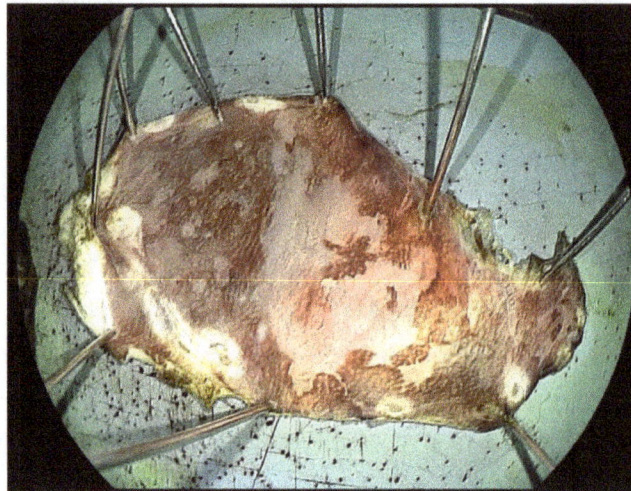

Figure 10. A macroscopic image of the resected specimen.

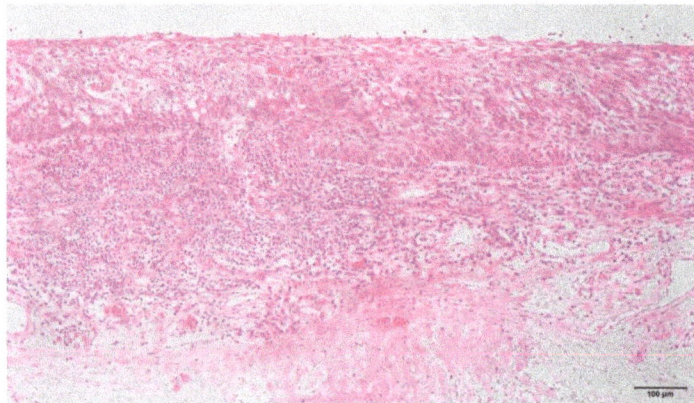

Figure 11. Histopathological examination revealed a diagnosis of squamous cell carcinoma with microinvasion beneath the epithelium.

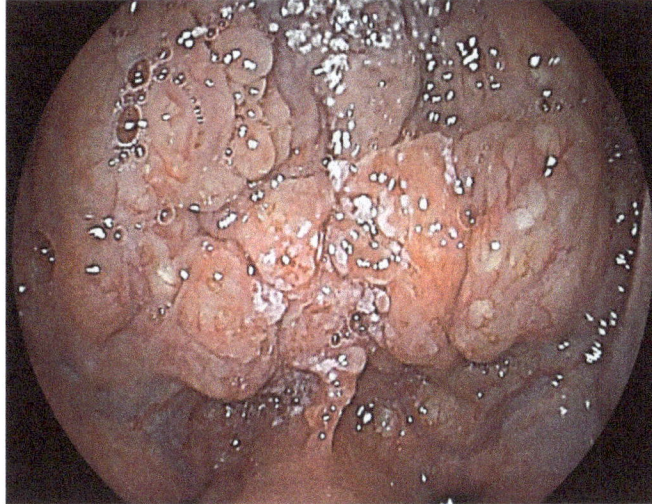

Figure 12. A case of superficial oropharyngeal cancer. The tumor observed using intra-oropharyngeal U-turn method.

5.1. Endoscopic features of superficial pharyngeal cancer

Recent advances in endoscopic procedures, such as magnifying endoscopy and the NBI system, have enabled precise observation of the oropharynx and hypopharynx [2, 5]. Mucosal redness, a pale and thickened mucosal apperance, white deposits and/or loss of the normal vascular pattern are important characteristics for diagnosing superficial carcinoma upon examination under white light (Figure 13). In addition, well demarcated areas covered with scattered dots observed on a closer observation of superficial microvascular structures and allows for the detection of a lesions at an earlier stages. The new transnasal endoscopy procedure with the BLI system enables physicians to easily observe the presence of scattered brown dots, contributing to the diagnosis of superficial cancers (Figure 14). Moreover, close BLI examinations using transnasal endoscopy enable the physician to obtain a mucosal diagnosis, even without magnification.

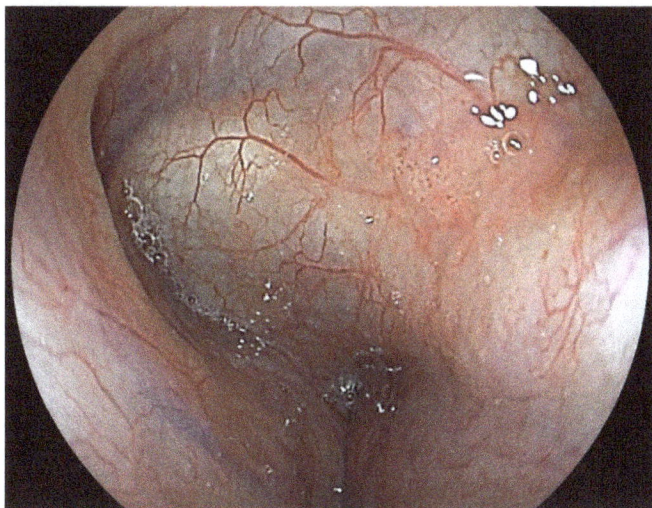

Figure 13. The white light image showed a 0-II b lesion of the right piriform sinus.

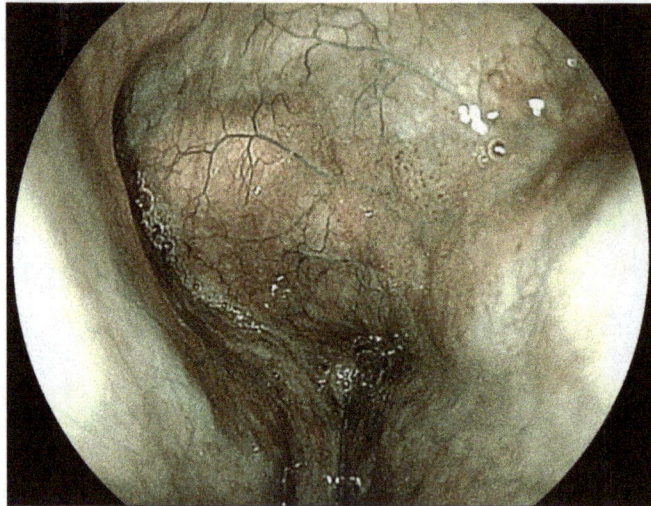

Figure 14. The close BLI image showed brown dots in the 0-II b lesion.

The modified Valsalva maneuver is also useful for detecting proximal invasion of the cervical esophageal cancer. This maneuver helps the physician to determine whether to preserve the patient's voice during surgery. On conventional screening, endoscopic images of hypopharyngeal cancer are often observed, however the distal part of the tumor is not visualized (Figure 15). A BLI endoscopic image obtained during the modified Valsalva maneuver using transnasal ESD is shown in Figure 16. The whole image of the tumor was able to observe (Figure 17). The entire tumor was observed, as indicated in Figure 17: the advanced cervical esophageal cancer had invaded the hypopharynx.

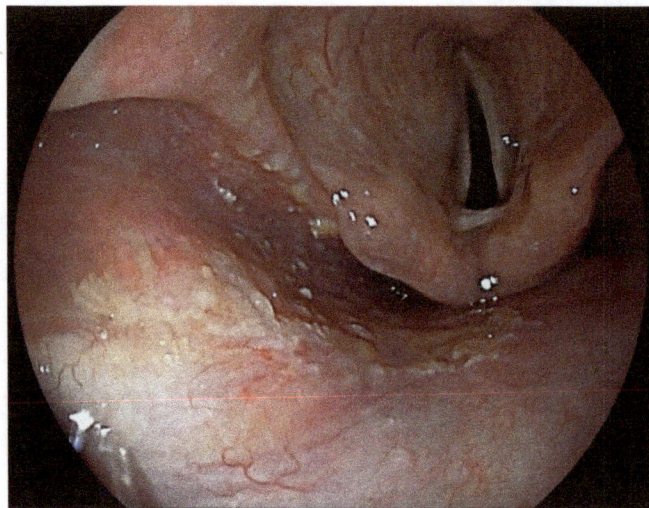

Figure 15. A reddish and irregular mucosa was shown in the hypopharynx. The distal part is not visualized.

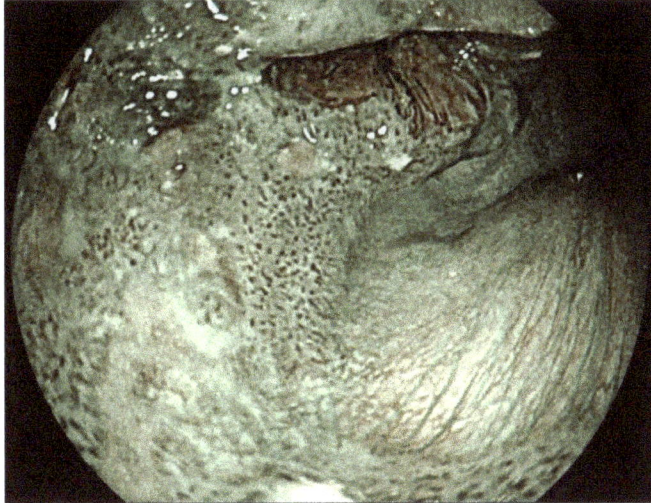

Figure 16. Advanced cancer was observed at the pharyngoesophageal junction using BLI during the trumpet maneuver.

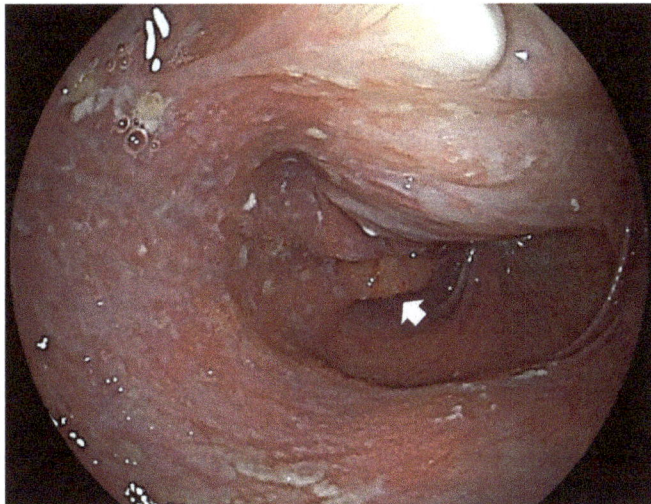

Figure 17. The advanced cervical esophageal cancer had invaded the hypopharynx (arrows).

6. Further research

It has been reported that the application of magnifying endoscopy with the NBI system drastically changes the diagnostic strategy for the early detection of early oropharyngeal and hypopharyngeal cancers. The development of transnasal endoscopy with the BLI system now enables the wider observation and can be used to obtain adequate information for diagnosing early cancers without magnification. The modified Valsalva maneuver and intra-oropharyngeal U-turn method using transnasal endoscopy are not popular in Japan as of yet, however these techniques are very easy to perform, and we expect that this method will become a standard procedure for observing the pharynx and orifice of the esophagus in the near future. Nevertheless, further studies, including randomized, prospective, multi-institutional joint trials comparing conventional endoscopy with the NBI system or transnasal endoscopy with the BLI system are required.

Transnasal endoscope technology is continually improving. From the viewpoint of early detection of pharyngeal cancer, we hope that transnasal endoscopy will become more widely adopted.

7. Conclusion

The significant progress achieved in the field of transnasal endoscopy rapidly within the last few years has improved the ability to observe the blind area typically noted during conventional screening. Therefore, transnasal endoscopy is expected to become a standard tool for screening of the upper gastrointestinal tract in the near future.

Author details

Kenro Kawada[1*], Tatsuyuki Kawano[1], Taro Sugimoto[2], Toshihiro Matsui[1], Masafumi Okuda[1], Taichi Ogo[1], Yuuichiro Kume[1], Yutaka Nakajima[1], Katsumasa Saito[1], Naoto Fujiwara[1], Tairo Ryotokuji[1], Yutaka Miyawaki[1], Yutaka Tokairin[1], Yasuaki Nakajima[1], Kagami Nagai[1] and Takashi Ito[3]

*Address all correspondence to: kawada.srg1@tmd.ac.jp

1 Department of Esophageal and General Surgery, Tokyo Medical and Dental University, Tokyo, Japan

2 Department of Otorhinolaryngology, Tokyo Medical and Dental University, Tokyo, Japan

3 Department of Human Pathology, Tokyo Medical and Dental University, Tokyo, Japan

References

[1] Slaughter DP, Southwick HW, Smejkal W. Field cancerization in oral stratified squamous epithelium; clinical implications of multicentric origin. Cancer 1953; 6: 963-968

[2] Muto M, Nakane M, Katada C et al. Squamous cell carcinoma in situ at oropharyngeal and hypopharyngeal mucosal sites. Cancer 2004; 101: 1375-1381.

[3]   Watanabe A, Tsujie H, Taniguchi M *et al*. Laryngoscopic detection of pharyngeal car-cinoma in situ with narrow band imaging. Laryngoscope 2006; 116: 650-654.

[4]   Gono K, Yamazaki K, Doguchi N *et al*. Endoscopic observation of tissue by narrow-band illumination. Opt Rev. 2003; 10: 211-215.

[5]   Muto M, Minashi K, Yano T, *et al*. Early detection of superficial squamous cell carci-noma in the head and neck region and esophagus by narrow band imaging: a multi-center randomized controlled trial. J Clin Oncol 2010; 28: 1566-1572.

[6]   Kawai T, Miyazaki I, Yagi K, *et al*. Comparison of the effects on cardiopulmonary function of ultrathin transnasal versus normal diameter transoral esophagogastro-duodenoscopy in Japan. Hepato-Gastroenterology 2007; 54: 770-774

[7]   Mori A, Ohashi N, Maruyama T, *et al*. Cardiovascular tolerance in upper gastrointes-tinal endoscopy using an ultrathin scope: prospective randomized comparison be-tween transnasal and transoral procedure. Dis Endosc 2008; 20: 79-83

[8]   Takezaki T, Shinoda M, Hotta S, *et al*. Subsite-specific risk factors for hypopharyng-eal and esophageal cancer (Japan). Cancer Causes Control 2000; 11: 597-608

[9]   Zeka A, Gore R, Kriebel D. Effets of alcohol and tabacco on aerodigestive cancer risks:a meta-regression analysis. Cancer Causes Control 2003; 14: 897-906

[10] Yokoyama A, Kato H, Yokoyama T, *et al*. Genetic polymorphisms of alcohol and al-dehyde dehydrogenases and glutathione S- transferase M1 and drinking, smoking, and diet in Japanese men with esophageal squamous cell carcinoma. Carcinogenesis 2002; 23: 1851-1859

[11] Yokoyama A, Yokoyama T, Muramatsu T, *et al*. Macrosytosis, a new predictor for esophageal squamous cell carcinoma in Japanese men. Cercinogenesis 2003; 24: 1773-1778

[12] Shimizu Y, Tsukagoshi H, Fujita M, *et al*. Head and neck cancer arising after endo-scopic mucosal resection for squamous cell carcinoma of the esophagus. Endoscopy 2003; 35: 322-326

[13] Muto M, Takahashi M, Ohtsu A, *et al*. Risk of multiple squamous cell caricinomas both in the esophagus and the head and neck region. Carcinogenesis 2005; 26: 1008-1012

[14] Muto M, Hhitomi Y, Ohtsu A, et al. Association of aldehyde dehydrogenase 2 gene-polymorphism with multiple oesophageal dysplasis in head and neck cancer pa-tients. Gut 2000; 47: 256-261.

[15] Yokoyama A, Omori T. Genetic polymorphisms of alcohol and aldehyde dehydro-genenases and risk for esophageal and head and neck cancers. Jpn J Clin Oncol 2003; 33: 111-121

[16] Yokoyama A, Yokoyama T, Kumagai Y, et al. Mean Corpuscular Volume, Alcohol Flushing and the Predicted risk of squamous cell carcinoma of the esophagus in cancer free Japanese men. Alcohol Clin Exp Res 2005; 29: 1877-1883

[17] Yokoyama T, Yokoyama A, Kato H, et al. Alcohol flushing, alcohol and aldehyde dehydorogenase genotypes, and risk for esophageal squamous cell carcinoma in Japanese men. Cancer Epidermiol Biomark Prev 2003; 12: 1227-1233

[18] Yoshida N, Yagi N, Yanagisawa A, Naito Y. Image-enhanced endoscopy for diagnosis of colorectal tumors in view of endoscopic treatment. *World J. Gastrointest. Endosc.* 4 ; 545-555, 2012

[19] Osawa H, Yamamoto H, Miura Y, et al. Blue laser imaging provides excellent endoscopic images of upper gastrointestinal lesions. Video Journal nad Encyclopedia of GI endoscopy 2014; 1: 607-610

[20] Kawada K, Okada T, Sugimoto T et al. Intraoropharyngeal U-turn method using transnasal esophagogastroduodenoscopy. Endoscopy 46; E137-8, 2014

[21] Kawada K, Okada T, Sugimoto T et al. Intra-oropharyngeal U-turn method with Trans-nasal Endoscopy (in Japanese with English abstract) J.Jpn Bronchoesophagol. Soc., 64:265-270, 2013

[22] Spraggs P D, Harries M L. The modified Valsalva maneuver to improve visualization of the hypopharynx during flexible nasopharyngoscopy. J. Laryngol. Otol. 1995; 109: 863-864.

[23] Purser S, Antippa P. Maneuver to assist examination of the hypopharynx. Head Neck 1995; 17: 389-393.

[24] Hillel AD, Schwartz A N. Trumpet maneuver for visualization and CT examination of the pyriform sinus and retrocricoid area. Head Neck 1989; 11: 231-6.

[25] Colquhoun-Flannery W, Davis A, Carruth J.A.S. Improving the endoscopic view of the hypopharynx with anterior neck traction during the trumpet manoeuvre. J. Laryngol. Otol. 2000; 114: 283-284.

[26] Williams R S, Lancaster J, Karagama Y *et al.* A systematic approach to the nasendoscopic examination of the larynx and pharynx. Clin. Otol. 2004; 29: 175-178.

[27] Kawada K, Kawano T, Nagai K, et al. Transnasal endoscopy for diagnosing superficial oro-hypopharyngeal cancer Stomach and Intestine (in Japanese with English abstract) 2010;45: 228-239

[28] Kawada K, Kawano T, Sugimoto T. Key points and techniques for trans-nasal endoscopic screening for superficial hypopharyngeal cancer. Treatment Strategies Gastroenterology 2013; 2: 42

[29] Tanaka T, Niwa Y, Tajika M, et al. Prospective evaluation of a transnasal endoscopy utilizing flexible spectral color enhancement (FICE) with the Valsalva maneuver for detecting pharyngeal and esophageal cancer. Hepatogastroenterology 2014; 61: 1627-34.

2

Endoscopy in Renal Cancer Organ Preservation Treatments

J.G. Calleary, T. Lee, B. Burgess, R. Hejj and P. Naidu

Abstract

This chapter traces the shift in treatment of localised renal cancer from major open surgery to endoscopic (ie laparoscopy) techniques. It also details the shift in treatment intent for localised Renal cancer toward Organ preservation. With advancement in technology and experience, the principles of endoscopic surgery have been adapted to treat renal malignancy with minimum complications and with maximal preservation of Renal function so much so that endoscopic techniques are seen as the "gold standard" by many. The chapter details these minimally invasive techniques of laparoscopic and Robotic partial nephrectomy and compares and contrasts both Oncological and Functional outcomes from both.

Keywords: Renal Cancer, Prostate cancer, Minimally invasive Surgery, Focal therapy, Partial Nephrectomy

1. Introduction

Urology is rapidly becoming a speciality where operative treatment of disease is primarily endoscopically administered The two last bastions of open surgical procedures in urology were reconstruction and radical surgical treatment of malignancy. In uro-oncology and in intra-abdominal reconstructive procedures such as Pelvi-Ureteric Junction (PUJ) obstruction, minimally invasive techniques are rapidly becoming the norm and indeed the debate is about which endoscopic technique results in the best outcomes [1]. From being the standard, open techniques are now limited to the worst locally advanced malignancies or revision reconstructive procedures. This review will chart the course of endoscopy in the treatment of localised RCC and especially in the era where organ preservation techniques have become paramount.

2. From open to Laparoscopic Radical Nephrectomy (LRN)

Perhaps the area which best illustrates this shift in emphasis in uro-oncology from open procedures to endoscopy is the treatment of localised Renal Cell Cancer. Robson et al. demonstrated improved survival established using open Radical Nephrectomy (all tissue within Gerotas fascia and ipsilateral adrenal and nodal tissue), and the technique became the gold standard treatment for localised renal cell cancer (T1–T2, see table 1 [2]. For about two decades, this remained the case, but there were concerns regarding complication rates and increased patient dissatisfaction, especially with flank incisions. An illustrative example of the latter is Chatterjee's work from 2004, which showed a 50% dissatisfaction rating vis-à-vis flank bulging and approximately 25% with ongoing wound pain [3].

In the early 1990's, the first laparoscopic procedures on the kidney were performed [4]. As experience with the technique grew and with favourable reports, it became the preferred choice. By mid to late 2000s, laparoscopic nephrectomy was the new gold standard after numerous studies demonstrated equivalent oncological outcomes in addition to enhanced patient experience. An example is the case-controlled study of Dunn et al. wherein equivalent short-term oncological outcomes were demonstrated in a comparative study of open and laparoscopic nephrectomy.

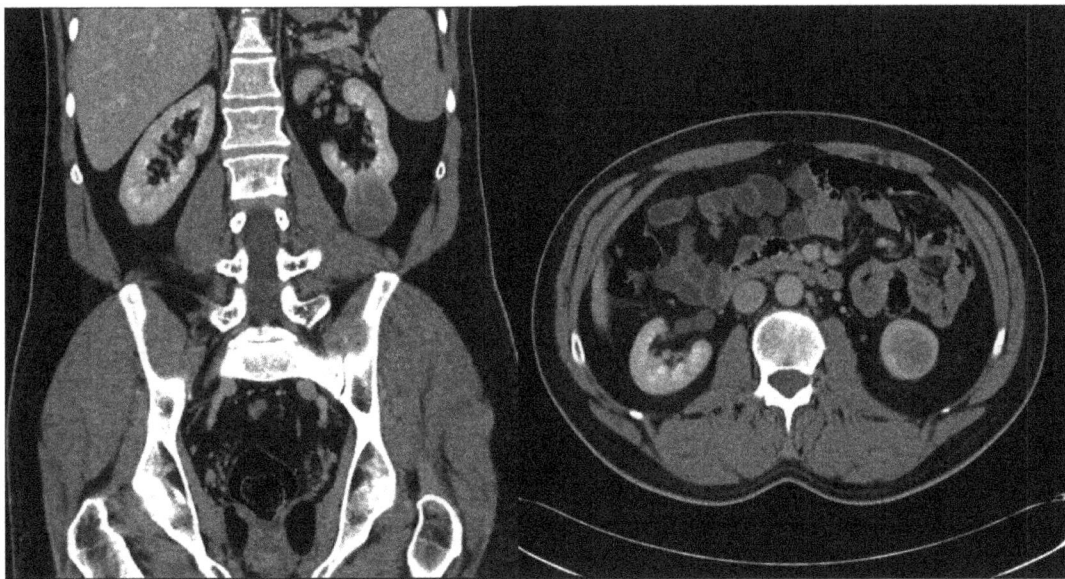

Figure 1. Two slices from a CT series to show a lesion treatable by partial nephrectomy (PN). This is a predominantly exophytic and polar lesion but it does cross the lower sinus line and probably involves the collecting system, thus making it a more complicated lesion than at first appearance.

However, laparoscopic nephrectomy was associated with more than a 50% reduction in blood loss, analgesic requirement, hospital stay and time to return to normal activities [5]. This low complication rate (eg bleeding rate of 2.8% and transfusion rate of 0.7%) was confirmed by a 2006 meta-analysis. The conversion rate was 2.5% and colonic injury was 1.5% [6]. This difference persists to the present day with Xu et al. showing a significant reduction in Claivan grade 2 complications, a 36% reduction in all complications and a 17% reduction in length of hospital stay [7]. Luo`s study published in 2010 confirmed the long-term oncological equivalence [8].

	Primary lesion
TX	Not assessable
T1a	0–4 cm diameter, limited to kidney
T1b	4–7 cm, limited to kidney
T2a	7–10 cm, limited to kidney
T2b	> 10 cm, limited to kidney.
T3a	Renal vein or segmental branch invasion
	Peri-renal / Renal sinus invasion confined to gerotas fascia
T3b	Invasion of IVC below diaphragm
T3c	Invasion of IVC above diaphragm
	Direct IVC wall invasion
T4	Invasion beyond Gerotas fascia
	Direct invasion of Ipsilateral Adrenal
	Regional Nodes
NX	Not assessed
N0	None
N1	Single node involved
N2	> single node involved
	Metastatic disease
M0	None
M1	Present

Table 1. TNM staging of Renal Cell Cancer (2009) – EAU Guidelines [9]

3. Organ preservation

As laparoscopic nephrectomy was becoming more widely practiced, two separate trends conspired against this endoscopic technique. The first was a stage migration of renal masses (i.e. presumed cancers) downward, which coincided with an increased incidence secondary to incidentally imaging (US and CT) detected lesions [10-11]. Allied to this was the increased identification of benign pathology in nephrectomy specimens performed for these small masses, which approached 20% in some series.

The second was an increasing realisation that the adverse effect of radical nephrectomy on renal function may result in reduced survival because of an association with cardiac mortality. Go et al. published a sentinel paper in the NEJM, which followed 120,295 adults over five years. Increased mortality, increased risk of vascular and cardiac disease and hospitalisations were significantly more common in those with chronic renal impairment (e GFR < 60 ml/min/ 1.73 m2) [12]. It was well documented that radical nephrectomy was associated with the development of renal failure. In 2006, Huang et al. demonstrated a reduction in the probability of developing new renal failure from 65% to 20% by the use of Nephron sparing Surgery (NSS) [13].

Studies like the above lead to an increasing search for alternatives to RN for T1a (< 4 cm) and T1b RCC (< 7 cm). NSS was the most extensively researched and in time has become a gold standard, especially for T1a lesions. It also led to the introduction of ablative technologies such as cryotherapy, HIFU (High-Intensity Focused Ultrasound) and RFA (Radio Frequency Ablation).

Partial Nephrectomy (table 2-3)

The aim of partial nephrectomy is the complete removal of the detected lesion with a margin of normal tissue of as little as 1 mm and as little damage to the remaining renal tissue as possible. Confirmation of a negative margin often requires frozen section analysis of the specimen. The initial indications for partial nephrectomy were tumours in a solitary kidney, multiple/ bilateral tumors or patients with poor renal function (table 3).

T stage	Recommendation
T 1a	Partial Nephrectomy (PN) is the preferred option
T 1b	Radical Nephrectomy (RN) or PN
T2	Radical Nephrectomy
	Partial Nephrectomy is associated with greater chance of local failure

Table 2. Accepted indications for PN

Absolute	Lesions in a single Kidney
	Bilateral synchronous lesions
	T1a lesions with low PADUA scores (see page 6)
Relative	T1b /T2 lesions with a normal contra-lateral Kidney but significant potential of future renal failure due to comorbidities
	Hereditary RCC
Elective	T1/ T2 lesion; other kidney normal, no "reno-toxic" comorbidity

Table 3. EAU guidelines for surgical treatment of localised Renal Cell Cancer (RCC) [9]

Traditionally, this involved dissection of the renal pedicle and subsequent clamping of the renal artery (± renal vein). This results in reduced blood loss and a reduced tissue tension, which makes dissection easier and improves visualisation. The perirenal fat is removed from the relevant area apart from directly over the lesion. The lesion is excised and the collecting system repaired. The kidney is then repaired and when done so satisfactorily, the clamp is removed.

Unfortunately, clamping is associated with ischaemia, which led to techniques to reduce the effects of ischaemia, and the concept of hypothermia following preconditioning prior to clamping with mannitol was introduced. The purported effect of mannitol is as promoter of renal vasodilation, thus promoting blood flow. It also prevents cast formation and decreases post-ischaemic swelling [14]. Hypothermia aims to get the renal core temperature to 15–20^{0}C and is achieved by cooling with ice slush for 10–15 minutes post clamping. This slows metabolism down to minimise the effects of ischaemia.

Initially this was thought to be possible only using open techniques, which meant a reduction in laparoscopic renal cancer procedures, although this tended to be mainly driven by academic centres. With time, the use of PN spread and Kim et al. using a US nationwide dataset showed the percentage of small renal masses treated by RN fell from 85% to 75% in the period from 2002 until 2008 [15].

The initial studies confirmed that OPN produces equivalent oncological outcomes compared to RN. Lau et al. showed equal cancer-specific survivals for both groups and metastatic disease in less than 5% of both RN and OPN groups in the case-controlled study of 164 patients in each group [16]. Similarly, Tan et al. showed excellent long-term cancer-specific survival again comparable to RN. Using the SEER database, they compared outcomes for 1925 PN against 5213 RN and showed similar RCC mortality from both PN (1.9%) and RN (4.3%) [17].

A significant proportion of the early debate in OPN focused on the question of the determinants of local recurrence and the potential effect on survival. One such risk is a positive surgical margin and Yossepowitch estimated that to happen in 2–8% of OPN [18]. Thankfully, this does not appear to have a survival impact, judging by the review of Van Popell and Joniou [19]. They have suggested that a 1 mm clear margin is enough to prevent local recurrence. An alternative technique practiced by some is lesional enucleation. This would be expected to be associated with greater local failure, but from the study of Minnervi et al., this would appear not to be the case [20]. Similarly, good oncological outcomes are achieved where PN is performed for lesions up to 7 cm [21].

Much of the early work on partial nephrectomy was done by the Cleveland Clinic group, especially by Novick and Gill. Some of their initial work confirmed the hypothesis that LRN was associated with significantly worse renal function (as measured by serum creatinine) at follow up albeit with reduced peri-operative complications in terms of bleeding, analgesia requirement and hospital stay. However, the two groups were not well matched as the LN group were significantly older, of greater comorbidity (as judged by ASA score) and had larger masses [22]. By the time Lesage`s review paper came out in 2007, the gap had narrowed and the complication rates were not significantly different, although there was a trend towards greater complications in the OPN groups. Importantly, the significantly increased risk of renal failure with RN compared to PN was confirmed [23]. Up to 22% of LRN patients had insufficiency at 10 years compared to at most 11.6% of the OPN group [16].

There are three factors, which contribute to renal function loss post any renal surgical intervention. These are pre-operative renal function (including comorbidity affecting renal function), the volume of excised/ damaged renal tissue and any intraoperative surgical ischaemia (be this warm or cold ischaemia). Of these, it is the ischaemia time which is the only variable open to surgical control. Warm ischaemia time (WIT) is defined as the length of time the blood supply is cut off or reduced at body temperature. Essentially, this equates to clamping time. Cold ischaemia time (CIT) is the time between when a tissue is cooled, has its blood supply reduced or cut off and is then re-warmed to body temperature [24].

It was because of the absolute centrality of clamping (and therefore a resultant ischaemic insult) to PN that the pendulum swung back to open surgery. This was the case even in centres that were pioneers in the field of PN and laparoscopic urology. IS Gill in an editorial in December 2012 stated of his time working with Dr. Novick at the Cleveland Clinic that *"never did we even discuss the possibility of doing major PN surgery without clamping the main renal artery"* [25].

As experience with PN grew and it became clear that PN was associated with superior functional and equivalent oncological outcomes, research shifted to focus on what if any was the limit of WIT and on methods to reduce ischaemic time. It is worth noting the primary tasks, which have to be completed during this time. These are removal of the lesion with a negative margin. The second is the repair of any collecting system injury, which may be checked by intravenous administration of indigo carmine and thirdly, the closure of the kidney using continuous sutures and adjunct measures. As can be imagined, the more complicated the lesion (larger, centrally placed or single kidney), the longer each step took, and hence, a greater potential for ischaemic injury.

The early animal and clinical studies suggested that 20 minutes of WIT and 120 min of CIT was the safe threshold above which irreversible renal damage was done [26]. This was not universally accepted and others argued that a WIT of up to 30 minutes was acceptable [27]. An elegant combined functional (MAG 3nuclear scan) and anatomical study (CT) from Japan would appear to suggest that the ideal time is around 25 minutes. In this study, Funahashi et al. used functional data from a MAG 3 study to show a net 25% drop in uptake at one week and more crucially that this drop had not recovered by six months. Importantly, the decreased uptake was globally seen and not limited to or concentrated on the operated site [28]. Becker et al. detail an excellent review on the topic of renal ischaemia in partial nephrectomy, which is worth reading as it details the pathophysiology, etc. Basically, the insult comes from a reperfusion injury brought on by free radical release, which, in turn, were formed by adenosine triphosphate breakdown due to vascular endothelial damage. It would also appear that, given that modern OPN is associated with WIT usually below 30 minutes, that there may be no benefit from cold ischaemia or indeed from mannitol. Where used, cold ischaemia is delivered using surface ice slush usually but can also be delivered using a retrogradely placed ureteric catheter or rarely by direct canulation of the renal artery [27].

Given this benchmark WIT of 20–25 minutes, it became crucial that techniques were developed to minimise WIT. The techniques considered were early unclamping, selective clamping or in select cases, control of the artery and vein with manual clamping of the hilum if necessary. This led to an upsurge in laparoscopic partial nephrectomy as the biggest fear amongst those offering LPN was to what extent the prolonged WIT of the early LPN experience had on renal outcomes. In a laparoscopic partial nephrectomy, there are three key steps. The first is lesion excision followed by accurate closure of the tumour bed and collecting system using two layers of interrupted sutures and thirdly, closure of the renal parenchyma. It is the latter that takes most time. Early unclamping is removal of the clamp once the lesion is excised and any repair required to the collecting system is finished. Any bleeding from the tumour bed can be controlled with separate sutures at that time. Nguyen and Gill dropped their WIT from a mean of 31.9 minutes to 13.9 minutes by this simple measure in a series of 100 consecutive LPN. There were more complications in the early unclamping group but this did not reach significance [29]. Similarly, a group from Europe in a cohort of 40 LPN demonstrated an equally impressive reduction in WIT from a mean of 27.2 minutes (± 5) to 13.7 (± 4), where two continuous sutures were used to close the tumour bed before unclamping and 10.3 (± 1.2), where one suture was used. In this study, there were no differences in blood loss, operative time or the need for transfusion between the control and early unclamping groups. Interestingly, the one major urinary leak happened in the control group and unfortunately required nephrectomy for management. The two vascular complications were also in the control group [30].

Selective arterial clamping (with laparoscopic bulldogs) appears to be more commonly studied in the minimally invasive PN series, especially in the robotic partial nephrectomy literature (RPN). The aim is to clamp the second-, third- or fourth-level branches within the renal sinus so that the area of ischaemia is limited to the renal mass only if possible or failing this that the area rendered ischaemic is a small as possible. It requires quite a sophisticated approach, which starts with 3D rendering of the kidney, its tumour and especially, its blood supply. The cross-sectional imaging used for this mapping is most commonly CT but can also be MRI. One- to three-mm slices are taken and processed using software, which provides the 3D reconstruction. The arterial and venous trees can then be mapped from the main artery and vein right up to the lesion. The level of the planned clamping is decided at this time and does not change unless due to unavoidable intraoperative reasons such as unexpected vessels. These images are thus available for review in theatre or in the case of robotic PN can be displayed on the operator's viewscreen.

Suitability for RPN/LPN and the extent of possible complications can be predicted using a variety of nephromotory scoring systems. One of the more commonly used is the Pre-operative Aspects And Dimensions Used for Anatomical (PADUA) system (table 4). It uses six characteristics to classify each lesion. These are relationship to the sinus line, location relative to renal border, relationship to renal sinus, collecting system involvement, the depth of penetration and the lesion size. The minimal score is 6 and the maximal score is 14. Not only can it be used to predict complexity (and thus suitability for PN) but it also correlates with complications. On this basis, lesions can be assigned to one of three groups, Low (6–7), intermediate (8–9) and

Anatomical feature	Scores 1	Scores 2	Scores 3
Sinus line	Entirely polar Crosses line < 50% Crosses > 50%	Between sinus lines	
Location vs. rim	Lateral border Endophytic near lateral border	Medial Border Endophytic near medial border	
Sinus located at lesion	None	Present	
Collecting system involvement	Not involved Dislocated i.e. compressed	Involved	
Depth of penetration into kidney	> 50% Exophytic	< 50% Exophytic	Endophytic
Size of lesion	< 4 cm	4–7 cm	> 7 cm

Table 4. PADUA score

high (>10) risk. Complications are significantly more likely to occur if the score is above 8. Using a baseline score of 6–7 as a comparator, those with a score of 8–9 had a 14-fold increased risk of complications and this increased to a 30-fold increased risk for score > 10 [31].

Shao et al. reported their experience of laparoscopic selective clamping in 125 patients over a two-year period and with 18 months of follow up. Visual clamping of the tumour vessel(s) was achieved in over 90% of cases, with the remainder requiring main artery clamping. The number of vessels clamped was totally dependent on tumour characteristics and this in turn predicted loss of renal function. Clamping of two or more vessels significantly increased the risk of bleeding and reduction in eGFR. Interestingly, they showed that posterior tumours were more likely to require 2 or more vessels clamped. This is slightly surprising given their approach to the kidney is retroperitoneal. Other factors predictive of multiple vessel clamping were size > 3 cm, endophytic lesions or lesions which were < 50% exophytic and lesions which involved both surfaces. Multiple vessel clamping in turn increases renal parenchymal tissue loss and thus renal function [32].

IS Gill is one of the "founding fathers" of PN and has been heavily involved in laparoscopic and robotic renal surgery. He has detailed his experience of LPN and his progression from full clamping through early unclamping, through selective clamping and finally to what he calls "zero ischaemia" [33-34]. This is the ultimate in selective clamping and entails clamping only the lesional vessel. As mentioned above, the preoperative lesional mapping is extremely important and this group uses 2–3 mm slices through the kidney and its vasculature. For their robotic work, the reconstructed images are displayed on the operating surgeons console. Putting this simply, the operating surgeon has a roadmap in front of them as they operate. Not only do they isolate the renal artery and its segmental branches but depending on tumour position, they can dissect third- and fourth-order branches. In addition to the highly detailed roadmap, the visual magnification from the use of MIS and the extra dexterity in tissue manipulation from using robotic instruments, this group uses two other adjunct techniques to minimise bleeding and clamping. The first was hypotensive anaesthesia. The second is to quantify the ischaemic area using either laparoscopic colour flow doppler ultrasound or more recently, intravenous indocyanine green [34-35].

Hypotensive anaesthesia involved controlled pharmacological lowering of systemic blood pressure. The aim is to avoid vasoconstriction of the arterial tree, thus maintaining perfusion in the setting of low pressure. Initially, the patient is given a mannitol solution followed by preloading with crystalloid. The required MAP of 60 mmHg is reached at the time at which the operator is dissecting the deep part of the lesion. It is achieved using a nitroglycerine infusion and isoflurane inhalation with heart rate support from a short-acting beta blocker. On removal of the lesion, the pressure is reversed. The advantage is that blood loss is minimised by reduced pressure while maintaining tissue oxygenation and thus preventing an ischaemic cascade. The disadvantage is that hypotension may trigger other end-organ failure and result in significant comorbidity. In their later experience, this group no longer used this technique. This is due to a combination of concern regarding the possibility of ischaemic complications such as myocardial infarction or cerebrovascular accidents and improved lesional vascular dissection helped in part by the adjunct technique described below [34-35].

Gill's group now uses indocyanine green as an adjunct to confirm devascularisation. This is used in conjunction with near-infrared fluorescence, which shows a black and white image with perfused areas being bright green. This group place the lesional vascular bulldog clamp. They then intravenously inject 7.5 mg of indocyanine green, switch to near infrared and confirm uptake by visualisation of the renal artery by its being outlined in green following which they visualise the lesion. If it is dark, then super-selective dissection has been successful; if not, they either search for an accessory vessel or convert the procedure to a standard clamped PN [35].

In their pilot study of 34 patients, some 80% underwent zero-ischaemia RPN. Most of the failures were due to persistent fluorescence, indicating accessory vessels. When paired with a cohort of "standard" clamped RPNs, the only differences were a longer operating time and better renal function in the zero-ischaemia group. None of the patients studied had a positive margin [35].

A very interesting by-product of the use of indocyanine green as a marker of devascularisation is that it appears to be poorly absorbed by RCC. Of 10 tumours, seven RCC appears were hypo-perfused, suggesting that this marker may have a further part to play in PN.

The previous ten paragraphs have described some of the techniques and strategies used by those at the cutting edge of partial nephrectomy to marry the enhanced patient experience of MIS with the improved functional outcomes from partial nephrectomy. These trail blazers describe a trifecta for minimally invasive PN of negative surgical margins, minimal loss of renal function and no urological complications. The question to be asked is can similar results be delivered by others.

The more widespread uptake of LPN started when the trail blazing units started to publish their experience. Initially, the lesions treated were the Anterior, polar and exophytic lesions, which scored a 6–7 using a PADUA system [31]. As experience was gained, units started doing more complicated lesions, while at the same time, experienced open surgeons with some laparoscopy skills began using robotic techniques. To this end, it can be difficult to compare OPN to LPN/ RPN as the number of centres publishing outcome data from LPN/RPN is very small. Amongst others to do such a comparative review was Van Poppel in a publication in 2010 [36]. This review looked at the published data at that time and as such was mainly, but not exclusively, from trail blazing units. The review has multiple tables which, for illustrative purposes, we have, somewhat crudely, condensed into two. The first (Table 5) attempts to summarise the oncological comparison. As would be expected, the mean follow-up is shorter and the mean lesion size is smaller for the LPN group. That said, the immediate (positive margins, local recurrence) oncological measure would appear to be equivalent. The inter-mediate performance comparator (% 5 year CSS – Cancer Specific Survival) would also suggest LPN provides an equivalent outcome.

	OPN	LPN
# Patients per quoted study	51–75	34–430
Mean size lesion (cm)	2.5–5.5	2.9–3.6
% Positive surgical margin	0– 5	0–2.9
% local recurrence	0–5.9	0–2.4
% 5 year CSS	89–98	91–100
% 10 year CSS	76–97	
Mean FU (months)	35–120	15–68

Table 5. Comparison of oncological outcomes of OPN (open partial nephrectomy) and LPN (laparoscopic partial nephrectomy) – modified from Van Poppel [36]

In partial nephrectomy, preservation of renal function and lack of urological complications are equally as important as excellent oncological outcomes. The second of the two tables (Table 6) summarises these outcomes from that Van Poppel publication. Some explanation of the table layout is required. The quoted studies had varying number of patients and hence the wide bands of reported complications. In an attempt to put each complication into context, the cumulative columns were constructed. Thus it can be seen that the operative and functional complications of LPN are equivalent to OPN [36].

One of the concerns expressed about the widespread expansion of LPN/RPN was that WIT times would increase as less experienced surgeons would prioritise tumour excision and renal repair. The accepted optimal WIT has been established at 20-30 minutes [26-28]. However it would appear from the "zero-ischaemia" work quoted above that each minute of WIT increases tissue loss [34-35]. One of the criticisms of MIS is the length of time it takes to become proficiently skilled in the procedure, the so-called learning curve. This is a controversial topic. One definition quoted is the number of cases to achieve a WIT of < 20 minutes. For robotic PN, Mottrie et al. put this at as little as 30–40 cases and based it on a single surgeon experience

	OPN		LPN	
	Range	Cumulative	Range	Cumulative
# Patients per quoted study	59–1029	2756	49–507	1679
% Overall complications	4.1–38.6	587 (21%)	9–33	337 (20%)
% Haemorrhage	0–7.5	88 (3%)	1.5 - 9.5	82 (5%)
% Urine leak	0.7–17.4	109 (4%)	1.4–10.6	57 (3%)
% sepsis	0 - 2.7	13 (0.4%)	0–2.5	11 (0.7%)
% Renal Failure	0–12.7	38 (1.4%)	0–2	12 (0.7%)

Table 6. Comparison of complications of OPN and LPN again modified from Van Poppel [36]

where the mean time for WIT in a group of 10 patients was less than 20 minutes. The caveat to this is that this group had significant robotic experience. However, the editorial comment accompanying their paper appeared incredulous that such a number could be quoted. The author of this editorial had > 400 LPNs under his belt. In LPN, the same debate seems to be taking place [37].

IS Gill suggests that it took him about 550 cases to become what he deemed to be proficient [33]. This is from one of the leading laparoscopic and robotic protagonists of PN. On the other hand, Springer et al. in their paper comparing OPN and LPN state that the fact that the two main surgeons had performed over 90 OPN and LPN each helped overcome the learning curve [38].

Their paper is worth summarising, representing as it does the experience of an early adapter of LPN where previously OPN was the procedure of choice. This group compared 140 consecutive LPNs (May 2005–November 2010) to a historic control group of 140 OPN (May 1999–April 2005). Overall, the oncological results, both in terms of positive margins (1.2 % LPN, 1.7 % OPN) and five-year CSS (91% LPN, 88% OPN), were identical and identical to the review by Van Poppel, which is tabulated above [36]. In addition, the functional outcomes were identical with approximately 5% of each group having post-operative complications. Hence, it would appear that the excellent results from LPN performed at centres of excellence are transferrable to the wider urological community.

This may be a moot point because of the rapid expansion in centres offering RAPN. Primarily, this is because robotics offers several significant advantages over "traditional" LPN. These are improved magnification, greater surgeon ergonomic comfort, instruments such as the endoWrist, which give greater degrees of movement facilitating easier dissection and suturing [35-37]. One of the latest meta-analyses on series comparing LPN and RPN is from Zhang et al. They identified seven valuable studies from an initial find of 569 studies on the topic. Unsurprisingly, there was no difference in tumour characteristics nor indeed in any discussed parameter apart from WIT. This was significantly shorter in the RAPN groups. While this is not a new finding, it is not universally found. It does appear to reaffirm the fears about LPN being associated with prolonged WIT. Looking at the tables in a little more detail, it becomes apparent that the series with larger numbers tended to have identical and more acceptable

	RPN		LPN	
	Ranges	Cumulative	Ranges	Cumulative
Numbers in quoted studies	11–220	425	14–102	341
Mean operating time in mins	152.17–233	176.2	117.5–226.5	194.35
Mean WIT mins	14.1–35.3	19.83	17.2–36.4	41.9
Mean blood loss mls	122.4–286.4	239.51	146.3–387.5	232.31
Conversion rate	N = 0–13 (0- 5.9%)	N = 18 4.24%	N = 0–5 (0–15%)	N = 12 3.52%
Positive margins	N = 0–18	N= 22 5.58%	N = 0–7	N = 11 3.49%
Complications	N= 0–45 (0–22%)	N = 69 (17.51%)	N= 0–17 (0–31%)	N = 55 (16.92%)
LOS days	2.51–6.1	4.98	2.7–6.8	4.48

Table 7. Comparison of complications and immediate oncological outcomes of RAPN (Robotic assisted) and LPN (Laparoscopic), modified from Zhang et al. [39] N refers to the total number of patients in the studies quoted

WIT for both RAPN and LPN. If 21 minutes is used as a marker for an acceptable WIT limit, four of the LPN and two of the RAPN trials are well above that limit. This is not discussed in the review but it may represent a learning curve effect or may reflect surgeons switching to the technically less demanding robotic approach [39]. Some evidence, albeit circumstantial, for the latter point is that having access to robotic technology increases the uptake of PN [40].

As can be seen from the preceding tables, it can be difficult to compare the MIS techniques for PN. In an effect to standardise reporting of outcomes, the MIC system was proposed and some groups have reanalysed their data accordingly. The MIC system is based on the trifecta discussed earlier. That is, negative surgical margins, WIT < 20 minutes and no significant complications. MIC is present when all three factors are present. Acceptability in terms of a study is where the global MIC score is > 80%. In their study, Porpiglia et al. showed increasing MIC with increasing experience and that acceptability was achieved after approximately 150 cases of LPN, i.e. the learning curve is 150 cases. The other factor negatively affecting MIC was increasing complexity of cases [41].

The future of endoscopically delivered NSS is secure and judging by recent publications describing MIS PN for increasingly more complex lesions, the focus will shift to which technique will become most practised. The debate is no longer about whether OPN is superior, it is now how about which of the endoscopic techniques will best achieve MIC.

4. Renal ablative therapies

Whilst most groups focused on organ preservation through PN other looked at the role of ablative technologies. The European Association of Urology guidelines suggest ablative therapies can be used for High risk patients who are keen to have definitive treatment. Two ablative techniques have entered main stream clinical practice and these are radiofrequency ablation (RFA) which uses heat energy and Cryotherapy (CA) which uses cold energy applied in a heat–thaw cycle to produce cell death. Tissue destruction happens when sufficient energy is applied at a rate equal to the rate thermal energy is removed (i.e. Heat sink). These techniques can be performed under general anaesthesia or sedation and in either an operating theatre (using ultrasound as the image guidance technique) or interventional radiology suite (using CT or MRI). Both require intensive imaging-based follow-up schedules as post-ablative biopsy histology is not very accurate. Failure (persistent contrast enhancement or growth on serial scans) or success (no contrast enhancement, lesion shrinkage) is based on cross-sectional imaging findings [42].

4.1. Cryotherapy Ablation (CA)

Cryotherapy has primarily been delivered laparoscopically. The principle is to deliver sufficient energy using freeze–thaw cycles to cause apoptosis and cell damage by mechanical and vascular means. The initial freeze cycle (using Argon gas) causes ice formation within the extracellular spaces. This acts as an osmotic agent and attracts fluid from the intracellular space. Freezing also causes mechanical cell damage. Thawing (using Helium gas) restores blood flow but damaged cells are released into the vasculature and result in thrombosis. The ideal freeze time appears to be 10 minutes for RCC based on basic science and clinical studies. The ideal tissue temperature is approximately -40⁰C. The margin of the iceball should be approx. 0.5 cm beyond the rim of the lesion [42].

Most of the studies on CA for localised RCC have involved a large proportion of small lesions < 3 cm and have at best short- to medium-term follow-up. The majority have performed laparoscopically. The initial oncological results seem encouraging with reported 3- and 5-year CSS equivalent to that of PN AT 98–100% and 92%, respectively. The downside is that there is a significant local failure rate of 10–20%. Aron et al. have 5-year follow-up on a group of 80 patients. Their 5-year CSS is 92% but the local recurrence rate is 14%. The definition of recurrence post CA is radiological because of the difficulty interpreting post CFA biopsy specimens. Exophytic, small (<3 cm) lesions along the lateral rim of the kidney are those with the best outcomes [43].

While CA appears to be an effective therapy, there are very few head-to-head trials comparing it to PN. One such trial was conducted by Tanagho et al., who compared CA to RAPN. This trial used the Clavien classification of complications, which standardises definitions and allows for more accurate reporting. Many criticisms of LCA trials had discussed complication reporting in addition to a more favourable lesional profile. They compared 267 patients treated by CA to 233 RAPN and the groups were matched for all matched characteristics. The immediate complication rate was equal (CA 8.6% vs. RAPN 9.4%). The renal preservation was significantly better for CA, but this was at the cost of a 12.7% local recurrence rate at approx. 40 months versus 0% for RAPN at a mean fu of approximately 22 months. That said, they conclude that CA is an excellent therapy [44].

4.2. Radio Frequency Ablation (RFA)

This is predominantly delivered percutaneously. A probe is advanced under screening into the lesion and heating begun using a high-frequency alternating current. This induces molecular oscillation, which leads to friction and cell death by coagulative necrosis. The temperature at the centre of the lesion lies between 50 and 120 °C depending on the interplay between device and patient factors. Device factors include the probe composition, its surface area, length and duration of use. Patient factors include the position of the lesion vis-à-vis the hilum (i.e. collecting system and major vessels), which can affect the heat sink principle as proximity to a major vessel results in greater heat dissipation, which in turn leads to less thermal injury to the lesion unless more energy is delivered. Depending on the tissue temperature, the destruction can be instantaneous or result in the triggering of an inflammatory cascade [42].

A recent report on 200 RFA in 165 patients is one of the largest to date and is unusual in that most of the treatments were performed under general anaesthesia. This may explain the technical success rate of 98.5% in a group of lesions of mean size 2.9 cm (range 1–5.6). For central lesions, they used cold pyeloperfusion to cool the upper ureter and collecting system via a retrogradely placed ureteric catheter. They also describe hydrodissection to move bowel within 1 cm of an exophytic lesion. This is achieved by the instillation of dextrose solution (i.e. nonconductive).

In terms of oncological outcomes, this group achieved a 97.9% CSS with exophytic and tumours < 3 cm doing best. Nine required retreatment and of those, six were tumour free after a further 1–2 treatments. From a functional outcome, Only 2% of their cohort had long-term renal function loss [45].

5. Conclusion

Open Radical Nephrectomy has gone from being the only therapy available to treat localised RCC to a therapy which is now rarely practised. Indeed, partial nephrectomy seems to be competing with ablative therapies for localised disease. This chapter has attempted to trace that change albeit trying to simplify the often crossing timelines between the various interventions. The place of endoscopy in organ preservation in localised RCC is however secure.

Author details

J.G. Calleary*, T. Lee, B. Burgess, R. Hejj and P. Naidu

*Address all correspondence to: johngcall@aol.com

Department of Urology, Pennine Acute Hospitals, North Manchester General Hospital, Crumpsall, Manchester, UK

References

[1] BLUS handbook of Laparoscopic and Robotic fundamentals. http: // www.aua.org/ common/pdf/education/BLUS-Handbook-pdf accessed Jan 15th 2015

[2] Robson CJ, Churchill BM, Anderson W. The results of radical nephrectomy for renal cell carcinoma. J Urol 1969;101: 297–301.

[3] Chatterjee S, Nam R, Fleshner N, Klotz L. Permanent flank bulge is a consequence of flank incision for radical nephrectomy in one half of patients. Urol Oncol 2004 Jan-Feb; 22(1): 36-39.

[4] Clayman RV, Kavoussi LR, Soper NJ. et al. Laparoscopic Nephrectomy: initial case report. J Urol 1991; 146(2): 278-282.

[5] Dunn MD, Portis AJ, Shalhav AL, Elbahnasy AM, Heidorn C, McDougall EM, Clayman RV: Laparoscopic versus open radical nephrectomy: a 9-year experience. J Urol 2000; 164:1153-1159.

[6] Pareek G, Hedican SP, Gee JR, et al. Meta-analysis of the complications of laparoscopic renal surgery: comparison of procedures and techniques. J Urol. 2006;175(4): 1208-1213.

[7] Xu H, Ding Q, Jiang HW. Fewer complications after laparoscopic nephrectomy as compared to the open procedure with the modified Clavien classification system--a retrospective analysis from southern China. World J Surg Oncol. 2014 Jul 31;12:242.

[8] Luo JH, Zhou FJ, Xie D, et al. Analysis of long-term survival in patients with localized renal cell carcinoma: laparoscopic versus open radical nephrectomy. World J Urol 2010; 28(3): 289-293.

[9] EAU guidelines. http: //www.uroweb.org/gls/pdf/10_Renal_Cell_Carcinoma_LR.pdf (accessed Jan 15th 2015).

[10] Hollingsworth JM, Miller DC, Daignault S, Hollenbeck BK. Rising incidence of small renal masses: a need to reassess treatment effect. JNCI Sep 20, 2006; 98(18):1331–1334.

[11] Chow WH, Devesa SS, Warren JL. et al. Rising incidence of renal cell cancer in the United States. *JAMA* 1999; 281(17):1628-1631.

[12] Go AS., Chertow GM., Fan D, McCulloch CE & Hsu CY. Chronic kidney disease and the risks of death, cardiovascular events, and hospitalization. *N. Engl. J. Med* 2004; 351: 1296–1305.

[13] Huang WC, Levey AS, Serio AM, et al. Chronic kidney disease after nephrectomy in patients with renal cortical tumours: a retrospective cohort study. Lancet Oncol. 2006 Sep; 7(9):735–740.

[14] Novick AC. Renal Hypothermia: in vivo and ex vivo. Urol Clin North Am 1983; 10:637-644.

[15] Kim, SP. *et al.* Contemporary trends in nephrectomy for renal cell carcinoma in the United States: results from a population based cohort. J. Urol. 2011;186: 1779–1785.

[16] Lau WK, Blute ML, Weaver AL, Torres VE, Zinke H. Matched comparison of radical nephrectomy vs nephron-sparing surgery in patients with unilateral renal cell carcinoma and a normal contralateral kidney. Mayo Clin Proc 2000; 79(12): 1236-1242.

[17] Tan HJ, Norton EC, Ye Z, Hafez KF, Gore JL, Miller DC. Long-term survival following partial versus radical nephrectomy among older patients with early-stage kidney cancer. JAMA 2012 April 18; 307(15).

[18] Yossepowitch O, Thompson RH, Leibovich BC *et al.* Positive surgical margins at partial nephrectomy: predictors and oncological outcomes. J. Urol. 2008; 179: 2158–2163.

[19] Van Poppel H, Joniau S. How important are surgical margins in nephron-sparing surgery? Eur. Urol. Suppl 2007; 6: 533–539.

[20] Minervini A, Tuccio A, Lapini A. *et al.* Review of the current status of tumor enucleation for renal cell carcinoma. Arch. Ital. Urol. Androl. 2009; 81: 65–71.

[21] Badalato GM, Kates M, Wisnivesky JP, Choudhury AR, McKiernan JM. Survival after partial and radical nephrectomy for the treatment of stage T1bN0M0 renal cell carcinoma (RCC) in the USA: a propensity scoring approach. BJUI 2011; 109: 1457-1462.

[22] Matin SF[1], Gill IS, Worley S, Novick AC. Outcome of laparoscopic radical and open partial nephrectomy for the sporadic 4 cm. or less renal tumor with a normal contralateral kidney. J Urol. 2002 Oct; 168(4 Pt 1):1356-1359; discussion 1359-1360.

[23] Lesage K, Joniau S, Fransis K, Van Poppel H. Comparison between open partial and radical nephrectomy for renal tumours: Perioperative outcome and health-related quality of life. Eur Urol 2007; 51: 614–620.

[24] NCI dictionary of cancer terms. Accessed on Jan 15th at www.cancer.gov/dictionary? cdrid = 630927.

[25] Gill IS. Towards the ideal partial nephrectomy. Eur Urol 2012: 62(6); 1009-1010.

[26] Simmons MN, Schreiber MJ, Gill I. Surgical renal ischemia: a contemporary overview. J Urol 2008; 180:19–30.

[27] Becker F[1], Van Poppel H, Hakenberg OW. et al. Assessing the impact of ischaemia time during partial nephrectomy. Eur Urol 2009 Oct; 56(4):625-634.

[28] Funahashi Y, Hattori R, Yamamoto T. et al. Ischemic renal damage after nephron-sparing surgery in patients with normal contralateral kidney. Eur Urol 2009; 55(1): 209-215.

[29] Nguyen MM, Gill IS. Halving ischemia time during Laparoscopic Partial Nephrectomy. The Journal of Urology 2008 ;179(2): 627-632.

[30] Baumert H, Ballaro A, Shah N. et al. Reducing warm ischaemia timeduring Laparoscopic Partial Nephrectomy: A prospective comparison of two renal closure techniques. Eur Urol 2007: 52; 1164–1169.

[31] Ficarra V, Novara G, Secco S, Macchi V. Preoperative aspects and dimensions used for an anatomical (PADUA) classification of renal tumours in patients who are candidates for nNephron-sparing surgery. Eur Urol 2009; 56(1): 786-793.

[32] Shao P, Tang L, Pu L. et al. Precise segmental renal artery clamping under the guidance of dual-source computed tomography angiography during laparoscopic partial nephrectomy. Eur Urol 2012, 62, 1001-1008.

[33] Gill IS, Kamoi K, Aron M, Desai MM. 800 Laparoscopic partial nephrectomy: a single surgeon series. J Urol 2010; 183: 34–41.

[34] Gill IS, Eisenberg MS, Aron M. et al. "Zero ischemia" partial nephrectomy: novel laparoscopic and robotic technique. Eur Urol 2011 Jan; 59(1):128-134.

[35] Borofsky MS, Gill IS, Hemal AK. et al. Near-infrared fluorescence imaging to facilitate super-selective arterial clamping during zero-ischaemia robotic partial nephrectomy. BJU Int 2013 Apr; 111(4): 604-610.

[36] Van Poppel H. Efficacy and safety of nephron-sparing surgery. International Journal of Urology 2010; 17, 314–326.

[37] Mottrie A, De Naeyer G, Schatteman P. et al. Impact of the learning curve on perioperative outcomes in patients who underwent robotic partial nephrectomy for parenchymal renal tumours. Eur Urol 2010; 58: 127-133. Discussion 133.

[38] Springer C, Hoda MR, Fajkovic H. et al. Laparoscopic vs open partial nephrectomy for T1 renal tumours: evaluation of long-term oncological and functional outcomes in 340 patients. BJUI 2012; 111: 281-288.

[39] Zhang X, Shen Z, Zhong S. et al. Comparison of peri-operative outcomes of robot-assisted vs laparoscopic partial nephrectomy: a meta-analysis. BJUI 2013; 112: 1133-1142.

[40] Kardos SV, Gross CP, Shah ND. et al. Association of type of renal surgery and access to robotic technology for kidney cancer: results from a population-based cohort. BJUI 2014; 114: 549–554.

[41] Porpiglia F, Bertolo R, Amparore D, Fiori C. Margins, ischaemia and complications rate after laparoscopic partial nephrectomy: impact of learning curve and tumour anatomical characteristics. BJUI 2013; 112: 1125–1132.

[42] Ramanathan R. Leveillee RJ. Ablative therapies for renal tumors. Ther Adv Urol 2010; 2(2): 51-68.

[43] Van Poppel HV, Becker F, Cadeddu et al. Treatment of localised Renal Cell Carcinoma. Eur Urol 2011; 60: 662–672.

[44] Tanagho YS, Bhayani SB, Kim EH, Figenshau RS. JEndourol 2013; 27(12): 1477-1486.

[45] Wah TM, Irving HC, Gregory W. et al. Radiofrequency ablation (RFA) of renal cell carcinoma (RCC): experience in 200 tumours. BJUI 2013; 112 (3): 416 – 428.

3

The Diagnosis and Treatment of Early-Stage Colorectal Cancer

Taku Sakamoto, Masayoshi Yamada,
Takeshi Nakajima, Takahisa Matsuda and
Yutaka Saito

Abstract

The introduction of colorectal endoscopic submucosal dissection (ESD) has expanded the applications for endoscopic treatment; as a result, lesions with low metastatic potential can be treated endoscopically regardless of the lesion size. The most attractive feature of ESD is the achievement of en bloc resection with a lower local recurrence rate in comparison to that of endoscopic piecemeal mucosal resection. However, in case of gastric cancers, ESD is not as widely applied to the treatment of colorectal neoplasms because of its technical difficulty, longer procedural time, and increased perforation risk. In the movement toward diversified endoscopic treatment strategies for superficial colorectal neoplasms, endoscopists who begin to perform ESD need to recognize the indications of ESD, as well as the technical issues and associated complications of this procedure.

Keywords: Superficial colorectal neoplasm, pit pattern, endoscopic submucosal dissection

1. Introduction

Endoscopic therapy is a major step forward in the management of early-stage gastrointestinal cancers. In the colorectum, lymph node metastasis always occurs only with deep invasion of the submucosa ($\geq$1000 μm), and lesions that are diagnosed as well-differentiated adenocarcinomas that are limited to the mucosa (intramucosal) or that superficially invade the submucosa (<1,000 μm from the muscularis mucosa) without lymphovascular invasion or a component with poor differentiation component (or both) are usually considered to not involve lymph node metastasis [1-3]. Among these factors, however, only the depth of invasion can be estimated by endoscopy prior to treatment. Thus, the depth of invasion must be accurately estimated before any therapeutic decision is made. Endoscopic resection plays two important roles in gastrointestinal surgery: achieving curative resection and allowing an accurate histological evaluation of lesions. As lesions measuring more than (or equal to) 10 mm have the potential for malignancy, they should be resected en bloc to avoid either residual or recurrent lesions (or both) [4].

Endoscopic submucosal dissection (ESD) is a state-of-the art technique for the treatment of large colorectal neoplasms that enables en bloc resection regardless of lesion size [5-8]. This chapter describes in detail the method for estimating depth invasion and ESD for colorectal neoplasms.

2. Diagnosis

Magnifying observation techniques, including chromoendoscopy and narrow-band imaging (NBI), have been recognized as high-precision methods for the diagnosis of depth invasion. With NBI, avascular or loose vascular findings are considered a key indicator of a submucosal and deep invasive cancer [9, 10]. However, NBI is a relatively new method with an unknown learning curve and different classifications, even within a single country like Japan. In contrast, pit pattern analysis using crystal violet staining has now become standardized due to its longer availability and one-to-one comparisons of endoscopic and pathological findings. In our view, pit pattern analysis is the most reliable predictor of depth invasion. During this analysis, each lesion should be confirmed to include a non-invasive pattern and Type V pit(s) with clearly demarcated areas, as this indicates that the lesion is suitable for endoscopic mucosal resection (EMR) or ESD with an estimated depth of invasion less than that of a submucosal invasive cancer [11].

In this section of the chapter, we will describe in order of the actual clinical process an endoscopic evaluation focused on the invasion depth of an early colorectal cancer, which is defined as confirmed cancer cells present in the mucosa or the submucosa, regardless of lymph node metastasis.

2.1. White-light non-magnifying endoscopy

The first diagnostic step is determination of the macroscopic lesion type. Most early-stage colorectal cancer lesions are classified as Type 0 according to Borrmann classification, which is equivalent to a superficial lesion in the Paris classification. In the latter classification, superficial lesions are divided into two groups: polypoid and non-polypoid lesions; in particular, non-polypoid lesions have received considerable attention, given their clinical importance. Non-polypoid lesions include superficial elevated (0-IIa), completely flat (0-IIb), and depressed (0-IIc) lesions. Moreover, a superficial-type lesion of size more than 10 mm with no increase in height is called a laterally spreading tumor (LST). LSTs can be further divided into two main classes: granular type (LST-G) and non-granular type (LST-NG) (Figure 1). We know that LST-NG tumors of size more than (or equal to) 20 mm and LST-G tumors of size more than (or equal to) 30 mm harbor a significantly higher likelihood of submucosal invasion [12]; therefore, a careful evaluation of morphological features is crucial for the depth diagnosis.

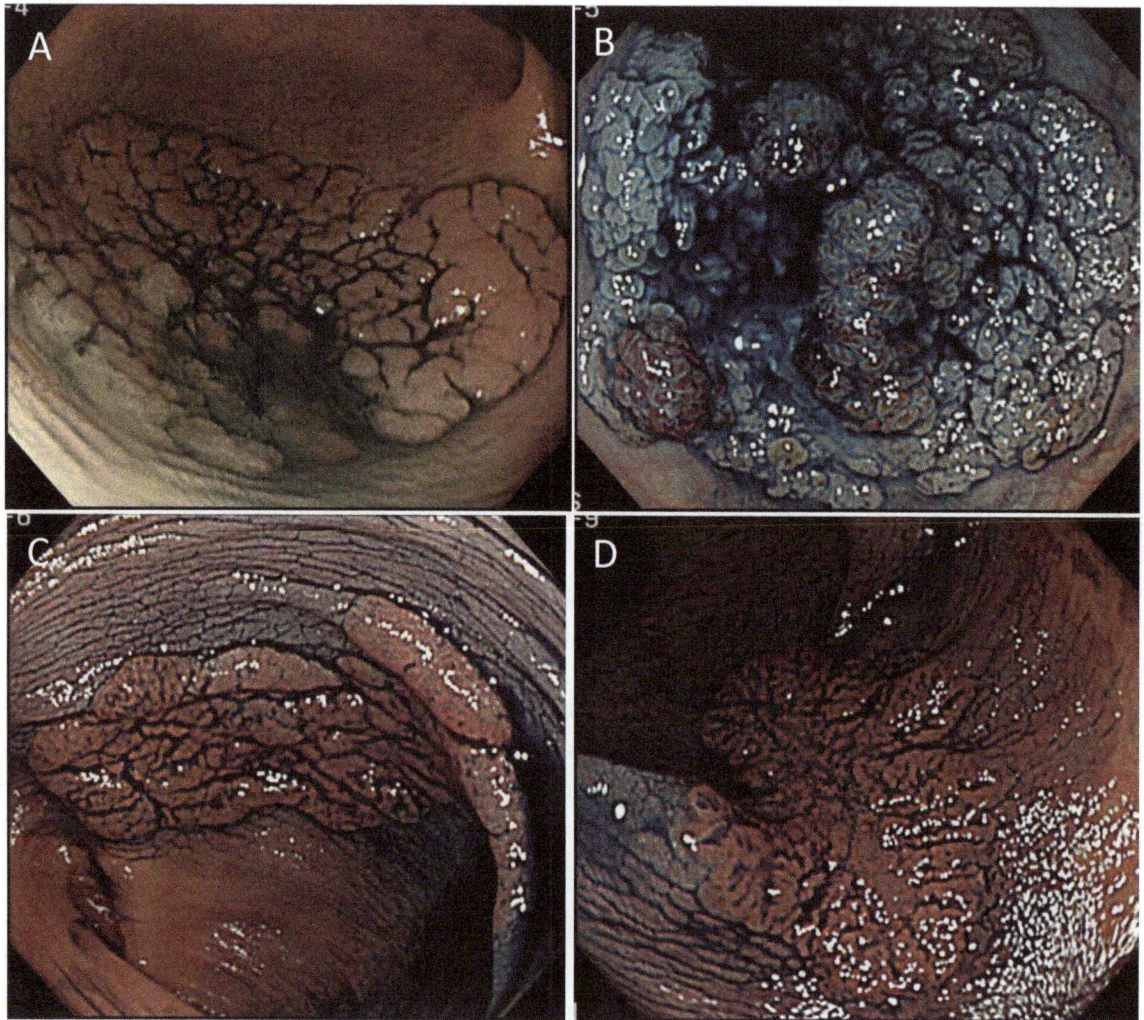

Figure 1. Subtypes of tumors with lateral spread. A: Laterally spreading tumor (LST), homogeneous granular type; B: LST, mixed granular type; C: LST, non-granular, flat elevated type; D: LST, non-granular, pseudodepressed type.

Some findings regarding the important conventional colonoscopic findings for determining the invasion depths of non-polypoid lesions have been reported in previous studies: redness, white spots (chicken-skin appearance), appearance of expansion, firm consistency, deep depression surface, irregular bottom of depression surface, and fold converging toward the tumor. Matsuda et al. verified these findings retrospectively to clarify the clinically important characteristics. White spots, redness, firm consistency, and a deep depressed area were significantly associated with an increased risk of submucosal deep invasion in a univariate analysis [13].

2.2. Narrow-band imaging with magnifying endoscopy

NBI is an innovative optical technology that uses interference filters for spectral narrowing of the bandwidth used in conventional white-light medical videoscopy. NBI allows a more detailed visualization of the mucosal architecture and capillary pattern without the need for dye spraying. Upon reviewing microvascular architecture using NBI, our institution identified four different patterns according to Sano classification [9]. By examining a lesion's microvessel pattern using NBI, invasion depth was subsequently classified as intramucosa/shallow submucosa (lack of uniformity and high vessel density; capillary pattern IIIA) or deep submucosa (nearly avascular or loose microvessel diameters; capillary pattern IIIB). Ikematsu et al. reported the diagnostic accuracy of this technique for determining the invasion depth as follows: the sensitivity, specificity, and diagnostic accuracy of capillary pattern IIIB for differentiating the intramucosa/shallow submucosa from deep submucosa were 84.8%, 88.7%, and 87.7%, respectively [9].

On the other hand, we assessed the interobserver agreement in terms of estimating the depth of invasion using NBI and pit pattern analysis and found substantial agreement with pit pattern analysis and moderate agreement for NBI with magnification [14]. Regarding the lower interobserver agreement in the interpretation of the NBI findings, we should remember that the NBI system is still a relatively new diagnostic method with an unknown learning curve; to complicate the matter, several different classifications for the evaluation of mucosal morphology in colorectal neoplasms have been proposed recently in Japan. Regarding a consensus on the microvascular architecture and classification of findings, there has not been sufficient discussion for the worldwide use of NBI to become a reality.

2.3. Pit pattern evaluation using crystal violet staining

According to the classification of colonic crypts described by Kudo and Tsuruta, type V pit patterns include areas of irregular crypts (type V_I) and apparently non-structured areas (type V_N). Type V_I pit patterns allow further subdivision into areas with mild irregularity (type V_I mild) and severe irregularity that show destroyed and severely damaged pits (type V_I severe). Type V_I severe pit patterns were defined by Tobaru et al. as areas containing pits with poor demarcation and those which contain faded or unstained stromal areas [15]. Regarding diagnostic standardization by magnifying chromoendoscopy, this classification should be directly linked to the choice of the most appropriate treatment. The depth of invasion of an early colorectal cancer is normally determined from the accumulated data of serial observations, which includes conventional imaging with no magnification. In this regard, Matsuda et al. described the clinical classification of an "invasive/non-invasive pattern" that incorporates conventional observations of lesion configuration, including depression, large nodules, and reddened areas (Figure 2) [13]. When differentiating between intramucosal/shallow submucosal lesions and deep submucosal lesions, an interpretation using this invasive pattern demonstrated a sensitivity of 85.6% and a specificity of 99.4%. In this report, the diagnostic accuracy was sufficient to demonstrate the efficacy of magnifying chromoendoscopy, and the clear advantage of this classification was directly reflected in the choice of treatment: endoscopic or surgical resection. Based on the pit pattern classification, the invasive pattern might include some cases classified as V_I severe and V_N pit patterns.

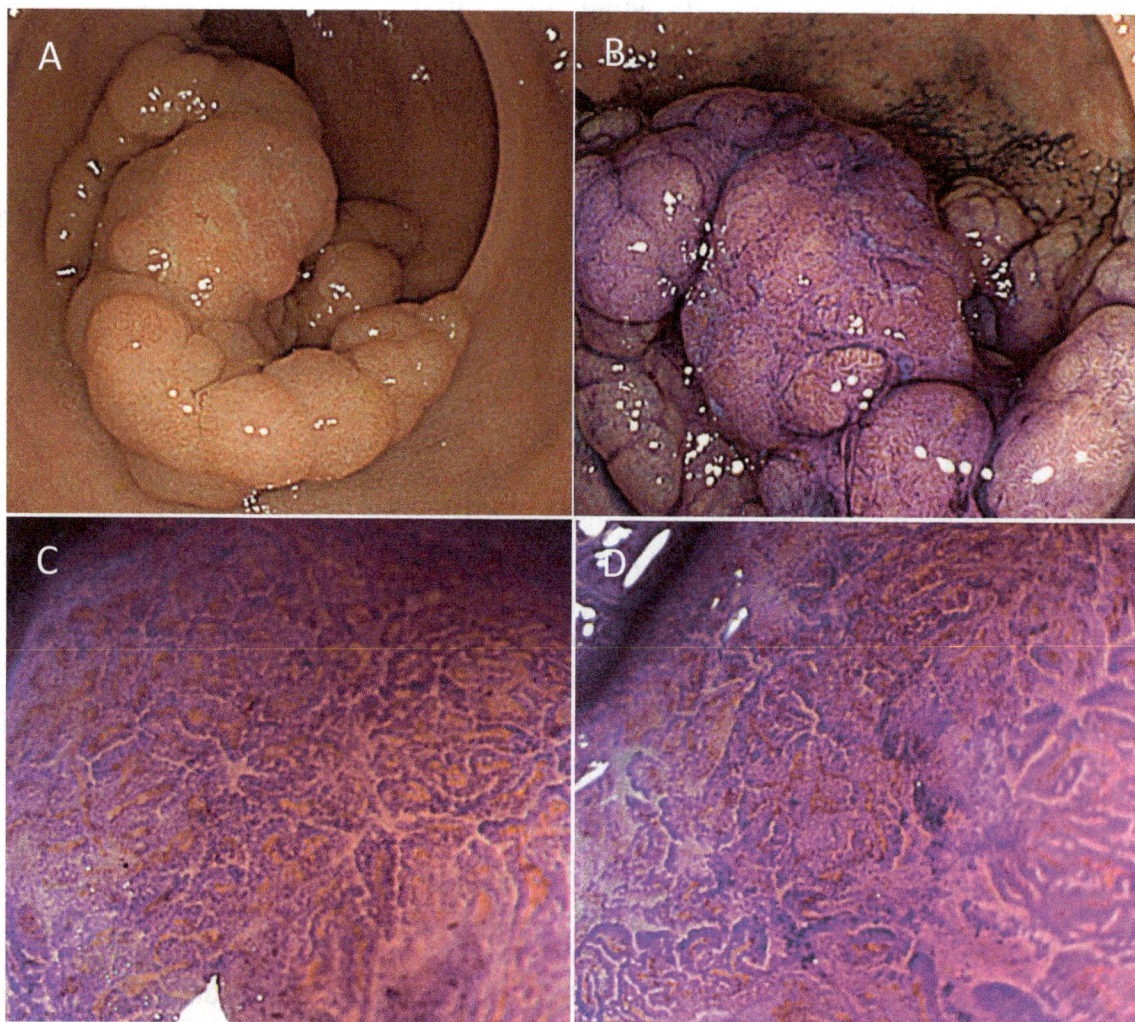

Figure 2. An invasive lesion exhibiting the "invasive pattern" visualized by magnifying chromoendoscopy with crystal violet staining. A: Large lesions with a reddish, protruding component; B: Depth diagnosis should focus on the reddish part; C, D: Reddish part displays a highly irregular type VI pit, which was demarcated as the reddish area.

2.4. Alternatives

2.4.1. Endoscopic ultrasonography

Data on the utility of high-frequency endoscopic ultrasonography (EUS) for the management of the malignant colorectal polyps is conflicting. Some previous reports have demonstrated the usefulness of EUS, in particular the advantages of high-frequency ultrasound for diagnosing the invasion depth of early colorectal cancer [16-19]. Hurlstone et al. reported that high-frequency ultrasound was superior to magnifying chromoendoscopy for determining depth invasion (accuracy of 93% vs. 59%, respectively). Matsumoto et al. also demonstrated the diagnostic superiority of EUS (probe-EUS) in their study (negative predictive value for deep invasion of 91% vs. 54%, respectively) [19]. In contrast, Fu et al. reported that there was no significant difference between magnifying chromoendoscopy and EUS for the preoperative staging of early colorectal cancer [20].

EUS is definitely very useful for determining the invasion depth or predicting submucosal fibrosis in flat or depressed lesions; however, its limited penetration depth is a recognized disadvantage. In particular, it might be difficult to accurately evaluate the invasion depth or submucosal fibrosis in protruding lesions. Moreover, the use of EUS to observe lesions located on the oral side of folds is also considered difficult.

2.4.2. Non-lifting sign

Uno et al. first described the "non-lifting sign" in 1994 [21]. Lesion observation during and after submucosal saline injection is a simple and crucial method for not only assessing the potential for deep invasion but also predicting the technical difficulty of endoscopic resection. Lesions may not lift as a result of submucosal fibrosis, a desmoplastic reaction, or the presence of large amounts of elastic fibers in vessels [22].

Regarding the diagnostic accuracy of the non-lifting sign for predicting deep invasion, Kobayashi et al. reported a sensitivity of 62% and specificity of 98%. However, magnifying chromoendoscopy displayed a sensitivity of 85% and specificity of 98% in the same study, resulting in a significant difference in sensitivity [23]. Therefore, despite its simplicity, the non-lifting sign could not reliably predict deep invasion when compared with a magnifying observation.

3. Indication of endoscopic treatment

In Japan, colorectal ESD has been covered under health insurance since 2012. Before 2012, the performance of colorectal ESD was allowed at only a restricted number of advanced medical centers that had been approved in 2009 by the Japanese Ministry of Health, Labor, and Welfare. From this, "The Colon ESD Standardization Implementation Working Group," a sub-organization of the "Gastroenterological Endoscopy Promotion Liaison Conference," produced a draft titled "Criteria of Indications for Colorectal ESD" [24]. In essence, ESD is indicated when lesions require en bloc resection for evaluation of histological features and for lesions whose resection using conventional EMR techniques is problematic. In other words, cancerous lesions that have the potential to invade the submucosal layer require treatment using ESD. In these cases, the size and morphology of the lesion are considered as critical factors. For example, a nodular mixed type LST of size more than (or equal to) 30 mm and an LST-NG of size more than (or equal to) 20 mm are considered to contain some risk of an invasive component. In addition, lesions for which resection is technically difficult via conventional EMR are also considered an indication for ESD; these include lesions exhibiting the non-lifting sign after submucosal injection, local recurrent lesions following previous treatment, and relatively large protruding-type lesions (except pedunculated polyps). In general, the en bloc resection of large neoplastic lesions (≥20 mm in size) via conventional EMR is technically difficult, and endoscopic piecemeal mucosal resection (EPMR) is typically applied. Undoubtedly, EPMR is an important method for removing lesions that harbor minimal potential for submucosal invasion, such as intramucosal neoplasms; however, it is crucial to recognize an important disadvantage of EPMR, specifically the increased risk of local recurrence. We previously reported that the removal of more than (or equal to) 5 specimens from a single patient is an independent risk factor for local recurrence following EPMR [25]. Moreover, colonoscopy with careful surveillance is required after multiple EPMR. Given the risk and occurrence of invasive recurrence in EPMR-treated patients, it is advisable to avoid such multiple resections and explore alternative treatment strategies.

4. Endoscopic submucosal dissection

Various treatment materials have been developed and applied in the context of ESD since the introduction of this technique. Hence, we introduce our ESD strategy as an example in this chapter.

4.1. Strategy

4.1.1. Preparation

A well-cleansed colon is a key element of safe ESD in preventing such adverse events such as bacterial peritonitis following iatrogenic perforation of the colonic wall. In our institution, patients generally receive 3 to 4 L of polyethylene glycol over 4 hours in the morning before ESD. Further, they also receive 1 g of cefmetazole in a 100-mL saline solution 20 to 30 minutes prior to ESD.

4.1.2. Sedation

Intravenous administration of an anti-peristaltic agent (10 mg of scopolamine butylbromide or 0.5 mg of glucagon) is mandatory, and intravenous administration of a sedative (2–3 mg of midazolam) and analgesic (15 mg of pentazocine) is provided as required during the procedure. Maintenance of conscious sedation during the procedure is essential, as patients are occasionally required to change position to enable the dissected part of the lesion to hang down due to gravity to improve identification of the submucosal layer.

4.1.3. Treatment devices

Here, we describe the equipment that is commonly used at our institution. ESD is done using a water jet endoscope (PCF-Q260JI and GIF-Q260J, Olympus Medical System Co., Tokyo, Japan). In cases in which handling the endoscope as the operator intended during the ESD procedure would be difficult due to the location of the lesion or paradoxical movements, a double-balloon colonoscope (EC-450BI, Fujifilm, Japan) is an available option for precise endoscope control [26].

A ball-tip bipolar needle knife with a water jet (Jet B knife, XEMEX Co., Tokyo, Japan) is used for both incision of the mucosa and dissection of the submucosa in the first step of the treatment. An important feature of this device is its use of a bipolar current system, which minimizes damage to deep tissue and decreases perforation risk [27]. Next, an insulation-tipped electrosurgical knife (IT knife nano, KD-612Q, Olympus Optical Co., Tokyo, Japan), fitted with a smaller insulation tip and short blade designed as a small disk to reduce burning of the muscular layer, is usually used to shorten the procedure time [28].

For distal attachment, we use a short-type ST hood (DH-28GR and 29CR, Fujifilm Medical Co., Tokyo, Japan) that facilitates broadening of the visual field of the operator and dissection of the submucosal layer due to its characteristic tapered configuration.

4.1.3.1. Electrosurgical current generator

The ERBE VIO 300 D (Erbe, Tubingen, Germany) is mainly used in our institution. Table 1 describes the output settings for ESD procedures.

	Device	Cut mode [E: effect]	Coagulation mode [E: effect]
Mucosal incision	Jet B knife	Dry Cut, [E]3 100 W	
Submucosal dissection	Jet B knife	Dry Cut, [E]3 100 W	Forced Coag, [E]2 50 W
	IT knife nano	Dry Cut, [E]3 100 W	Swift Coag, [E]2 50 W
Hemostasis	Hemostat-Y		Bipolar, [E]5 25 W

Table 1. Output setting of VIO 300D for colorectal ESD at the National Cancer Center Hospital, Tokyo, Japan

4.1.3.2. Submucosal injection

ESD procedures are critically dependent on the maintenance of suitable submucosal elevation by injection. We therefore prefer solutions for submucosal injection which enable a longer period of submucosal elevation. Two solutions are used in our center, as follows: glyceol (10% glycerin and 5% fructose; Chugai Pharmaceutical Co., Ltd., Tokyo, Japan) mixed with small quantities of indigocarmine and epinephrine, and a 0.4% sodium hyaluronate solution (MucoUp; Seikagaku Corp, Tokyo, Japan) [29]. In practice, a small amount of Glyceol is first injected into the submucosal layer to confirm the appropriate submucosal layer elevation; MucoUp is subsequently injected into the properly elevated submucosal layer, after which an additional small amount of Glyceol is injected to flush any residual of MucoUp [30].

4.1.4. Carbon dioxide insufflation

Carbon dioxide (CO_2) gas should be used for colonic lumen insufflation, as previously confirmed [31, 32]. CO_2 insufflation reduces the risk of pneumoperitoneum in cases of perforation, and also reduces the development of abdominal conditions pre- or post-treatment (or both).

4.1.5. ESD technique

In this section, the key points of the ESD technique performed at our institution are described (Figure 3).

The process begins in the retroflex view because endoscope handling can be better stabilized than is achievable with the forward view. After ensuring suitable submucosal elevation via injection, the initial mucosal incision is produced with the Jet B knife from the lesion's distal aspect.

In cases where a retroflex view is difficult to obtain, the tunneling method described by Yamamoto is a useful approach [33]. Briefly, incision and trimming of the mucosa are commenced from the distal aspect of the lesion until the last tissue segment is approached. Incision of the mucosa and dissection of the submucosa are then continued from the lesion's proximal aspect.

In most cases, insertion of the tip of the endoscope into the submucosal layer immediately after the initial mucosal incision is difficult. For these, trimming of the mucosa is performed. As the space for dissection is inadequate for continuation of submucosal dissection during trimming, the submucosal layer is gently and carefully cut near the mucosal layer.

Once the submucosal layer is secure in the visual field, submucosal dissection is furthered with the Jet B knife. One advantage of ESD is the clear visualization of structures in the submucosal layer, such as vessels and fibrosis. This allows the prevention of bleeding by pre-coagulation of the involved vessels. Cutting devices are used to perform pre-coagulation for thin-walled vessels; for thick-walled or pulsatile vessels, however, coagulation forceps should be used. In our center, we use Hemostat-Y forceps (H-S2518, Pentax Co., Tokyo, Japan) in bipolar mode (25 W) for the control of visible bleeding and minimization of any risk of burning of the muscle layer. In ESD, adjustment of the cutting line during submucosal dissection is also possible. In adenomatous lesions, the line of incision can be located near the mucosal layer to minimize perforation risk. In contrast, for potentially submucosal invasive cancer-type lesions, which require R0 resection, the line of incision should be located in the deeper tissues, for example near the muscularis propria, notwithstanding that the risk of perforation is increased.

Once an adequate visual field has been obtained as described, dissection is continued using the IT knife nano. The usable section of this "blade"-type knife is longer than that of other "needle"-type knives and can therefore reduce procedure time compared to those done without this knife. During the entire procedure, submucosal injection should be repeated whenever necessary to ensure suitable submucosal elevation.

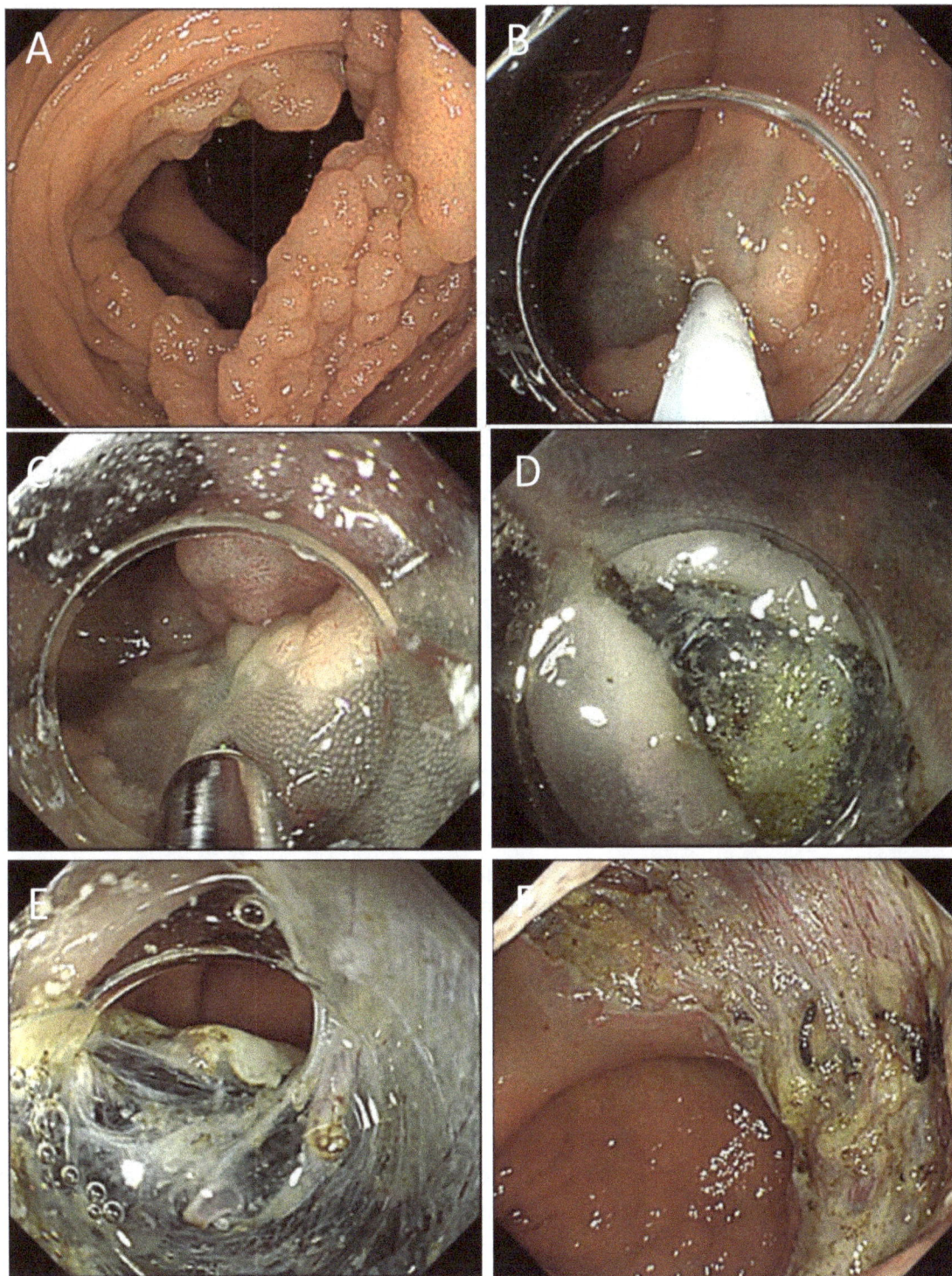

Figure 3. A case of ESD performance. A: Flat elevated lesion (85 mm) located in the ascending colon. It was impossible to maintain the retroflex view for this lesion. B, C: The submucosal injection of glyceol and first circumferential incision were initiated from the oral side of the lesion with a forward view. The first cut was made with a Jet B knife. D: After the first circumferential incision, it was difficult to slide the top of the short-type ST hood into the submucosal layer. Next, the visual field was broadened by carefully cutting the blue-colored submucosal layer near the mucosa (white dotted line). E: After step D, the top of the short-type ST hood slid easily into the submucosal layer, which became easier to cut. Here, the IT knife nano was useful and easily and quickly dissected the submucosal layer. F: En bloc resection was achieved without any adverse events during a period of 180 minutes.

Following the completion of colorectal ESD, a routine colonoscopic review is done to identify possible perforations or exposed vessels, and minimum coagulation is conducted with hemostat-Y forceps on visible but non-bleeding vessels to minimize the risk of bleeding after the operation.

4.2. Alternative technique

Hybrid ESD, which was first reported as "endoscopic resection with local injection of hypertonic saline–epinephrine" by Hirao et al. in 1986, is considered an alternative to ESD. This procedure could enable en bloc resection or at least reduce the number of piecemeal resections for large colorectal neoplasms in a manner that is both safe and relatively rapid. The technique is simple; the first step is a circumferential incision of the mucosa, followed by placement of a snare around the mucosa via the circumferential incision, and tightening of the snare (Figure 3) [34, 35]. However, there are some limitations associated with this technique. From our limited experience, lesions of size more than (or equal to) 35 mm and LST-NG pseudo-depressed–type tumors are often difficult to treat via en bloc resection, and we consider hybrid ESD to be most suitable for lesions measuring 20 to 30 mm.

4.3. Outcomes

In Japan, The Japan Society for Cancer of the Colon and Rectum conducted a multicenter observation study of all patients treated via conventional endoscopic resection and ESD for colorectal neoplasms of size more than 20 mm from October 2007 to December 2010 [36]. A total of 816 lesions were treated via ESD, and the short-term outcomes were as follows. The mean lesion diameter was approximately 40 mm. En bloc resection was achieved in more than 90% of cases regardless of lesion size, with a perforation rate of 2.0% and delayed bleeding rate of 2.2%. No perforation cases required emergency surgery and all were treated conservatively by endoscopic closure; nothing per os, antibacterial therapy. Hence, most iatrogenic perforations are very small and can be closed by endoscopic clip placement.

4.4. Training for ESD

Given the high risk of complications that arise from the anatomical characteristics of the colon, ESD requires a high level of skill and experience in endoscopy. A better understanding of the learning curve for ESD is therefore required to standardize training, and to achieve a more global acceptance of this technique. At our institution, endoscopists who will begin using ESD must meet the following prerequisites to perform colorectal ESD: a high level of skill in the non-loop insertion colonoscopy technique (more than 10 cases of total colonoscopy completed within 5 minutes without any abdominal discomfort), skill in conventional EMR or EPMR techniques, experience with more than 20 gastric ESD cases, and assistance in more than 20 colorectal ESDs conducted by experienced endoscopists [37]. In Western countries, however, gastric cancer is less common than colorectal cancer, and the introduction of trainees to ESD using colorectal lesion resection as a first step might be difficult. When required, trainees should start clinical training in colorectal ESD with lower rectal lesions, which carry a lower risk of perforation and a similar setting to gastric lesions.

We reported the short-term outcomes of colorectal ESD performed by less-experienced endoscopists [37, 38]. In terms of the learning curve, the endoscopists could perform the technique safely and independently after preparatory training and experience of 30 or more cases. On the other hand, most LST-G tumors of size less than (or equal to) 40 mm could be treated safely within a 120-minute procedure time without any adverse events. Therefore, we recommend that an LST-G tumor of size less than 40 mm is likely suitable for introducing trainees to ESD.

5. Conclusion

Various treatment materials have been developed and applied to ESD since the introduction of this technique. Of note, ESD is reliable for the en bloc resection of large colorectal superficial neoplasms. It has a better success rate than EPMR and enables more accurate pathological evaluations. In addition, colorectal ESD reduces unwanted surgery for mucosal carcinomas and improves the overall quality of life of patients with lesions in the lower rectum. Nevertheless, the technical difficulty of ESD and the complications associated with it, including iatrogenic perforation, have held back its wider global adoption. We consider that adoption of this technique will improve in future following further development of treatment devices with improved safety and reduced technical difficulty. However, there is no exact standardized procedure for ESD, and it is important to continue efforts toward improving the safety and technical ease of the procedure.

Author details

Taku Sakamoto*, Masayoshi Yamada, Takeshi Nakajima, Takahisa Matsuda and Yutaka Saito

*Address all correspondence to: tasakamo@ncc.go.jp

Endoscopy Division, National Cancer Center Hospital, Tokyo, Japan

References

[1] Morson BC, Whiteway JE, Jonse EA, et al. Histopathology and prognosis of malignant colorectal polyps treated by endoscopic polypectomy. Gut. 1984;25:437-444.

[2] Fujimori T, Kawamata H, Kashida H. Precancerous lesion of the colorectum. J Gastroenterol. 2001;36:587-594.

[3] Ikematsu H, Yoda Y, Matsuda T, et al. Long-term outcomes after resection for submucosal invasive colorectal cancers. Gastroenterology. 2013;144:551-559.

[4] Sakamoto T, Matsuda T, Nakajima T, et al. Clinicopathological features of colorectal polyps: Evaluation of the 'predict, resect and discard' strategies. Colorectal Dis. 2013;15(6):e295-e300.

[5] Saito Y, Uraoka T, Matsuda T, et al. Endoscopic treatment of large superficial colorectal tumors: A case series of 200 endoscopic submucosal dissections (with video). Gastrointest Endosc. 2007;66:966-973.

[6] Fujishiro M, Yahagi N, Kakushima N, et al. Outcomes of endoscopic submucosal dissection for colorectal epithelial neoplasms in 200 consecutive cases. Clin Gastroenterol Hepatol. 2007;5:678-683.

[7] Tanaka S, Oka S, Kaneko I, et al. Endoscopic submucosal dissection for colorectal neoplasia: Possibility of standardization. Gastrointest Endosc. 2007;66:100-107.

[8] Saito Y, Uraoka T, Yamaguchi Y, et al. A prospective, multicenter study of 1111 colorectal endoscopic submucosal dissections (with video). Gastrointest Endosc. 2010;72:1217-1225.

[9] Ikematsu H, Matsuda T, Emura F, et al. Efficacy of capillary pattern type IIIA/ IIIB by magnifying narrow band imaging for estimating depth of invasion of early colorectal neoplasms. BMC Gastroenterol. 2010;10:33.

[10] Hayashi N, Tanaka S, Hewett DG, et al. Endoscopic prediction of deep submucosal invasive carcinoma: Validation of the narrow-band imaging international colorectal endoscopic (NICE) classification. Gastrointest Endosc. 2013;78:625-632.

[11] Matsuda T, Fujii T, Saito Y, et al. Efficacy of the invasive/non-invasive pattern by magnifying chromoendoscopy to estimate the depth of invasion of early colorectal neoplasms. Am J Gastroenterol. 2008;103:2700-2706.

[12] Uraoka T, Saito Y, Matsuda T, et al. Endoscopic indications for endoscopic mucosal resection of laterally spreading tumors in the colorectum. Gut. 2006;55:1592-1597.

[13] Matsuda T, Parra-Blanco A, Saito Y, et al. Assessment of likelihood of submucosal invasion in non-polypoid colorectal neoplasms. Gastrointest Endosc Clin N Am. 2010;20:487-496.

[14] Sakamoto T, Saito Y, Nakajima T, et al. Comparison of magnifying chromoendoscopy and narrow-band imaging in estimation of early colorectal cancer invasion depth: A pilot study. Dig Endosc. 2011;23:118-123.

[15] Tobaru T, Mitsuyama K, Tsuruta O, et al. Sub-classification of type VI pit patterns in colorectal tumors: Relation to the depth of tumor invasion. Int J Oncol. 2008;33:503-508.

[16] Saitoh Y, Obara T, Einami K, et al. Efficacy of high-frequency ultrasound probes for the preoperative staging of invasion depth in flat and depressed colorectal tumors. Gastrointest Endosc. 1996;44:34-39.

[17] Turuta O, Kawano H, Fujita M, et al. Usefulness of the high-frequency ultrasound probe in pretherapeutic staging of superficial-type colorectal tumours. Int J Oncol. 1998;13:677-684.

[18] Hurlstone DP, Brown S, Cross SS, et al. High magnification chromoscopic colonoscopy or high frequency 20 MHz mini probe endoscopic ultrasound staging for early colorectal neoplasia: A comparative prospective analysis. Gut. 2005;54:1585-1589.

[19] Matsumoto T, Hizawa K, Esaki M, et al. Comparison of EUS and magnifying colonoscope for assessment of small colorectal cancers. Gastrointest Endosc. 2002;56:354-360.

[20] Fu KI, Kato S, Sano Y, et al. Staging of early colorectal cancers: Magnifying colonoscopy versus endoscopic ultrasonography for estimation of depth of invasion. Dig Dis Sci. 2007;53:1886-1892.

[21] Uno Y, Munakata A. The non-lifting sign of invasive colon cancer. Gastrointest Endosc. 1994;40:485-489.

[22] Moss A, Bourke MJ, Williams SJ, et al. Endoscopic mucosal resection outcomes and prediction of submucosal cancer from advanced colonic mucosal neoplasia. Gastroenterology. 2011;140:1909-1918.

[23] Kobayashi N, Saito Y, Sano Y, et al. Determining the treatment strategy for colorectal neoplastic lesions: Endoscopic assessment or the non-lifting sign for diagnosing invasion depth? Endoscopy. 2007;39:701-705.

[24] Saito Y, Kawano H, Takeuchi Y, et al. Current status of colorectal endoscopic submucosal dissection in Japan and other Asian countries: Progressing towards technical standardization. Dig Endosc. 2012;24 Suppl 1:67-72.

[25] Sakamoto T, Matsuda T, Otake Y, Nakajima T, Saito Y. Predictive factors of local recurrence after endoscopic piecemeal mucosal resection. J Gastroenterol. 2012;47:635-640.

[26] Ohya T, Ohata K, Sumiyama K, et al. Balloon overtube-guided colorectal endoscopic submucosal dissection. World J Gastroenterol. 2009;15:6086-6090.

[27] Nonaka S, Saito Y, Fukunaga S, et al. Impact of endoscopic submucosal dissection knife on risk of perforation with an animal model-monopolar needle knife and with a bipolar needle knife. Dig Endosc. 2012;24:381.

[28] Hotta K, Yamaguchi Y, Saito Y, Takao T, Ono H. Current opinions for endoscopic submucosal dissection for colorectal tumors from our experiences: Indications, technical aspects and complications. Dig Endosc. 2012;24 Suppl 1:110-116.

[29] Uraoka T, Fujii T, Saito Y, et al. Effectiveness of glycerol as a submucosal injection for EMR. Gastrointest Endosc. 2005;61:736-740.

[30] Yamamoto H, Kawata H, Sunada K, et al. Successful en bloc resection of large superficial tumors in the stomach and colon using sodium hyaluronate and small-caliber-tip transparent hood. Endoscopy. 2003;35:690-694.

[31] Saito Y, Uraoka T, Matsuda T, et al. A pilot study to assess the safety and efficacy of carbon dioxide insufflation during colorectal endoscopic submucosal dissection with the patient under conscious sedation. Gastrointest Endosc. 2007;65:537-542.

[32] Kikuchi T, Fu KI, Saito Y, et al. Transcutaneous monitoring of partial pressure of carbon dioxide during endoscopic submucosal dissection of early colorectal neoplasia with carbon dioxide insufflation: A prospective study. Surg Endosc. 2010;24:2231-2235.

[33] Monkemuller K, Wilcox CM, Munoz-Navas M, eds. Interventional and Therapeutic Gastrointestinal Endoscopy. Front Gastrointest Res. Basel; Karger; 2010. Vol 27, pp 287-295.

[34] Terasaki M, Tanaka S, Oka S, et al. Clinical outcomes of endoscopic submucosal dissection and endoscopic mucosal resection for laterally spreading tumors larger than 20 mm. J Gastroenterol Hepatol. 2012;27:734-740.

[35] Sakamoto T, Matsuda T, Nakajima T, et al. Efficacy of endoscopic mucosal resection with circumferential incision for patients with large colorectal tumors. Clin Gastroenterol Hepatol. 2012;10:22-26.

[36] Nakajima T, Saito Y, Tanaka S, et al. Current status of endoscopic resection strategy for large, early colorectal neoplasia in Japan. Surg Endosc. 2013;27:3262-3270.

[37] Sakamoto T, Saito Y, Fukunaga S, et al. Learning curve associated with colorectal endoscopic submucosal dissection for endoscopists experienced in gastric endoscopic submucosal dissection. Dis Colon Rectum. 2011;54:1307-1312.

[38] Sakamoto T, Sato C, Makazu M, et al. Short-term outcomes of colorectal endoscopic submucosal dissection performed by trainees. Digestion. 2014;89:37-42.

4

Minimally Invasive Transcanal Endoscopic Ear Surgery

Lela Migirov and Michael Wolf

Abstract

Endoscopes have rapidly become widely accepted in the performance of ear surgery. Current chapter describes surgical technique and benefits and limitations for endoscopic eradication of cholesteatoma, endoscopic tympanoplasty, endoscopic stapedotomy and endoscopic cochlear implantation.

Minimally invasive endoscopic and endoscope-assisted surgical techniques are increasingly being employed in the surgical management of cholesteatoma. Endoscopic surgeries distinctly reduced residual cholesteatomas and the indications of later tympanotomy thanks to the good visualization of residual cholesteatoma sites, such as the anterior and posterior epitympanic spaces, sinus tympani, facial recess, and hypotympanum. Minimally invasive transcanal endoscopic approach can be applied as for primary cholesteatomas as well as for revision of CWU cases, when residual/recurrent cholesteatoma is confined to the middle ear, and in CWD or radical cavities, when residual/recurrent disease is hidden in the supratubal recess, sinus tympani or under pseudo-membrane in the large mastoid cavities.

The use of endoscopes in myringoplasty is especially helpful in patients with narrow external canals, anterior defects and bone overhang, when perforation's margins are barely, if at all, visible under a microscope.

The transcanal endoscopic stapedotomy can be beneficial in improving the visibility and accessibility of the stapes and the oval window niche, avoiding manipulation of the chorda tympani nerve and blind fracture of the stapedial crurae.

An endoscopic cochlear implantation involves entering the middle ear by means of endoscopic transcanal tympanotomy and insertion of the electrode array into the scala tympani via the round window under direct endoscopic control. The main benefits of the endoscopic transcanal approach to cochlear implant are improving the visibility and accessibility of the round window membrane, obviating the need to divide the chorda tympani nerve in order to obtain adequate exposure of the middle ear structures, and eliminating the risk of the facial nerve injury since it is not in the direction of drilling.

Keywords: endoscopic surgery, approach, tympanoplasty, stapedectomy, cochlear implant

1. Introduction

The introduction of endoscopes completely changed the surgical approach to the middle ear pathologies. Management of cholesteatoma continues to pose a surgical challenge, and the choice of surgical technique depends on the extension of the disease, the surgeon's own experience and skills, published data, and the patient's socioeconomic circumstances. Minimally invasive endoscopic and endoscope-assisted surgical techniques are increasingly being employed in the surgical management of cholesteatoma.

2. Endoscopic surgery for cholesteatoma

Exclusive transcanal endoscopic approach (TEA) can be used for the resection of a primary cholesteatoma or for endoscopic revision of an accessible residual/recurrent cholesteatoma in the post-mastoidectomy cavity. In endoscope-assisted ear surgery (EAES), the endoscopes are introduced intraoperatively for completion of surgery performed under a microscope.

Endoscopic ear surgery (EES) and EAES distinctly reduced residual cholesteatomas and the indications of later tympanotomy thanks to the good visualization of residual cholesteatoma sites, such as the anterior and posterior epitympanic spaces, sinus tympani, facial recess, eustachian tube and hypotympanum [1-10]. Moreover, it was found that retraction pockets extending into the facial recess may be more readily removed by using endoscopes than by converting to an intact canal wall mastoidectomy with a facial recess approach [10,11].

The vast majority of cholesteatomas starts to develop in the middle ear and its extensions, and only later involves the mastoid cavity. Thus, the most logical access to a cholesteatoma has not yet advanced to the mastoid is the transcanal approach. However, the endoscopic approach depends on the experience and skills of the surgeon. In addition, otosurgeons are accustomed to using both hands at surgery while in the EES one hand is occupied with the endoscope and the other performs the manipulations for the eradication of the pathology, suctioning, hemostasis and subsequent reconstructions [10].

A cholesteatoma is defined as being accessible with TEA when it does not extend beyond the level of the lateral semicircular canal [11]. In case of cholesteatoma inaccessible even with angled instruments under direct vision of angled endoscopes traditional mastoidectomy is performed. The optimal surgical approach to residual/recurrent cholesteatoma is a controversial issue since residual lesions can be missed and cholesteatoma tends to recur despite the variety of surgical options. The common sites of residual lesions and recurrences are sinus tympani, attic, anterior epitympanic space, facial recess and the supratubal region, and they can all be visualized and accessed using the TEA [3,5-7,12-26].

Preoperative assessment includes otoscopy and pure tone audiometry in all patients. Recent studies have shown that non-echo planar (non-EPI) diffusion-weighted (DW) magnetic resonance imaging (MRI) can accurately predict the presence and extent of cholesteatoma in both primary and residual cases [27-31]. The size of lesion determined by the non-EPI DW images correlated well with intra-operative findings, with error margins lying within 1 mm [28-31]. Non-EPI DW MRI can distinguish cholesteatoma from other tissues and from mucosal reactions in the middle ear (ME) and mastoid, and it can also demonstrate the extent of the lesion [27-31]. Thus, we prefer performing the non-EPI DWI MRI prior to primary cholesteatoma surgery as well as before revision procedures [31]. Non-EPI DW images allow avoiding the irradiation, and this point is extremely important for all patients, especially children [32]. The choice of approach as in primary as well as in revision surgery depends on the extent of disease and on the preoperative otoscopic and radiological findings (Figures 1-8). We already found that cholesteatoma < 8 mm in size and confined to the ME or its extensions can be eradicated with a minimally invasive TEA, while endoscope-assisted retroauricular mastoidectomy is the preferable procedure for larger lesions [31].

Many primary and some residual/recurrent lesions can be accessed with endoscopes. However, prior to undergoing the intervention, all the patients are informed of the possibility of extending their surgery to a transmastoid approach in the event that the cholesteatoma could not be satisfactorily eradicated by the transcanal endoscopic approach.

2.1. Surgical technique

The operating room setup, instrumentation and surgical technique were similar to those proposed by Tarabichi [11-14]. Rigid 3-mm diameter, 0°, 30° and 45° endoscopes, angled picks and forceps and routine otologic micro-instruments are used for all the TEA procedures (the list of the instruments can be seen in the web site of the International Working Group on Endoscopic Ear Surgery). A wide posterior tympanomeatal flap was elevated via the external auditory canal and then transposed inferiorly in cases of cholesteatoma situated in the middle ear (ME) under a closed or perforated tympanic membrane (TM). If needed, the scutum was removed with a bone curette until the cholesteatoma extension and the mastoid antrum could be visualized. The malleus and incus are removed when they are involved in the cholesteatoma or when they limit access to cholesteatoma in the anterior or posterior epitympanic space. When present, the stapes is left intact and meticulously and gently cleaned when it is involved with the cholesteatoma. Scutumplasty is done with tragal cartilage, and TM defects are reconstructed with the palisade technique and perichondrium in the relevant cases. In certain cases, cholesteatoma can be assessed and removed using the endoscopes directly from the radical cavity or from the mastoid cavity remaining after a canal-wall-down (CWD) procedure.

An operating microscope is used when the surgeon needs both hands to complete the removal of the cholesteatoma from the facial nerve or stapes footplate, and occasionally for ossicular chain reconstruction (OCR). Operative time depends on the extension of the disease, ossicular involvement in cholesteatoma and whether OCR is required.

Post-operative follow-up recommendations included repeated clinical examinations, and all the patients are encouraged to perform non-EPI DWI MRI at approximately one year following surgery. Second-look procedures or secondary OCRs usually are planned according to the clinical and MRI findings and the postoperative audiometric results. Whatever the etiology of cholesteatoma, scutumplasty with cartilage yielded good results in terms of prevention of postoperative retraction pockets.

EES has several advantages as compared to traditional mastoidectomy. This is a minimally invasive surgical approach in terms of incision, bleeding, drilling, postoperative pain and healing, and it is curative in terms of the radical eradication of the pathology including hidden areas poorly accessible and thus overlooked by a microscope. In the TEA, bony work can be circumvented leading to a decrease of possible intraoperative complications. This is functional surgery since scutumplasty and reconstruction of the tympanic membrane lead to conditions favorable to the introduction of the water into the external auditory meatus, and primary ossicular chain reconstruction can be done at the same setting. The patient can be discharged on the same day or on the day after surgery, and the hospital stay can be shortened compared to at least 2 days postoperative admission for uneventful retroauricular mastoidectomy. In contrast to mastoidectomy, the EES can be performed under local anaesthesia, and there is no need for postoperative wound care. Post-EES healing time is usually painless and is shorter compared to mastoidectomy. The set-up time and costs of the endoscopic procedure are comparable with mastoidectomy and even less since there is no need in drilling, cotton material and cauterization for hemostasis, suturing of the wound, bandage and postoperative wound care. The endoscopes and video-cameras are in routine use for endoscopic sinus surgery and thus are already available in most departments. The routine otologic micro-sets should be completed with some angled picks and forceps.

Although mastoidectomy is a procedure that is familiar to all otosurgeons, it can be complicated by accidental trauma to middle cranial fossa dura, dural exposure in the tegmen and sinodural angle, and brain herniation into the mastoid cavity. Dural and tegmen defect due to dural tears and cerebrospinal fluid leakage may result in pneumocephalus, brain herniation, subdural empyema, epidural or brain abscess [33-39]. In addition to primary cholesteatoma cases, minimally invasive TEA can be applied for revision of canal-wall-up (CWU) cases, when residual/recurrent cholesteatoma is confined to the middle ear, and in CWD or radical cavities, when residual/recurrent disease is hidden in the supratubal recess, sinus tympani or under pseudo-membrane in the large mastoid cavities, when access to cholesteatoma via external ear canal is difficult using the operating microscope due to the limited axis of work [24]. The TEA can be one of the options for eradication of residual/recurrent lesions in addition to traditional CWU and CWD techniques. The TEA avoids drilling in the mastoid region, thereby obviating the risk of dural injury and postoperative intracranial complications. Pre-operative non-EPI DWI MRI can predict cholesteatoma extension and is essential in planning revision surgery for residual/recurrent lesions. Screening with non-EPI DWI MRI at one year postoperatively is highly recommended to rule out residual disease, especially in patients who underwent CWU mastoidectomies.

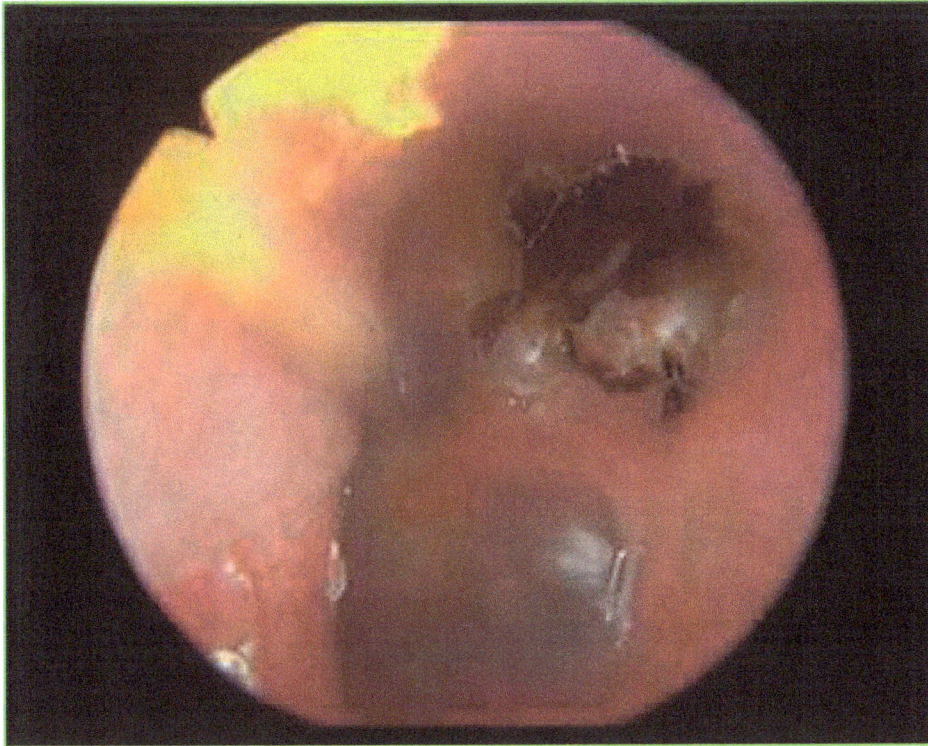

Figure 1. A view (with a 0° endoscope) of a left ear primary retraction pocket cholesteatoma.

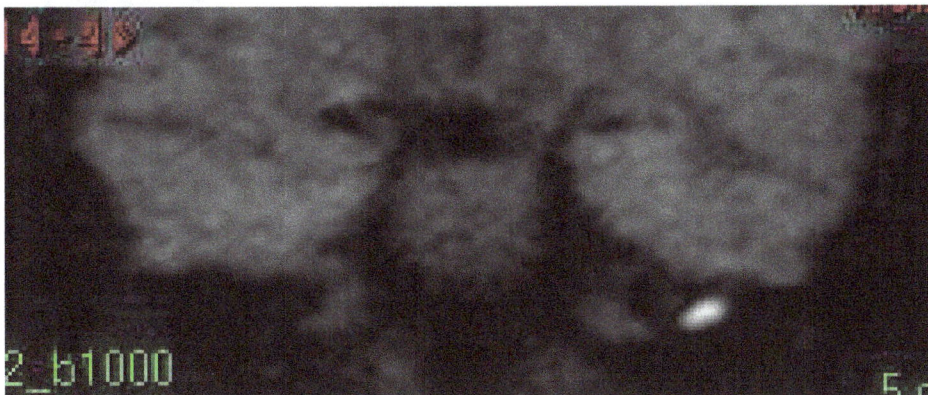

Figure 2. Non-EPI DW coronal images of the same patient presented in Figure 2 shows a 7-mm hyperintense lesion in the left attic (it was managed with TEA).

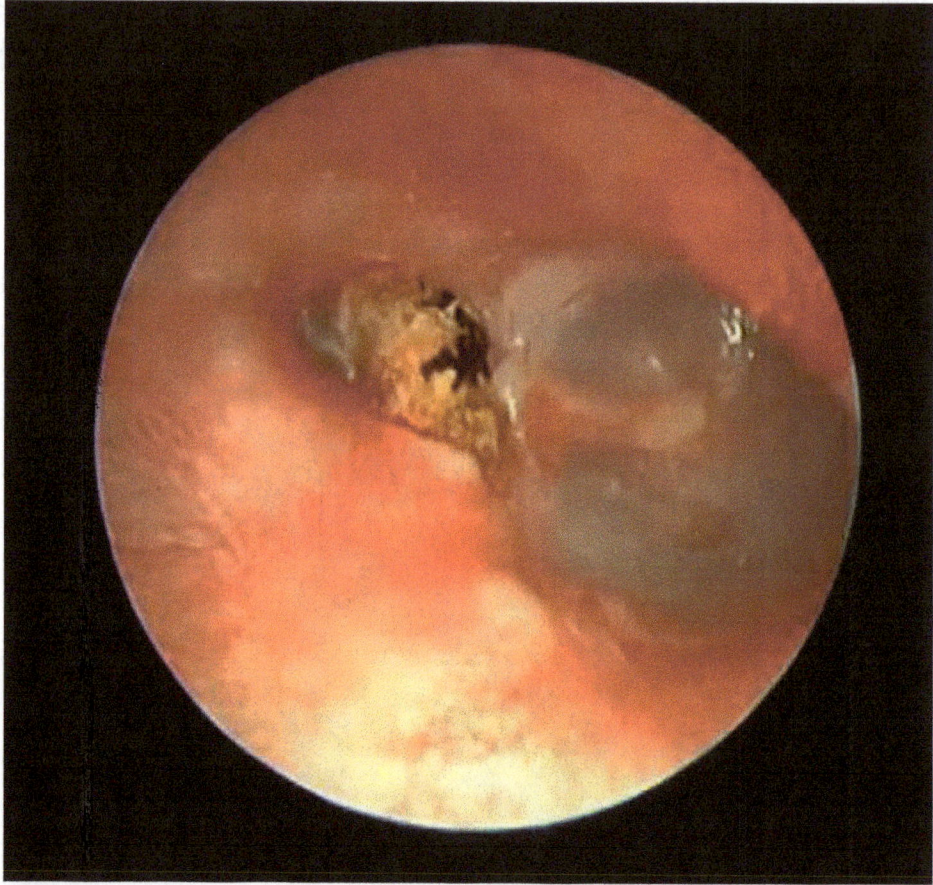

Figure 3. Endoscopic view of right ear primary retraction pocket cholesteatoma extended to the mastoid cavity.

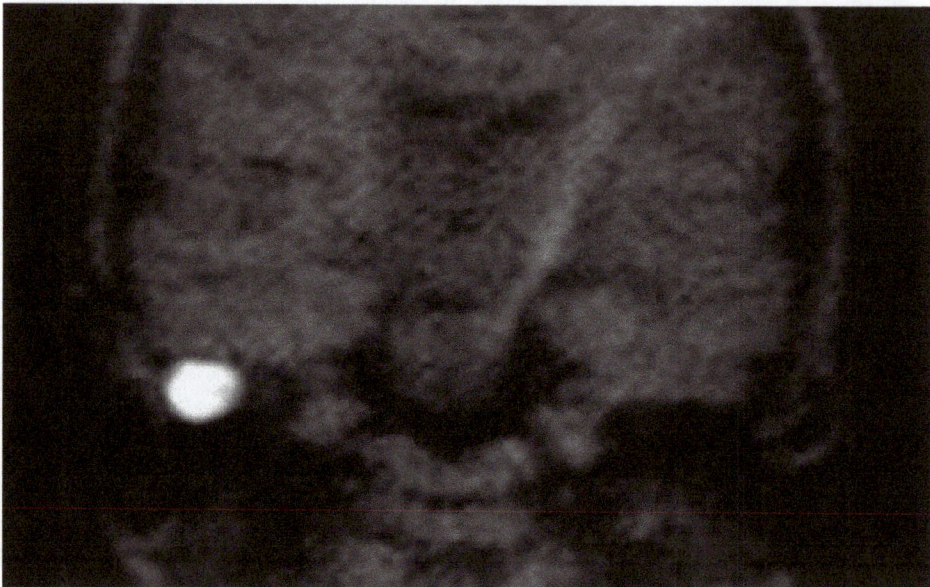

Figure 4. Non-EPI DW coronal images of the same patient presented in Figure 3 shows a hyperintense lesion occupied whole mastoid cavity (it was managed with CWD mastoidectomy).

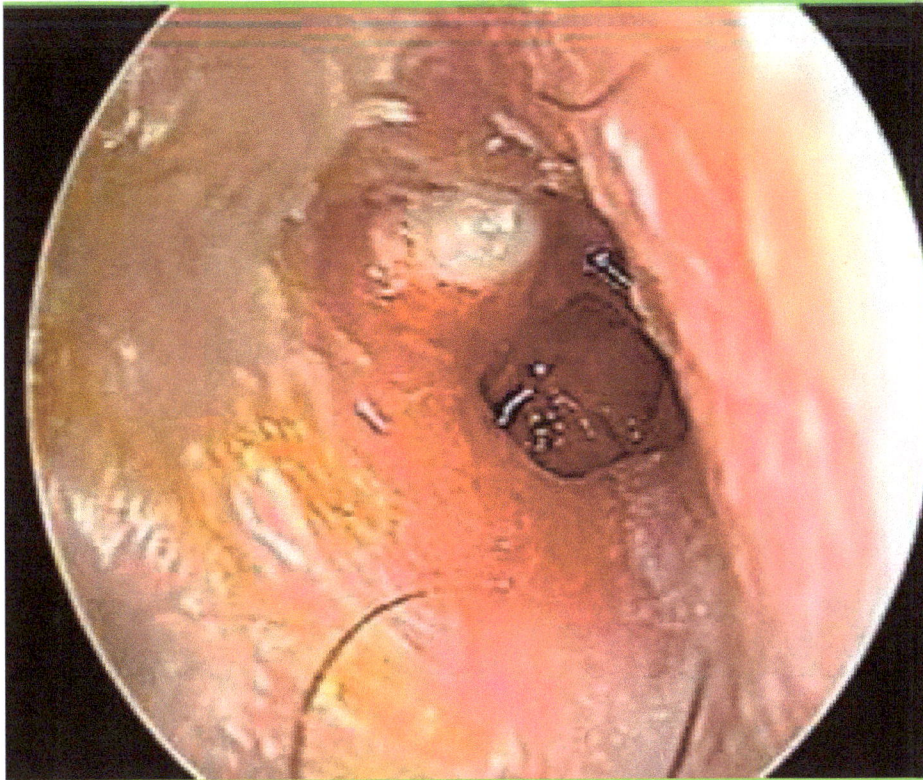

Figure 5. Endoscopic view of right ear residual cholesteatoma presented 1 year after CWU mastoidectomy.

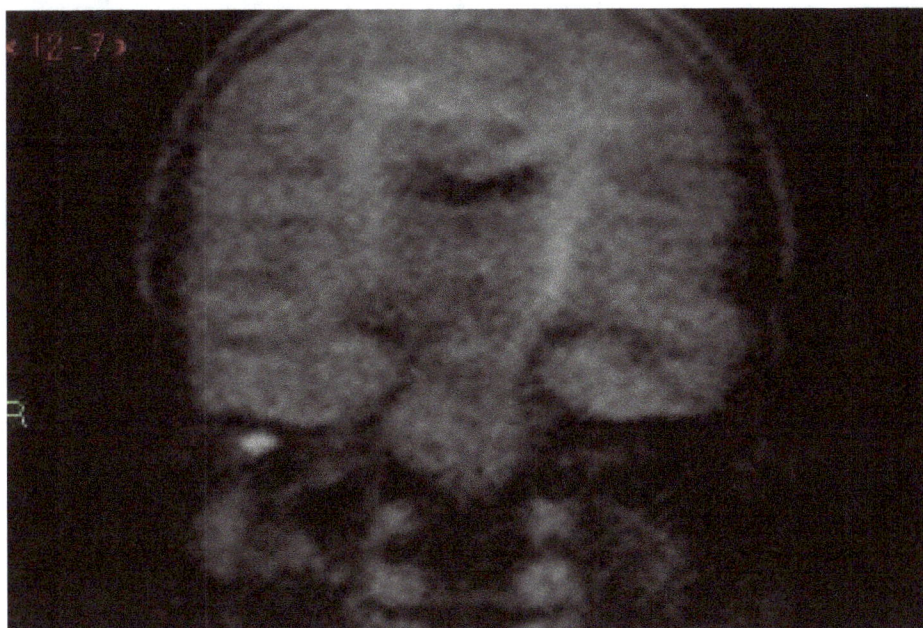

Figure 6. Non-EPI DW coronal images of the same patient presented in Figure 5 shows a 6-mm hyperintense lesion in the right attic (it was managed with TEA).

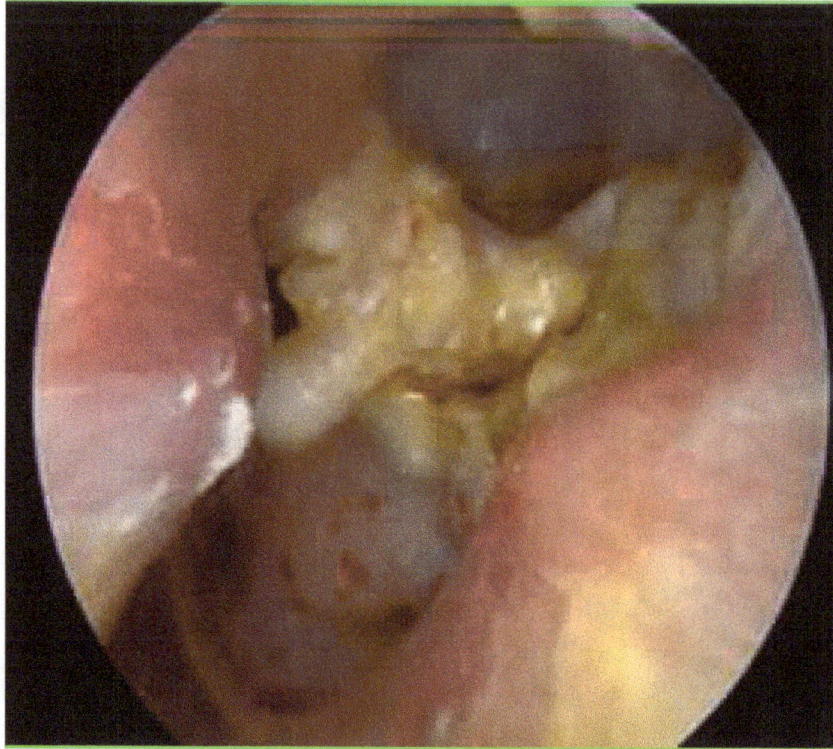

Figure 7. Endoscopic view of left ear recurrent cholesteatoma presented 2.5 years after CWD mastoidectomy.

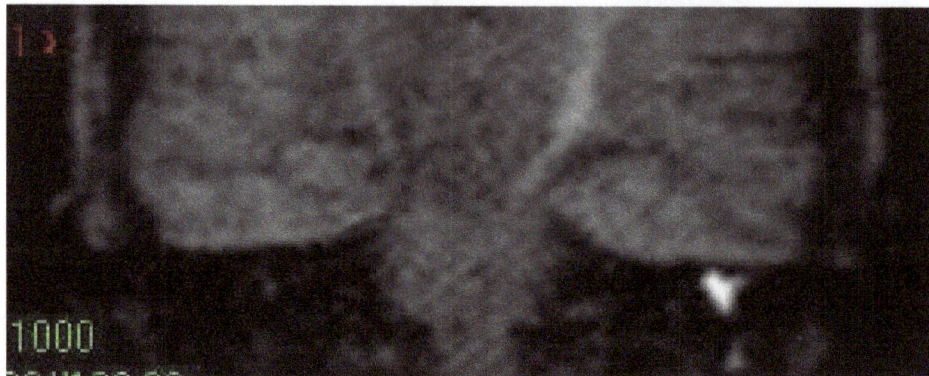

Figure 8. Non-EPI DW coronal images of the same patient presented in Figure 7 shows a 9-mm hyperintense lesion in the left middle ear with an extension to the mastoid (it was managed with TEA).

3. Endoscopic myringoplasty

Recently, different endoscopes have been used in the performance of ear surgery in general and myringoplasty in particular, and the surgical success of endoscope-assisted myringoplasty ranges between 80 and 100 % [40-46]. Myringoplasty can be technically difficult, especially in pediatric patients, due to the narrowness of the external auditory canal and the generally small size of the ear [46]. Moreover, temporalis fascia grafts and myringoplasties for anterior perforations are more likely to fail in children [40-43,47,48]. Surgical management of anterior perforations requires total exposure of the anterior angle, but a microscope may fail to provide a view of the anterior edge in 73 % of perforations that can, however, be entirely exposed with an endoscope [44]. As a result, drilling of the anterior part of an external auditory canal is usually unavoidable for the repair of anterior perforations when only a microscopic approach is employed [47].

3.1. Surgical technique

Transcanal endoscopic myringoplasties are performed under local or general anesthesia with a chondro-perichondrial graft that is harvested from the tragus and placed medial to the tympanic membrane remnants, utilizing the underlay technique and 14-mm length, 3-mm diameter, 0° and 30° endoscopes (Figures 9 and 10). Tympanomeatal flap is elevated using the 0° endoscope in all the cases, and the 30° endoscope can be utilized for better visualization of anterior perforations. The margins of perforations are freshened using the 0° or 30° endoscopes. A microscope is used for removal of the sclerotic plaques and releasing adhesions surrounding the ossicles when bimanual manipulations are needed.

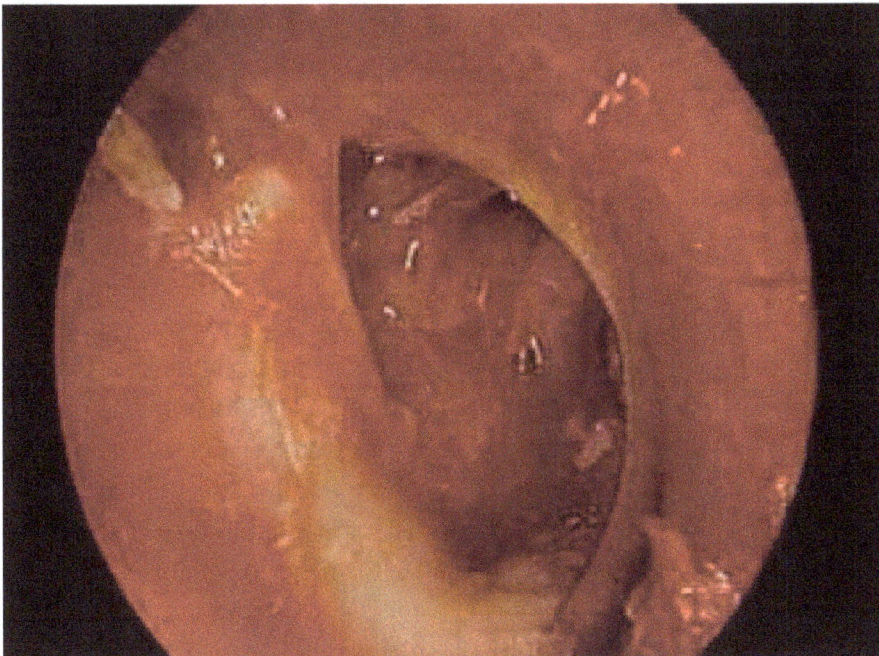

Figure 9. Endoscopic view of a large anterior perforation in the right tympanic membrane.

We found that an endoscope is very effective in ensuring satisfactory approximation of graft material to the perforation margins in small, medium-sized, large and subtotal perforations as well. The transcanal endoscopic myringoplasty had, in our hands, a 100% rate of surgical success for closure of tympanic membrane defects. This technique is especially helpful in patients with narrow external canals, anterior defects and bone overhang, when perforation's margins are barely, if at all, visible under a microscope. The choice of chondro-perichondrial graft material and the meticulous removal of myringosclerotic plaques can enhance the surgical outcome of endoscopic myringoplasty performed by an experienced otologist.

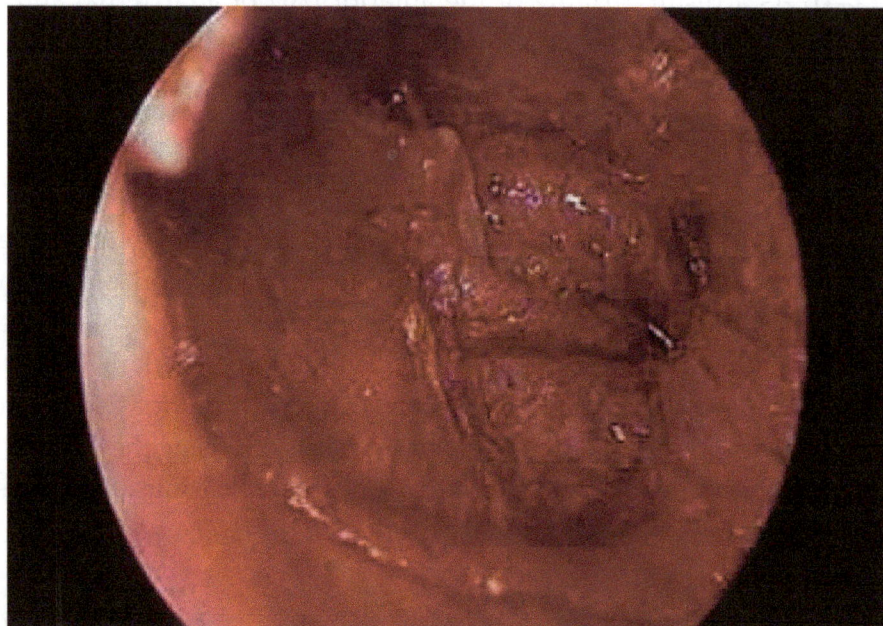

Figure 10. Endoscopic view of the same ear as in Figure 9 at the end of the myringoplasty.

4. Endoscopic stapedotomy

Stapedotomy can be technically difficult and challenging due to anatomic variations in size, configuration, shape or irregularity of the external ear canal. The stapes and oval window niche (OWN) can be obscured by the scutum. Excessive removal of the bone for better visualization of the middle ear (ME) structures can rarely result in subluxation of the incus [49-51]. When the posterior part of the bony annulus is removed to visualize the stapes, the chorda tympani nerve (CTN) can be occasionally touched, stretched, manipulated or transected and result in 20-60% of postoperative taste disorders or tongue symptoms [52-57]. The existing data indicate that the CTN should be preserved whenever possible, especially if surgery is bilateral [53,54,57,58]. Bilateral CTN damage can result in transient or permanent bilateral ageusia of the anterior two-thirds of the tongue, as well as a decreased resting salivary flow rate. In addition, the patients may suffer from transient or persistent, distressing xerostomia or tactile dysguesia [58-60]. However, damage to the CTN and subluxation of the ossicles or stapes fracture significantly decreases in the hands of an experience surgeon.

Endoscopic stapedotomy was introduced in our department with the intent to avoid injury to the CTN when attempting to achieve visibility of the ME structures. The CTN was preserved in all cases, and our preliminary audiometric results were comparable with the others [61-63].

4.1. Surgical technique

The position of the patients is the same as for routine otomicroscopic ear surgeries. The external ear canal is injected with lidocaine 1% with 1:100.000 epinephrine. A fully endoscopic trans-canal procedure was undertaken using rigid endoscopes 3 mm diameter, 14-cm length, 0° and 30°. Angled picks and curved scissors and forceps are used in addition to the routine otologic micro-instruments. A posterior tympanomeatal flap is elevated transmeatally with the 0° endoscope and then transposed anteriorly. All the surgeries are performed with a 0° endo-scope, while a 30° endoscope can be required to better visualize the OWN, the anterior crus of the stapes, the tympanic portion of the facial nerve and the pyramidal eminence in some cases due to bony overhang in the posterior tympanum. Stapes fixation is confirmed by gentle testing of ossicular chain mobility. The stapes tendon is cut with curved micro-scissors and the stapes is separated from the incus in the incudo-stapedial joint. The anterior and posterior stapedial crus are carefully fractured and the superstructure is removed. The distance between the footplate and medial surface of the long process of the incus was measured to determine the required prosthesis size. The hole in the footplate is created with a Skeeter microdrill using a 0.5-mm diameter diamond burr. A platinum/fluoroplastic piston prosthesis (0.4-mm diameter, 4.5/4.75-mm length) is placed into this hole and fitted along the long process of the incus (Figures 11-14). The appropriate ossicular chain movement with the replaced stapes is ensured by malleus palpation. The tympano-meatal flap is repositioned, and the external auditory canal is filled with Gelfoam® soaked in ear drops containing antibiotics.

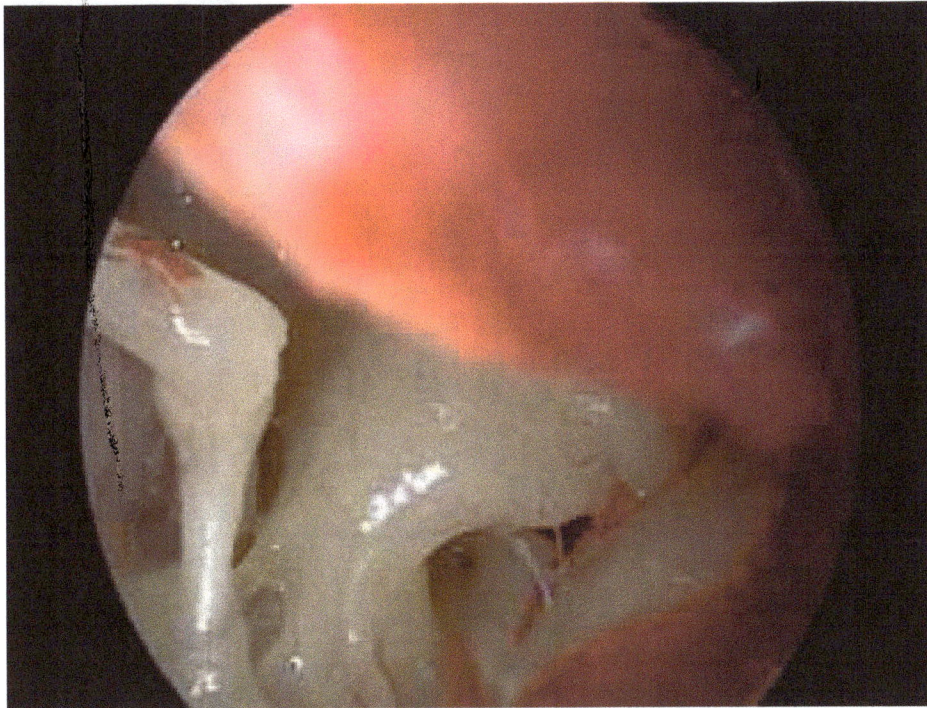

Figure 11. Endoscopic view of the right middle ear after an elevation of the tympano-meatal flap. Good access to the stapes and oval window niche was achieved without removal of the scutum and without touching the chorda tympani nerve.

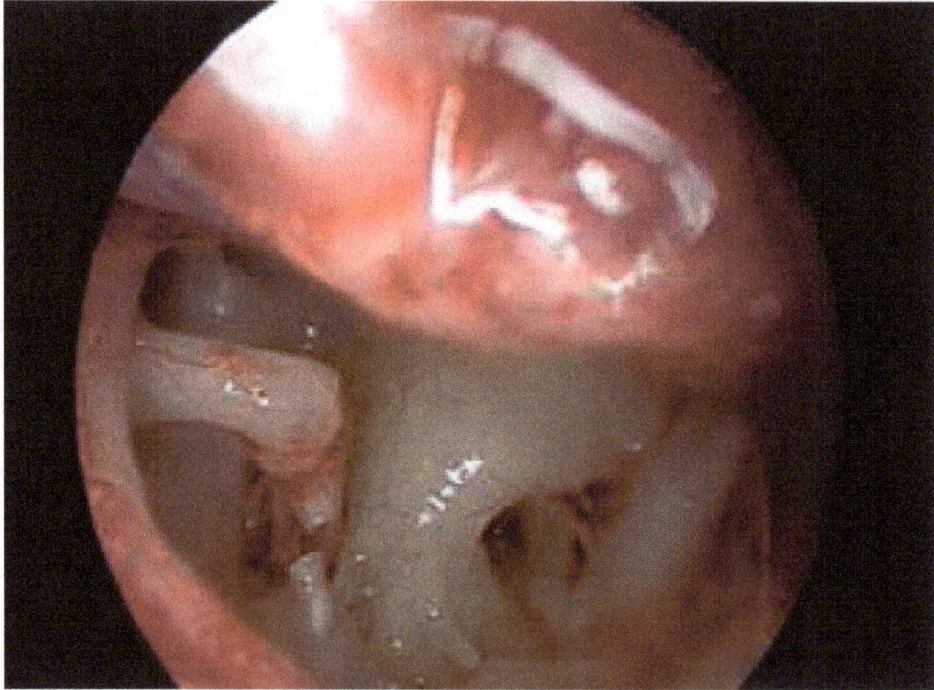

Figure 12. Endoscopic view of the right ear: cutting of the stapedius.

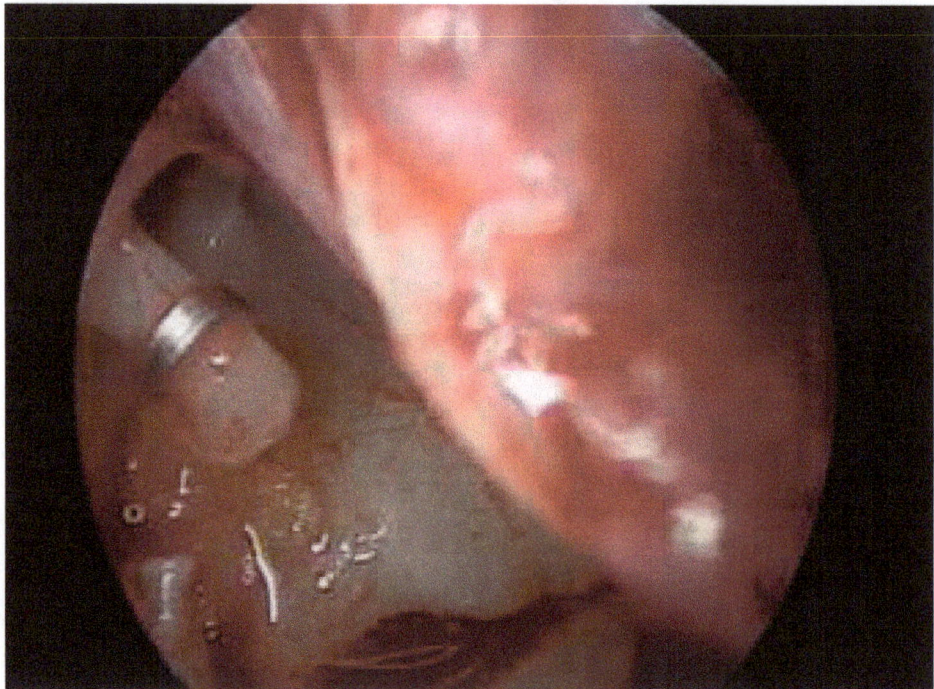

Figure 13. Endoscopic view of piston prosthesis placed in the hole that was created in the footplate and covered with a small piece of fat.

The possible benefits of ES are excellent visibility and accessibility of the stapes and the OWN, and avoiding manipulation of the CTN and blind fracture of the stapedial crurae. Assistance in using the operating microscope can be required when there is the need for two-hand manipulations for proper placing and coupling of the prosthesis, especially during the surgeon's initial endoscopic procedures. Finally, right-handed surgeon (L.M.) found that the axis of work was initially more comfortable when performing surgery on right ears and that the relative difficulty in creating a hole in the footplate and positioning the prosthesis in left ears could be overcome with more training.

Transcanal fully endoscopic stapedotomy can be utilized in patients with unfavorable external or middle ear anatomy, in candidates for revision or bilateral stapedotomy, in patients with already impaired taste sensation, with food-, smell- or taste-related occupations, and in those for whom the taste of food contributes appreciably to their quality of life.

5. Endoscopic cochlear implantation

Recent developments in cochlear implant electrode array design and modifications of surgical techniques have resulted in improved post-implantation performance by minimizing intra-cochlear damage during implantation [64]. However, electrodes and the surgical procedures used for their insertion still produce intracochlear trauma. An optimal site for cochleostomy in terms of avoiding insertion trauma during cochlear implantation (CI) has not yet been established. Some authors recommend the insertion of the electrode array through the cochleostomy corresponding to the antero-inferior margin of the round window membrane (RWM), while others contend that atraumatic insertion can be achieved directly through the RWM by removing the antero-inferior overhang of the RW niche, drilling down the crista fenestra, and incising the most lateral aspect of the RWM before insertion [64]. Regardless of the site of electrode insertion, the first step is achieving adequate exposure of the RWM in order to facilitate minimally invasive surgery. However, the topographical relationships among the facial nerve (FN), CTN, and RW showed that the widest route of approach through the facial recess (FR) frequently did not point directly towards the RW, but rather towards the basal turn at the promontory [65]. RWM insertion using the FR approach can be more challenging in pediatric patients, with the visibility of the RWM being limited in 11%-22 % of children even after an "optimal" posterior tympanotomy. An extended membranous cochleostomy or conventional bony cochleostomy may be required in some of these cases [66]. Moreover, the access to the RWM may be compromised in an FR approach due to the bony overhangs, abnormal course of the FN, jugular bulb location or abnormalities, anteriorly located sigmoid sinus, narrow FR and an undeveloped mastoid [67-70].

An endoscopic CI involves entering the ME by means of endoscopic transcanal tympanotomy and insertion of the electrode array into the scala tympani via the RW under direct endoscopic control [71,72]. Limited access to the ME structures can result in electrode misplacement, damage to the FN and injury to the CTN when a CI is carried out with an FR approach [73-78]. Indeed, bilateral sacrificing of the CTN due to a narrow FR in bilaterally implanted children can lead to morbidity that has not yet been investigated in depth. One of the reasons for incorrect electrode insertion using the microscopic approach through the FR can be the presence of a wide subcochlear canaliculus that could be mistaken with the RW niche [72]. Our experience as well as findings of our colleagues showed that the direct visualization of the RWM using a transcanal endoscopic approach permits electrode insertion through the RWM into the scala tympani with less drilling of the niche comparing to the FR technique [72].

5.1. Surgical technique

The procedures are performed with the patients under general anesthesia. The position of the patients, the skin incisions and the drilling of the implant wells are the same as for routine otomicroscopic CI. The external ear canal is injected with lidocaine 1% with 1:100.000 epinephrine. Cortical mastoidectomy until visualization of the incus is performed. A 6 o'clock vertical incision is made in the meatal skin, and a posterior tympano-meatal flap is elevated transmeatally to expose the ME cavity using a rigid 0° endoscope 3 mm in diameter and 14 cm in length held manually, and then transposed anteriorly. The CTN and body of the incus are exposed. Visualization of the incus body serves as a target for drilling and preventing injury to the FN which is located medial to it. The RWM is incised, and the electrodes are passed through the tunnel from the mastoid to epitympanum, medial to the CTN and lateral to the incus into the RW (Figure 15). The tympano-meatal flap is repositioned, and the external auditory canal is filled with Gelfoam® soaked in ear drops containing antibiotics. The surgical procedure can be modified in some procedures as follows: instead of inserting the electrodes through a tunnel that could limit the angle of insertion, an open groove is drilled starting superiorly and laterally to the CTN and ending in the mastoid region. The electrodes are passed through the groove medially to the CTN and laterally to the incus into the scala tympani through the RW, which is then covered with a small piece of temporalis fascia. The groove is filled with bone dust that had been collected during the drilling of the implant well, and covered with a large piece of fascia prior to repositioning of the tympano-meatal flap, aiming to prevent extrusion of the electrode array into the external auditory canal or tracking of the canal skin into the mastoid with cholesteatoma formation. All patients routinely receive intravenous ceftriaxone intra-operatively, followed by a course of oral cephalexin during the first postoperative week.

Fully endoscopic CI with complete electrode insertion via the RW was found more feasible for insertion of Concerto (Medical Electronics, Innsbruck, Austria) electrode followed by HiRes90K (Advanced Bionics Corporation, California, USA) and Nucleus 24 Contour Advance (Cochlear Corporation, Australia) [71].

The main benefits of the TEA to CI are improving the visibility and accessibility of the RWM, obviating the need to divide the CTN in order to obtain adequate exposure of the ME structures, and eliminating the risk of FN injury since the FN is not in the direction of drilling. The open groove technique was used several times in the past by the first author in cases of low-set dura and anteriorly based sigmoid sinus. A follow up of these patients showed that there is no protrusion of the electrode over a period of at least 5 years when the groove is filled with bone dust and is covered with intact skin.

A good knowledge of the endoscopic anatomy of the middle ear and a good practical knowledge of the endoscopic technique are essential to ensure a safe endoscopic CI with good outcome. An assistance of another surgeon may be required for holding the endoscope during the insertion of the electrode by a right-handed surgeon in the right cochlea and in removal of stylet, when relevant. Moreover, modern electrodes designed for hearing preservation by all companies are very thin and there is the need in bimanual manipulations for their safe and slow insertion requiring the help of an assistant in holding the endoscope. An angle of electrode insertion seems more comfortable in the transcanal approach compared to the epitympanic root of insertion. Right-handed surgeons (e.g. the first author) found that the axis of work was initially more comfortable when performing surgery on left ears and that the relative difficulty in electrode insertion in right ears could be overcome with more training [71]. Complete electrode insertion is achievable into the scala tympani via the round window both in children and adults. This technique can be used as a first surgical option or complementarily to the traditional posterior tympanotomy approach in patients with undeveloped or anomalous mastoid, narrow facial recess, anteriorly based sigmoid sinus, abnormal course of the facial nerve, high jugular bulb, malformed cochlea or distorted anatomy of the middle ear. The main limitation of an endoscopic CI is that it is a difficult one-hand surgery, technically possible only for highly skilled otosurgeons with extensive experience in performing classic aproaches as well as various endoscopic ear procedures. In endoscopic CI, one hand is occupied by the endoscope while the other performs manipulations during endoscopic CI including suctioning, hemostasis and subsequent introduction of the electrode into the cochlea [71]. The lack of stereoscopic vision was not considered to be a drawback by the first author in any surgery.

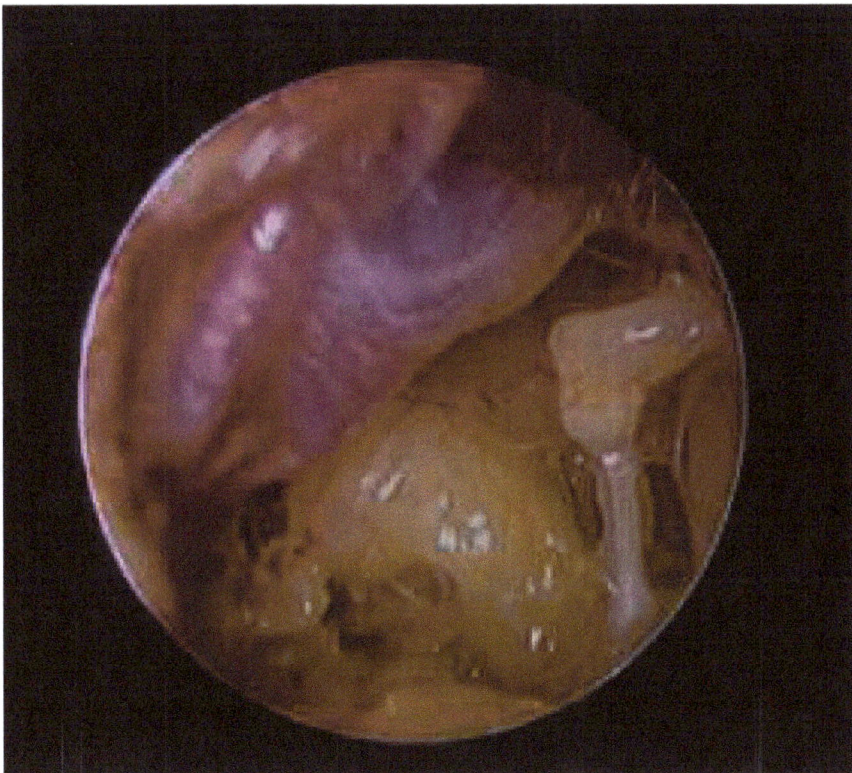

Figure 14. Wide exposure of the middle ear after elevation of the tympano-meatal flap in an endoscopic transcanal cochlear implantation (left ear).

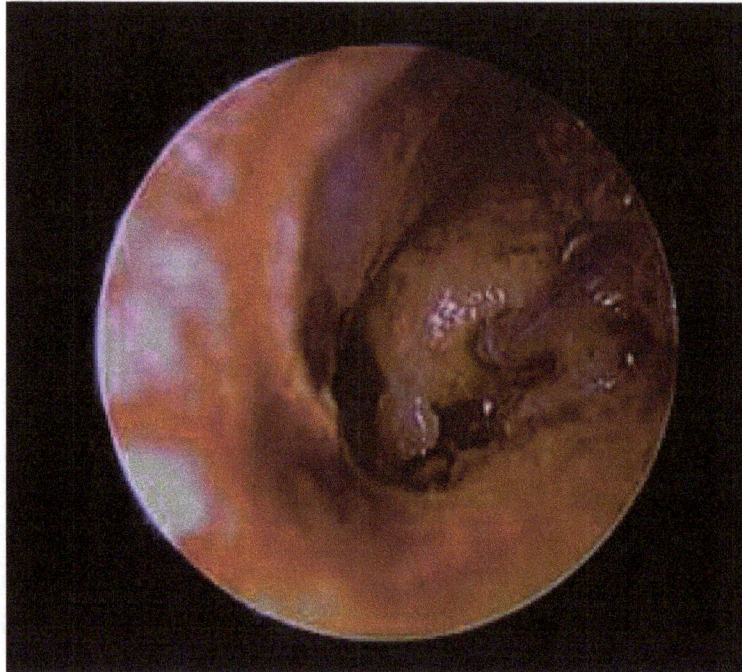

Figure 15. An electrode array passing through the tunnel medial to the chorda tympani nerve and lateral to the incus into the cochlea via the round window in an endoscopic transcanal cochlear implantation (the same ear as in Figure 14).

6. Conclusion

The transcanal endoscopic approach is minimally invasive surgery that can be successfully applied for various ear pathologies. Knowledge on middle ear anatomy, ear radiology and an experience in classic techniques is essential before starting the endoscopic approach. The assistance of an operating microscope may be required when there is the need for two-hand manipulations in dissection of the cholesteatoma from the dehiscent facial nerve, ossicles, stapes footplate, and in some cases of ossicular chain reconstruction, introduction of the electrode array into the cochlea. In inexperienced hands, the endoscopic approach can be associated with complications due to direct trauma from the tip of the endoscope to the facial nerve, the ossicular chain and a low-lying tegmen.

Author details

Lela Migirov* and Michael Wolf

*Address all correspondence to: migirovl@gmail.com

Department of Otolaryngology- Head and Neck Surgery, Sheba Medical Center, affiliated to the Sackler School of Medicine, Tel Aviv University, Israel

References

[1]   Thomassin JM, Korchia D, Doris JM. Endoscopic-guided otosurgery in the prevention of residual cholesteatomas. Laryngoscope 1993;103:939-943.

[2]   Good GM, Isaacson G. Otoendoscopy for improved pediatric cholesteatoma removal. Ann Otol Rhinol Laryngol 1999;108:893-896.

[3]   Badr-El-Dine M. Value of ear endoscopy in cholesteatoma surgery. Otol Neurotol 2002;23:631–635.

[4]   El-Meselaty K, Badr-El-Dine M, Mandour M, Mourad M, Darweesh R. Endoscope affects decision making in cholesteatoma surgery. Otolaryngol Head Neck Surg 2003;129:490-496.

[5]   Ayache S, Tramier B, Strunski V. Otoendoscopy in cholesteatoma surgery of the middle ear. What benefits can be expected? Otol Neurotol 2008;29:1085-1090.

[6]   Migirov L, Shapira Y, Horowitz Z, Wolf M. Exclusive endoscopic ear surgery for acquired cholesteatoma: preliminary results. Otol Neurotol 2011;32:433-436.

[7]   Presutti L, Marchioni D, Mattioli F, Villari D, Alicandri Ciufelli M. Endoscopic management of acquired cholesteatoma: our experience. J Otolaryngol 2008;37:481-487.

[8]   Bottrill ID, Poe DS. Endoscope-assisted ear surgery. Am J Otol 1995;16:158-163.

[9]   Marchioni D, Mattioli F, Alicandri-Ciufelli M, Presutti L. Transcanal endoscopic approach to the sinus tympani: a clinical report. Otol Neurotol 2009;30:758-765.

[10] Tarabichi M. Endoscopic middle ear surgery. Ann Otol Rhinol Laryngol 1999;108:39-46.

[11] Tarabichi M. Endoscopic management of limited attic cholesteatoma. Laryngoscope 2004;114:1157-1162.

[12] Tarabichi M. Transcanal endoscopic management of cholesteatoma. Otol Neurotol 2010;31:580-588.

[13] Tarabichi M. Endoscopic management of acquired cholesteatoma. Am J Otol 1997;18:544-549.

[14] Tarabichi M. Endoscopic management of cholesteatoma: long-term results. Otolaryngol Head Neck Surg 2000;122:874-881.

[15] Wilson KF, Hoggan RN, Shelton C. Tympanoplasty with intact canal wall mastoidectomy for cholesteatoma: long-term surgical outcomes. Otolaryngol Head Neck Surg 2013;149:292-295.

[16] Tomlin J, Chang D, McCutcheon B, Harris J. Surgical technique and recurrence in cholesteatoma: a meta-analysis. Audiol Neurootol 2013;18:135-142.

[17] Stew BT, Fishpool SJ, Clarke JD, Johnson PM. Can early second-look tympanoplasty reduce the rate of conversion to modified radical mastoidectomy? Acta Otolaryngol 2013;133:590-593.

[18] Stankovic M. The learning curve in revision cholesteatoma surgery. Am J Otolaryngol 2013; 34:65-71.

[19] Drahy A, De Barros A, Lerosey Y, Choussy O, Dehesdin D, Marie JP. Acquired cholesteatoma in children: strategies and medium-term results. Eur Ann Otorhinolaryngol Head Neck Dis 2012; 129:225-229.

[20] Gaillardin L, Lescanne E, Morinière S, Cottier JP, Robier A. Residual cholesteatoma: prevalence and location. Follow-up strategy in adults. Eur Ann Otorhinolaryngol Head Neck Dis 2012;129:136-140.

[21] Minovi A, Venjacob J, Volkenstein S, Dornhoffer J, Dazert S. Functional results after cholesteatoma surgery in an adult population using the retrograde mastoidectomy technique. Eur Arch Otorhinolaryngol 2014;271:495-501.

[22] Osborn AJ, Papsin BC, James AL. Clinical indications for canal wall-down mastoidectomy in a pediatric population. Otolaryngol Head Neck Surg 2012;147:316-322.

[23] Vercruysse JP, De Foer B, Somers T, Casselman JW, Offeciers E. Mastoid and epitympanic bony obliteration in pediatric cholesteatoma. Otol Neurotol 2008;29:953-960.

[24] Migirov L, Yakirevitch A, Wolf M. The utility of minimally invasive transcanal endoscopic approach for removal of residual/recurrent cholesteatoma: preliminary results. Eur Arch Otorhinolaryngol. 2014 Nov 21. [Epub ahead of print]

[25] Marchioni D, Mattioli F, Alicandri-Ciufelli M, Presutti L. Transcanal endoscopic approach to the sinus tympani: a clinical report. Otol Neurotol 2009;30:758-765.

[26] James AL. Endoscopic middle ear surgery in children. Otolaryngol Clin North Am 2013; 46:233-244.

[27] De Foer B, Vercruysse JP, Spaepen M, Somers T, Pouillon M, Offeciers E, Casselman JW. Diffusion-weighted magnetic resonance imaging of the temporal bone. Neuroradiology 2010;52:785-807.

[28] Dhepnorrarat RC, Wood B, Rajan GP. Postoperative non-echo-planar diffusion-weighted magnetic resonance imaging changes after cholesteatoma surgery: implications for cholesteatoma screening. Otol Neurotol 2009;30:54-58.

[29] Profant M, Sláviková K, Kabátová Z, Slezák P, Waczulíková I. Predictive validity of MRI in detecting and following cholesteatoma. Eur Arch Otorhinolaryngol 2012;269:757-765.

[30] Edfeldt L, Strömbäck K, Danckwardt-Lillieström N, Rask-Andersen H, Abdsaleh S, Wikström J Non-echo planar diffusion-weighted MRI increases follow-up accuracy

after one-step step canal wall-down obliteration surgery for cholesteatoma. Acta Otolaryngol 2013;133:574-583.

[31] Migirov L, Wolf M, Greenberg G, Eyal A. Non-EPI DW MRI in planning the surgical approach to primary and recurrent cholesteatoma. Otol Neurotol 2014;1:121-125.

[32] Brenner DJ, Hall EJ. Computed tomography-an increasing source of radiation exposure. N Engl J Med 2007;357:2277-2284.

[33] Garap JP, Dubey SP. Canal-down mastoidectomy: experience in 81 cases. Otol Neurotol 2001;22:451-456.

[34] De Corso E, Marchese MR, Scarano E, Paludetti G. Aural acquired cholesteatoma in children: surgical findings, recurrence and functional results. Int J Pediatr Otorhinolaringol 2006;70:1269-1273.

[35] Wormald PJ, Nilssen EL. Do the complications of mastoid surgery differ from those of the disease? Clin Otolaryngol Allied Sci 1997;22:355-357.

[36] Wootten CT, Kaylie DM, Warren FM, Jackson CG. Management of brain herniation and cerebrospinal fluid leak in revision chronic ear surgery. Laryngoscope 2005;115:1256-1261.

[37] Dubey SP, Jacob O, Gandhi M. Postmastoidectomy pneumocephalus: case report. Skull Base 2002;12:167-173.

[38] Migirov L, Eyal A, Kronenberg J. Intracranial complications following mastoidectomy. Pediatr Neurosurg 2004;40:226-229.

[39] Moore GF, Nissen AJ, Yonkers AJ. Potential complications of unrecognized cerebrospinal fluid leaks secondary to mastoid surgery. Am J Otol 1984;5:317-323.

[40] Usami S, Iijima N, Fujita S, Takumi Y: Endoscopic-assisted myringoplasty. ORL J Otorhinolaryngol Relat Spec 2001; 63:287-290.

[41] Karhuketo TS, Ilomäki JH, Puhakka HJ: Tympanoscope-assisted myringoplasty. ORL J Otorhinolaryngol Relat Spec 2001;63:353-357; discussion 358.

[42] Konstantinidis I, Malliari H, Tsakiropoulou E, Constantinidis J: Fat myringoplasty outcome analysis with otoendoscopy: who is the suitable patient? Otol Neurotol 2013;34:95-99.

[43] Yadav SP, Aggarwal N, Julaha M, Goel A: Endoscope-assisted myringoplasty. Singapore Med J 2009;50:510-512.

[44] Ayache S: Cartilaginous myringoplasty: the endoscopic transcanal procedure. Eur Arch Otorhinolaryngol 2013;270:853-860.

[45] Raj A, Meher R: Endoscopic transcanal myringoplasty-A study. Indian J Otolaryngol Head Neck Surg 2001;53:47-49.

[46] Mohindra S, Panda NK: Ear surgery without microscope; is it possible. Indian J Oto-laryngol Head Neck Surg 2010; 62:138-141.

[47] Halim A, Borgstein J: Pediatric myringoplasty: postaural versus transmeatal approach. Int J Pediatr Otorhinolaryngol 2009;73:1580-1583.

[48] Castro O, Pérez-Carro AM, Ibarra I, Hamdan M, Meléndez JM, Araujo A, Espiña G: Myringoplasties in children: our results. Acta Otorrinolaringol Esp 2013; 64: 87-91. [Article in English, Spanish]

[49] Gołabek W, Szymański M, Siwiec H, Morshed K. Incus subluxation and luxation during stapedectomy. Ann Univ Mariae Curie Sklodowska Med 2003;58:302-305.

[50] Lesinski SG. Causes of conductive hearing loss after stapedectomy or stapedotomy: a prospective study of 279 consecutive surgical revisions. Otol Neurotol 2002; 23:281-288.

[51] Malafronte G, Filosa B. Fisch's reversal steps stapedotomy: when to use it? Otol Neurotol 2009; 30:1128-1130.

[52] Miuchi S, Sakagami M, Tsuzuki K, Noguchi K, Mishiro Y, Katsura H. Taste disturbance after stapes surgery--clinical and experimental study. Acta Otolaryngol Suppl 2009;562:71-78.

[53] Guder E, Böttcher A, Pau HW, Just T. Taste function after stapes surgery. Auris Nasus Larynx 2012;39:562-566.

[54] Clark MP, O'Malley S. Chorda tympani nerve function after middle ear surgery. Otol Neurotol 2007;28:335-340.

[55] Michael P, Raut V. Chorda tympani injury: operative findings and postoperative symptoms. Otolaryngol Head Neck Surg 2007;136:978-981.

[56] Saito T, Manabe Y, Shibamori Y, Yamagishi T, Igawa H, Tokuriki M, et al. Long-term follow-up results of electrogustometry and subjective taste disorder after middle ear surgery. Laryngoscope 2001;111(11 Pt 1):2064-2070.

[57] Yung M, Smith P, Hausler R, Martin C, Offeciers E, Pytel J, et al. International Common Otology Database: taste disturbance after stapes surgery. Otol Neurotol 2008;29:661-665.

[58] Guinand N, Just T, Stow NW, Van HC, Landis BN. Cutting the chorda tympani: not just a matter of taste. J Laryngol Otol 2010;124:999-1002.

[59] Chen JM, Bodmer D, Khetani JD, Lin VV. Tactile dysgeusia: a new clinical observation of middle ear and skull base surgery. Laryngoscope 2008; 118:99-103.

[60] Mandel L. Hyposalivation after undergoing stapedectomy. J Am Dent Assoc 2012;143:39-42.

[61] Migirov L, Wolf M. Endoscopic transcanal stapedotomy: how I do it. Eur Arch Oto-rhinolaryngol. 2013;270:1547-1549.

[62] Poe DS. Laser-assisted endoscopic stapedectomy: a prospective study. Laryngoscope 2000;110 (5 Pt 2 Suppl 95):1-37.

[63] Nogueira Júnior JF, Martins MJ, Aguiar CV, Pinheiro AI. Fully endoscopic stapes surgery (stapedotomy): technique and preliminary results. Braz J Otorhinolaryngol 2011;77:721-727 [Article in English, Portuguese].

[64] Skarzynski H, Lorens A, Matusiak M, Porowski M, Skarzynski PH, James CJ. Partial deafness treatment with the nucleus straight research array cochlear implant. Audiol Neurootol 2012;17:82-91.

[65] Hamamoto M, Murakami G, Kataura A. Topographical relationships among the facial nerve, chorda tympani nerve and round window with special reference to the approach route for cochlear implant surgery. Clin Anat 2000;13:251-256.

[66] Leong AC, Jiang D, Agger A, Fitzgerald-O'Connor A. Evaluation of round window accessibility to cochlear implant insertion. Eur Arch Otorhinolaryngol 2013;270:1237-1242.

[67] Song JJ, Park JH, Jang JH, Lee JH, Oh SH, Chang SO, Kim CS. Facial nerve aberrations encountered during cochlear implantation. Acta Otolaryngol 2012;132:788-794.

[68] Leung R, Briggs RJ. Indications for and outcomes of mastoid obliteration in cochlear implantation. Otol Neurotol 2007;28:330-334.

[69] Kuhn MA, Friedmann DR, Winata LS, Eubig J, Pramanik BK, Kveton J, Kohan D, Merchant SN, Lalwani AK. Large jugular bulb abnormalities involving the middle ear. Otol Neurotol 2012;33:1201-1206.

[70] Jang JH, Song JJ, Yoo JC, Lee JH, Oh SH, Chang SO. An alternative procedure for cochlear implantation: transcanal approach. Acta Otolaryngol 2012;132:845-849.

[71] Migirov L, Shapira Y, Wolf M. The feasibility of endoscopic transcanal approach for insertion of various cochlear electrodes: a pilot study. Eur Arch Otorhinolaryngol. 2014 Mar 12. [Epub ahead of print]

[72] Marchioni D, Grammatica A, Alicandri-Ciufelli M, Genovese E, Presutti L. Endoscopic cochlear implant procedure. Eur Arch Otorhinolaryngol 2014;271:959-966.

[73] Orús Dotú C, Venegas Pizarro Mdel P, De Juan Beltrán J, De Juan Delago M. [Cochlear reimplantation in the same ear: findings, peculiarities of the surgical technique and complications]. Acta Otorrinolaringol Esp 2010;61:106-117. [Article in Spanish]

[74] Mouzali A, Ouennoughi K, Haraoubia MS, Zemirli O, Triglia JM. Cochlear implant electrode array misplaced in Hyrtl's fissure. Int J Pediatr Otorhinolaryngol 2011;75:1459-1462.

[75] Nevoux J, Loundon N, Leboulanger N, Roger G, Ducou Le Pointe H, Garabédian EN. Cochlear implant in the carotid canal. Case report and literature review. Int J Pediatr Otorhinolaryngol 2010;74:701-703.

[76] Hara M, Takahashi H, Kanda Y. The usefulness of reconstructed 3D images in surgical planning for cochlear implantation in a malformed ear with an abnormal course of the facial nerve. Clin Exp Otorhinolaryngol 2012;5 Suppl 1:S48-52.

[77] Wagner JH, Basta D, Wagner F, Seidl RO, Ernst A, Todt I. Vestibular and taste disorders after bilateral cochlear implantation. Eur Arch Otorhinolaryngol 2010;267:1849-1854.

[78] Brito R, Monteiro TA, Leal AF, Tsuji RK, Pinna MH, Bento RF. Surgical complications in 550 consecutive cochlear implantation. Braz J Otorhinolaryngol 2012;78:80-85. [Article in English, Portuguese]

5

Endoscopic Management of Pediatric Airway and Esophageal Foreign Bodies

Phillip L. Chaffin, Jonathan M. Grischkan,
Prashant S. Malhotra and Kris R. Jatana

Abstract

The use of endoscopy is critical to the management of pediatric tracheobronchial and esophageal foreign bodies. Children may present with nonspecific symptoms, and the diagnosis can be difficult when the ingestion or aspiration events go unwitnessed. Advances in endoscopic techniques and the use of optical graspers in the removal of foreign bodies in children have helped decrease morbidity and mortality. In this chapter, the history, clinical presentations, workup, and management for pediatric aerodigestive foreign bodies are discussed.

Keywords: foreign body, pediatric airway, esophagus, endoscopic, aspiration, ingestion

1. Introduction

The history of endoscopic management of pediatric foreign bodies was predated by significant innovations allowing for the evolution of adult and pediatric bronchoesophagology. Prior to these advances, tracheotomy was the accepted method for successful removal of airway foreign bodies [1]. In 1806, Philipp Bozzini, reported using the "lichtleiter" or "light conductor" to visualize the upper esophagus using candle illumination [2]. While his instruments and methods did not gain wide acceptance during his lifetime, they set the stage for further innovations that occurred over the ensuing decades. Desormeaux, a urologist, is credited with coining the term "endoscopy" in 1867 [3] and is considered by most to be the "Father of

Endoscopy" [4]. Kussmaul is credited with performing the first direct esophagoscopy, and his student Killian further explored these techniques and instrumentation. Mikulicz further refined the techniques and instrumentation of esophagoscopy, bringing it into more common use [5].

In 1895, Alfred Kirstein, a laryngologist in Berlin who was familiar with the work of Kussmaul and Mikulicz, was the first to directly visualize the larynx and trachea [6]. Killian became interested in Kirstein's achievements and began to practice laryngoscopy on cadavers and tracheotomized patients. In 1897, he was the first to remove a foreign body from the right mainstem bronchus of an adult via the translaryngeal route. His contributions and achievements have prompted many to consider him the "Father of Bronchoscopy" [7]. Following these innovations, tracheoscopy and bronchoscopy became accepted surgical techniques.

Chevalier Jackson became interested in laryngology while studying medicine in Pennsylvania and eventually furthered his studies in London. After learning the techniques of his mentors and as an instrument maker, he created an esophagoscope allowing for direct visualization of the esophagus. With this design, he was successful in removing esophageal foreign bodies from both adults and children. Jackson further refined his technique and the instruments he used, eventually developing the largest endoscopy clinic in the world [5]. Through the innovations of Jackson and his predecessors, the techniques for removal of esophageal and airway foreign bodies was perfected, reducing the mortality from foreign body ingestion or aspiration from more than 50% to less than 2% [5].

2. Endoscopic equipment

Modern endoscopic equipment is available in various sizes and configurations to accommodate patient age and size, and the use of flexible vs. rigid endoscopic equipment are both available (Figure 1). There are some clear advantages to the use of rigid bronchoscopy for removal of a tracheobronchial foreign body. The scope is designed to have ventilating ports so the anesthesia circuit can be directly attached for active ventilation and control of the airway during the procedure.

Flexible bronchoscopy can be done with insufflation techniques in the oropharynx or through the scope, but the channel on the scope is small, thus limiting flow of gas. Alternatively, the flexible scope can be passed through a secured endotracheal tube (Figure 2). If the foreign body cannot fit through the endotracheal tube, then this creates a problem for removal with the tube in place. The foreign body forceps have more limited sizes with flexible bronchoscopy, and there is also less control of the scope itself since it can bend to various configurations. Certainly in our experience, flexible bronchoscopy can be a useful adjunct to removal of foreign bodies, as it can give more distal visualization of the lower airways for small food particles, like nuts, that may fall further than the rigid scopes can reach. Such smaller, distal airways can be irrigated with saline and additional attempts using flexible or rigid bronchoscopy can then be utilized to remove these small fragments using endoscopic optical graspers or suction.

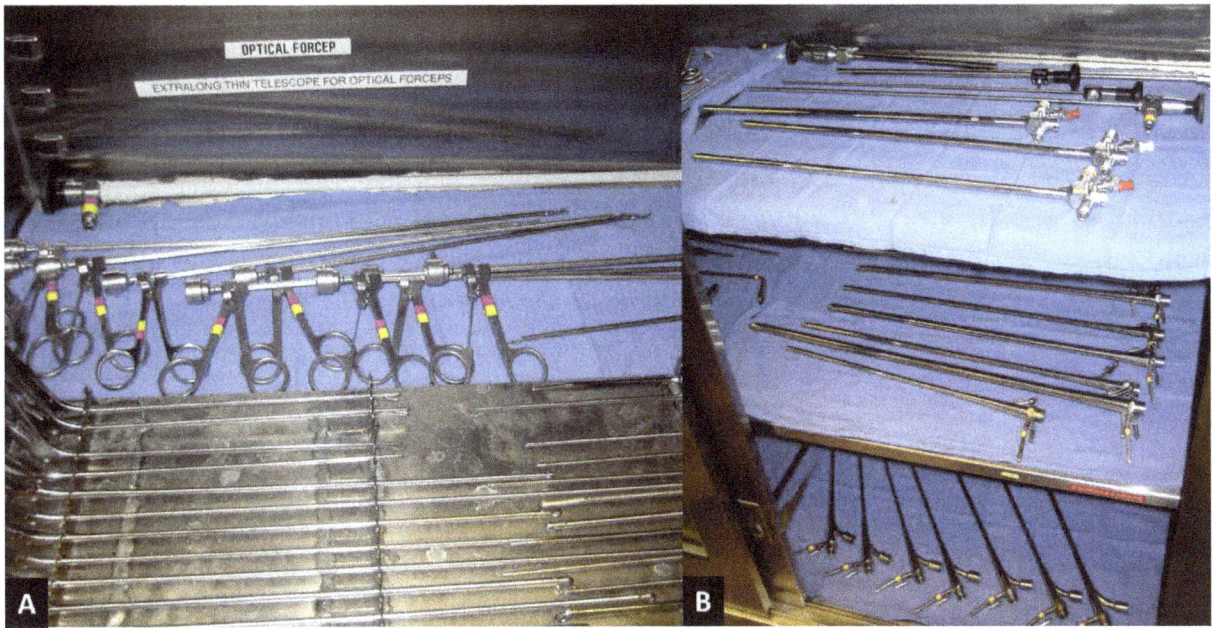

Figure 1. A) Various non-optical and optical graspers used for removal of foreign bodies from the aerodigestive tract. B) Rigid, ventilating bronchoscopes of various sizes. Selection depends on the age of the patient and size of the airway.

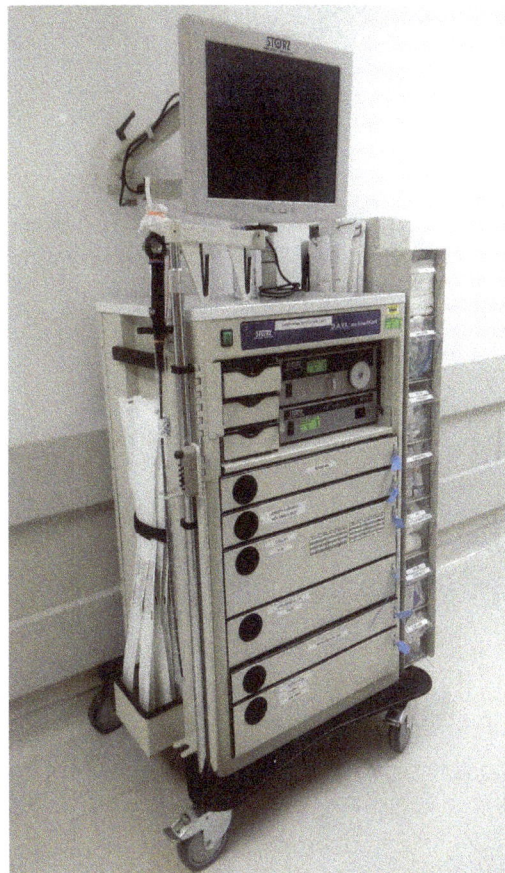

Figure 2. Flexible bronchoscopy cart setup.

For esophagoscopy, the use of the rigid scope allows for use of the same endoscopic optical graspers used in airway cases. While many esophageal foreign bodies are safely removed with flexible endoscopy, the rigid scope does not require insufflation of the esophagus with air and using rigid equipment, more direct visualization of the insertion through the upper esophageal sphincter can be made. There are fewer options for types of graspers available for the flexible esophagoscope. In our opinion, the endoscopic optical graspers themselves used through the rigid scope allow for enhanced visualization and easier foreign body removal (Figure 3).

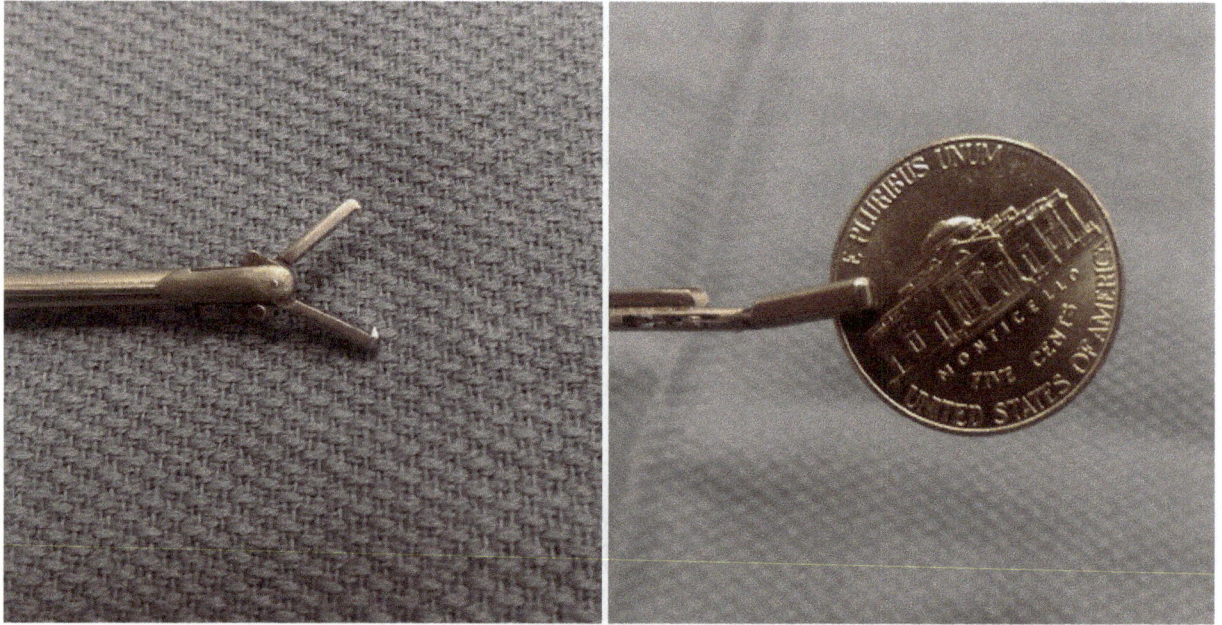

Figure 3. An example of an endoscopic, optical coin grasper, with a fine tooth at the tip, which allows the coin to pivot or swivel through the path of least resistance through the esophagus during removal.

3. Relevant airway anatomy

The upper aerodigestive tract extends from the lips and nasal vestibule to the upper esophagus and trachea and mainstem bronchi. It can be divided into anatomic subsites, including the nasal cavity, nasopharynx, oropharynx, hypopharynx, larynx, trachea, bronchi, and esophagus.

With regard to the nasal cavity, foreign bodies typically get lodged between the inferior turbinate and the septum. As the nasal cavity is part of the airway, care must be taken during removal attempts in the office setting to avoid converting this upper airway foreign body into a lower airway foreign body.

Several differences between the adult and pediatric airway exist that the endoscopist should consider when evaluating and treating patients with aerodigestive foreign bodies. First, the infantile larynx is positioned much higher in the neck. Additionally, the neonatal larynx is approximately one-third the size of the adult larynx, with the narrowest portion being at the level of the cricoid cartilage and not at the level of the glottis, as in adults [8]. A small reduction in the size of the pediatric airway can have significant and devastating consequences. The size of the airway must be kept in mind when choosing the appropriate size of the bronchoscope. As a general rule, the largest size ventilating scope that can be placed based on age of the child and size of subglottis, allows for optimal ventilation, visualization, and endoscopic removal.

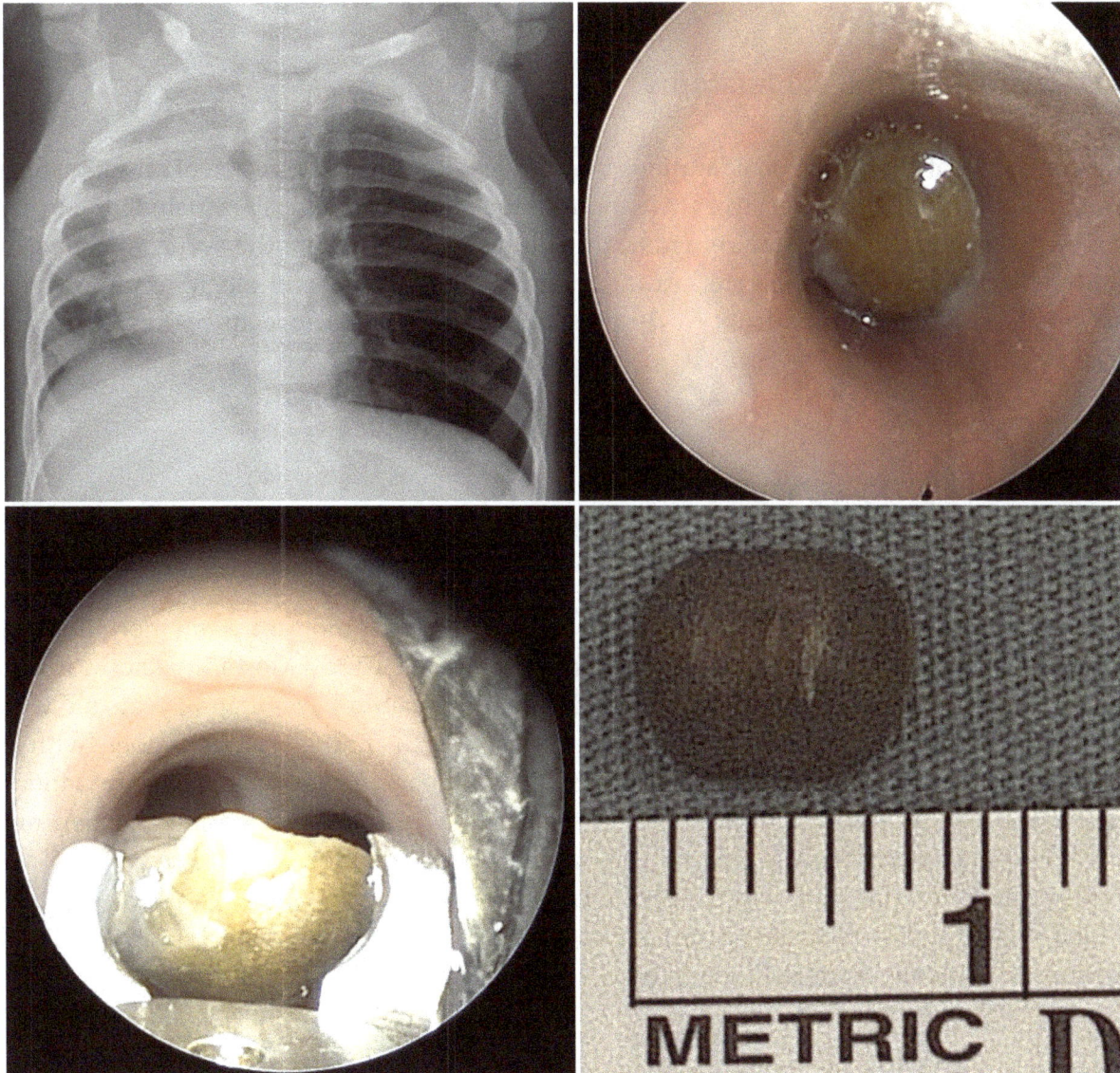

Figure 4. A 13-month old presented to the emergency room with wheezing and coughing. The child had reportedly put something into its mouth earlier that day. An A-P plain film showed hyperinflation of the left lung with right-sided mediastinal shift. There was no radiopaque foreign body noted on the plain film. Direct laryngoscopy with rigid bronchoscopy revealed a left mainstem foreign body, consistent with half of a wooden bead that was removed with an endoscopic optical forceps.

The presence of a foreign body within the tracheobronchial tree can lead to a ball-valve effect, resulting in early hyperinflation of the lung ipsilateral to the foreign body (Figure 4). Over time, the obstructed lung segment becomes atelectatic. In addition to its physical obstruction, the presence of a foreign body disrupts the normal mucociliary clearance of the tracheobronchial tree. These factors can contribute to the rapid accumulation of secretions and subsequent superimposed pneumonia [9].

The right mainstem bronchus creates a more obtuse angle with the trachea when compared to the left mainstem bronchus, leading to a higher incidence of right-sided airway foreign bodies [10].

4. Relevant esophageal anatomy

There are several anatomic considerations that can lead to arrested passage of an esophageal foreign body through the digestive tract and into the stomach. These sites include the upper esophageal sphincter or cricopharyngeus, the mid-esophagus where the aortic arch crosses, and the lower esophageal sphincter. Additionally, there are a few pathologic conditions that can predispose pediatric patients to dysphasia and esophageal foreign bodies, including vascular rings and slings.

5. Pediatric airway foreign bodies

5.1. Epidemiology

Airway foreign bodies represent an important cause of pediatric morbidity and mortality both in developed and developing countries. According to the US CDC's Morbidity and Mortality Weekly Report, nonfatal choking-related episodes among children less than 14 years old were responsible for approximately 17, 000 emergency room visits in the year 2001 alone, with an estimated rate of 29.9 episodes per 100, 000 children. The incidence was greatest in patients less than 1 year old (140.4 per 100, 000) and steadily declined with increasing age. Seventy-seven percent of patients presenting with chocking-related symptoms were three years old or younger. In their data, there was a higher incidence in males (55.1%) and a higher incidence of food-related substances when compared to nonfoods (59.5% vs. 31.4%, 9% unknown) [11]. The most commonly aspirated foreign bodies include round, hard foods such as nuts, seeds, beans, corn, and berries [12].

In Tan et al.'s 10-year retrospective review of children treated for airway foreign bodies via bronchoscopy, they reported a male preponderance (63.7%) in a series of 135 cases. Three quarters of their patients were under 3 years of age [13]. Both of these trends mirror that of other published series [14–16]. Tan proposed that the higher incidence of foreign body aspiration in younger children was due to their poor oro-motor control and their lack of dentition, in addition to their propensity to explore the world with their mouths.

Prior to the advent of modern endoscopic techniques, the reported mortality from aspirated foreign bodies was as high as 50% or greater [5]. Following the advent of endoscopic techniques and increased public awareness, the mortality rate of patients with foreign bodies is approximately 1% [17]. The total number of foreign body--related deaths in the United States is estimated to be between 500 and 2000 [13].

The nasal cavity is the most common sub-site for foreign bodies when considering the entire upper aerodigestive tract, accounting for approximately two-thirds of all foreign bodies. In Chinski's study of aerodigestive tract foreign bodies in Argentina, 1559 nasal foreign bodies were reported. The most common objects found in the nose in decreasing order were pearls, stationery, food, seeds/nuts/beans, pins/nails/metal, other inorganic materials and stones, followed by other less common items, including 1 button battery and 11 magnets [18]. The majority of nasal foreign bodies occur on the patient's right side, with this trend increasing with the patient's age [19]. Interestingly, some studies have demonstrated a decreased incidence of nasal foreign bodies during the summer months [20]. Others have commented on the increased incidence of nasal foreign bodies during the months of January, March, April, and October, coinciding with the months near Christmas, Easter, and Halloween when children are exposed to more toys and treats [19].

5.2. Clinical evaluation

5.2.1. Nasal foreign bodies

Many nasal foreign bodies are asymptomatic, presenting only because their placement was witnessed or admitted (Figure 5). Unwitnessed or untreated nasal foreign bodies may present with a variety of symptoms, including unilateral purulent rhinorrhea or nasal obstruction, halitosis, epistaxis, sinusitis, or a combination of these symptoms [19, 21]. A nasal septal hematoma should be differentiated from a nasal foreign body (Figure 6). In a European study assessing complications and hospitalizations due to nasal foreign bodies, Gregori et al. demonstrated that battery nasal foreign bodies were more likely to experience complications and require hospitalizations when compared to many other types of nasal foreign bodies [21]. As with other studies regarding aerodigestive foreign bodies, they reported a fairly high incidence of children placing nasal foreign bodies while under adult supervision (38%).

5.2.2. Laryngeal and tracheobronchial foreign bodies

Foreign bodies of the laryngotracheobronchial tree can present with varying degrees of airway symptoms depending on their location, shape, size relative to airway, and chronicity.

Larnygeal Foreign Bodies

Foreign bodies of the larynx, while infrequent, are associated with the most devastating outcomes. In addition to more common symptoms associated with foreign bodies of the trachea and bronchi, these patients are more likely to present with hoarseness, aphonia, drooling, stridor, and drooling. Complete obstruction can cause cyanosis, respiratory distress, and respiratory arrest followed by death. Persistent irritation can lead to significant laryngeal edema that can persist and cause significant symptoms even after foreign body removal [10, 22].

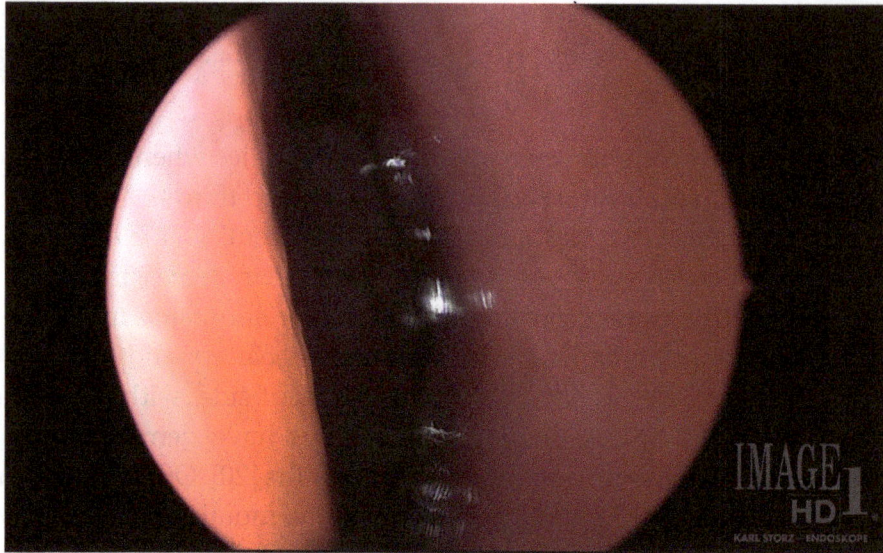

Figure 5. Right nasal foreign body, a piece of broken glass, placed by a 5-year old boy. This was removed in the operating room, instead of clinic setting, due to sharp edges and risk of bleeding following removal.

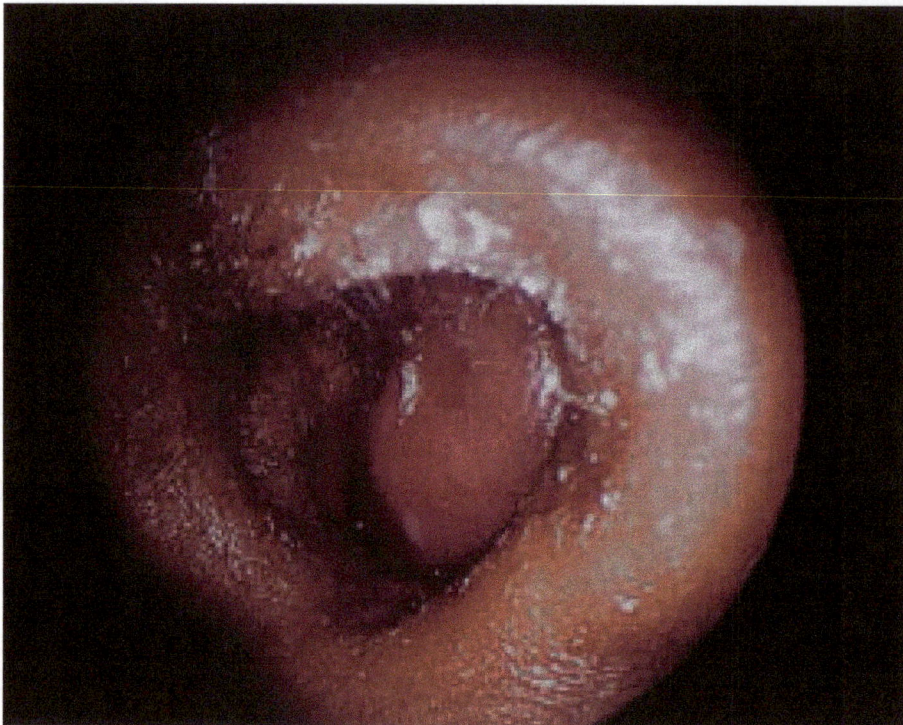

Figure 6. Right nasal septal hematoma after nasal trauma could be mistaken for a foreign object; the mucoperichondral flap is fluctuant to palpation with a cotton tip applicator. Surgical drainage is the required treatment to prevent abscess formation and cartilage necrosis.

Tracheal Foreign Bodies

Patients with tracheal foreign bodies may present with biphasic stridor, a dry cough with an associated "sharp crack" or "slap" when a moving foreign body impacts the subglottis. Patients may place themselves in the "tripod" position, leaning forward with elbows or hands on their knees. There may also be a dramatic shift in symptoms when the patient changes positions, owing to the mobility of the foreign body [22].

Bronchial Foreign Bodies

In Tan et al.'s series, the most common presenting symptoms of tracheobronchial foreign bodies were "choking, coughing, gagging" with 91.8% of patients presenting in this manner. This was followed by "wheezing" in 84.4% of patients and finally the classic triad of "coughing, wheezing, and reduced breath sounds" in only 57% of patients. Less common symptoms reported in their series included fever, pneumonia, stridor, chest pain, blood stained mucous, restlessness, throat discomfort, sternal discomfort, increased seizure episodes, and nose bleed [13].

5.3. Radiographic evaluation

A thorough history and physical exam are paramount in the evaluation of a child with suspected foreign body and can frequently lead to a diagnosis without the need for further diagnostic workup or imaging. Traditionally, plain film radiography has been advocated for patients with suspected foreign body aspiration. A-P and lateral plain films may reveal a radiopaque foreign body within the tracheobronchial tree. Additionally, sequelae from the presence of the foreign body may be recognized, including air-trapping with associated mediastinal shift, atelectasis, or pneumonia from long-standing foreign body. Decubitus films may demonstrate lack of dependent mediastinal shift on the side ipsilateral to the foreign body [23].

The use of plain film radiography does not need to be routinely employed in patients where there is a high index of suspicion for foreign body based on history and physical examination. In a 6-year retrospective review of 93 cases of possible airway foreign body cases, Silva et al. reported a imaging study sensitivity and specificity of 74% and 45%, respectively [24]. In a series of 232 patients with pre-operative radiography in whom foreign bodies confirmed via bronchoscopy, 110 had plain film imaging that was considered normal by the surgeon (47%). For patients with radiology reports, 42% of patients with bronchial foreign bodies and 81% of patients with tracheal foreign bodies had negative imaging reports. The same study did note that patients with long-standing foreign bodies are more likely to have positive findings on plain film radiography when compared to patients with foreign bodies that have been present for less than 24 h [25]. In their retrospective reviews, neither Assefa nor Brown found sufficient evidence to support the routine use of decubitus films in the identification of airway foreign bodies, citing the lack of sensitivity [23, 26].

Some studies have reported on the diagnostic utility of CT imaging and CT virtual bronchoscopy, with reported sensitivities and specificities ranging from 90% to100% [27, 28]. Foreign bodies that are radiolucent on plain films may be identified on CT. The risks of ionizing radiation and the inability to concurrently diagnose and treat foreign body aspiration should be recognized when considering these modalities.

Despite negative imaging studies, if the history is concerning for possible aspiration, then endoscopic evaluation should still be considered given the potential morbidity and mortality of airway foreign bodies.

5.4. Airway foreign body removal

Nasal foreign bodies can frequently be managed in the clinic if the object is in the anterior nasal cavity. After removal, confirmation using nasal endoscopy can ensure that no additional retained foreign body is present. Objects that are difficult to grasp or that are posterior within the nasal cavity may require sedation or a general anesthetic removal. If the object is round, using a right angle probe behind it and pulling anterior is safest, to avoid propelling the object into the pharynx or causing it to be aspirated into the lower tracheobronchial tree. Other upper airway foreign bodies require direct laryngoscopy and removal with endoscopic visualization of the pharynx and larynx (Figure 7). These are considered an emergency as they can potentially lead to lower airway obstruction if the object is aspirated. When done in the operating room, the endoscopist must be prepared for emergent bronchoscopy, should the object fall distally during induction of anesthesia. Thorough discussion with the anesthesia team on the plan prior to induction must take place. All potential non-optical and optical graspers should be available to quickly use as needed. In addition, instrumentation for emergent tracheostomy placement should be immediately available should the need arise. Figures 8-14 demonstrate a variety of cases where endoscopic management was performed.

5.4.1. Anesthetic considerations

The choice of anesthetic technique should be based on a discussion between the surgeon and anesthesiologist. Pediatric airway and esophageal foreign body removal is performed under general anesthesia. Anesthetic induction can be achieved either by inhalation of volatile anesthetic gas or intravenous medications. Anesthesia can then be maintained with spontaneous ventilation or paralysis with control of the airway. This choice is surgeon and anesthesiologist dependent, but should be agreed upon prior to the start of the procedure.

Especially in the case of tracheobronchial foreign bodies, constant and deliberate communication regarding the airway should be maintained between the surgical and anesthesia teams. This situation represents a true "shared airway"[29, 30].

An age-appropriate size bronchoscope and one size smaller should always be set up for tracheobronchial foreign bodies. A back-up fiberoptic light source is helpful in case one fails during the procedure. Given that the rigid bronchoscope itself is a means of ventilation, strategic use of the instrument during the procedure is important. For example, if the oxygen saturations drop, the telescope can be removed and this increases the ventilating diameter, and therefore the volume of airflow through the bronchoscope tube with occlusion of the proximal end with a cap. The mouth and nose can be manually sealed around the scope to create some "positive pressure" as needed. Optical graspers of various shapes can be easily passed through the bronchoscope while maintaining ventilation, and foreign bodies can be removed under direct endoscopic visualization. The surgeon must ensure all equipment is functional, available, and all desired instruments fit through the bronchoscope size selected prior to the patient's anesthetic induction.

Tracheostomy is rarely required; however, equipment should be immediately available for obtaining an emergent surgical airway in the management of airway foreign bodies. This is always discussed with the parents during the informed consent process.

5.4.2. Adjunctive procedures

In the rare case where the foreign body cannot be removed endoscopically, additional interventions may be required. As a temporizing measure, the use of extracorporeal membrane oxygenation (ECMO) may allow oxygenation in a case of inability to ventilate [31]. This is a highly specialized technique that is not available in all centers. It allows oxygenation of the blood and maintenance of circulation until a definitive plan for removal can be facilitated.

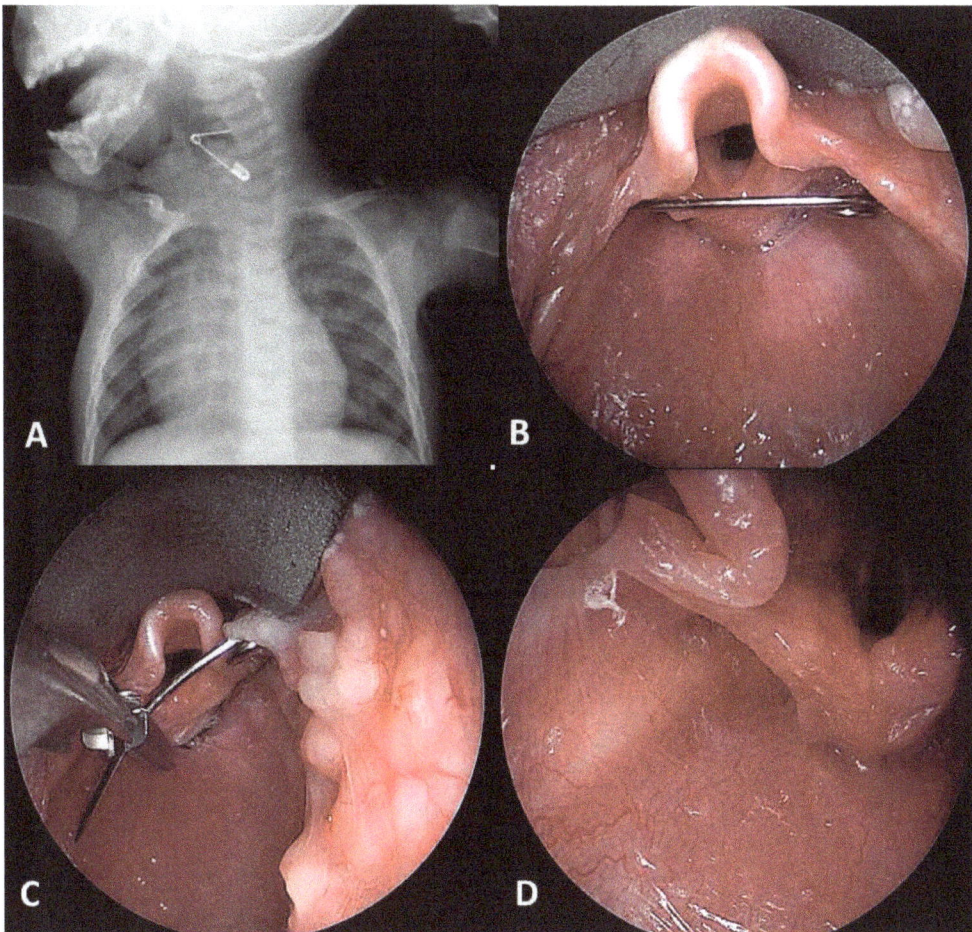

Figure 7. An 11-month old with an open safety pin in the upper airway. The patient presented with irritability and drooling of several hours duration, and the mother felt the child might have put something into its mouth. A-P and lateral plain films confirmed the diagnosis.

In cases where the foreign body cannot be removed endoscopically, open approaches may be required [32]. Cervical esophagostomy for proximal esophageal foreign bodies, or thoracotomy with bronchotomy, may be required for tracheobronchial foreign bodies. In these rare cases, close collaboration with pediatric thoracic surgeons or pediatric surgeons is required.

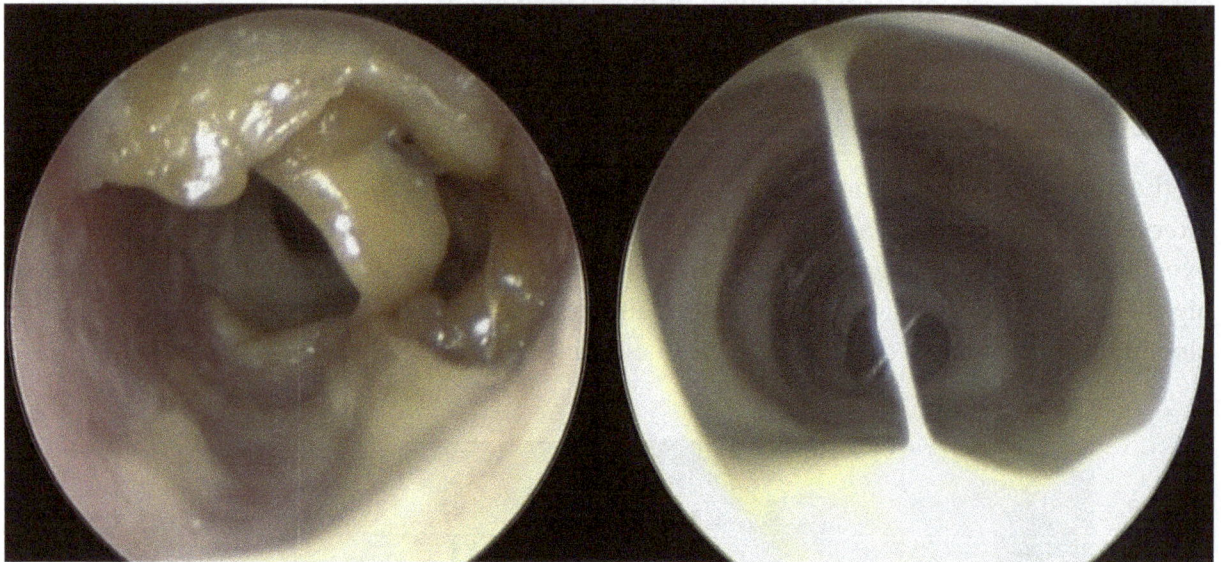

Figure 8. A 9-year-old patient presenting with cough and stridor with concurrent fever. Direct laryngoscopy with rigid bronchoscopy revealed bacterial tracheitis. Tracheal casts can cause airway symptoms similar to aspirated foreign bodies.

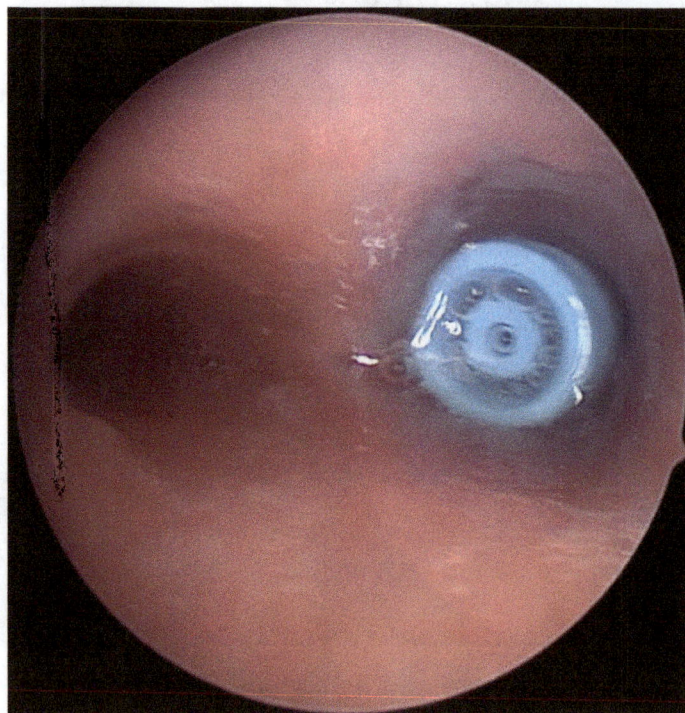

Figure 9. A 12-month old presented to the Emergency Department with increased work of breathing and stridor after reportedly having swallowed a piece of a pen. Plain film imaging was unrevealing. Given the clinical presentation, the patient underwent direct laryngoscopy with rigid bronchoscopy, revealing a plastic foreign body in the right mainstem bronchus.

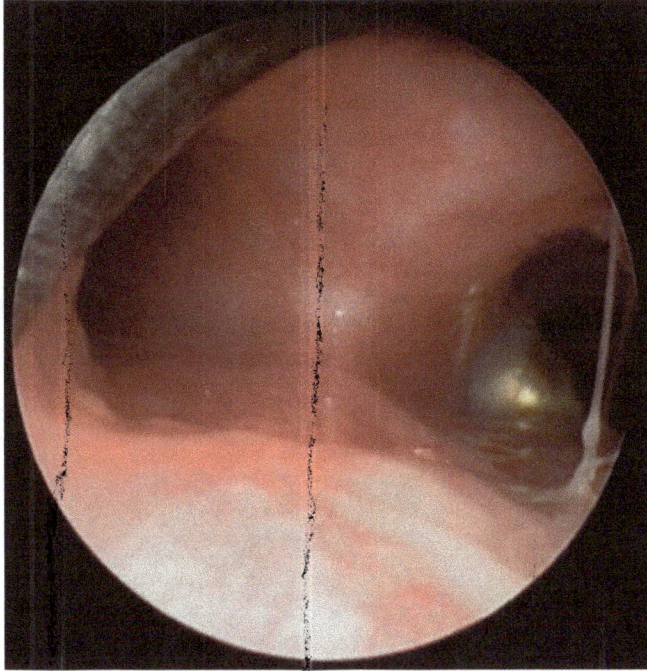

Figure 10. A 12-month old presenting with respiratory symptoms and concern for foreign body aspiration. Direct laryngoscopy with rigid bronchoscopy confirms a high-powered magnet sphere within the right mainstem bronchus. Another was trapped in the esophagus directly behind this. This has the potential to cause a tracheoesophageal fistula given magnetic strength and tissue necrosis between the two magnets. Severe injuries are more common in the lower gastrointestinal tract causing perforation when more than one of these is swallowed (this child had additional magnetic spheres in the small bowel which caused transmural necrosis and perforation requiring repair).

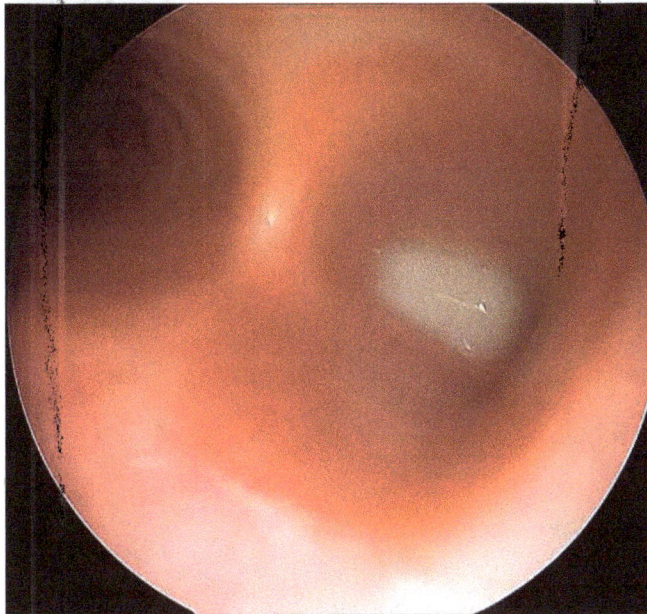

Figure 11. While having a tooth extracted at a dentist office, this child accidently aspirated the tooth, found in the right mainstem bronchus.

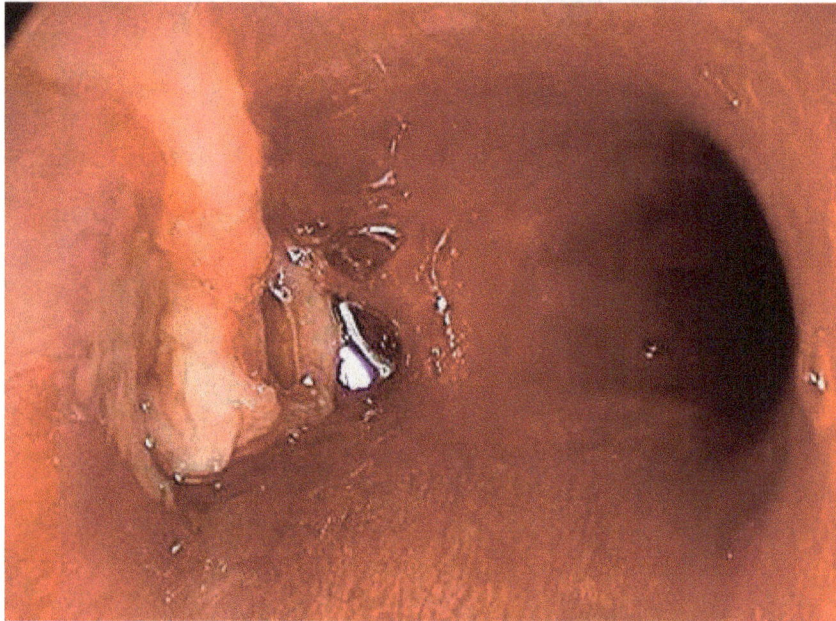

Figure 12. Plastic bronchitis in a patient with congenital heart disease, showing a cast in the left bronchial tree.

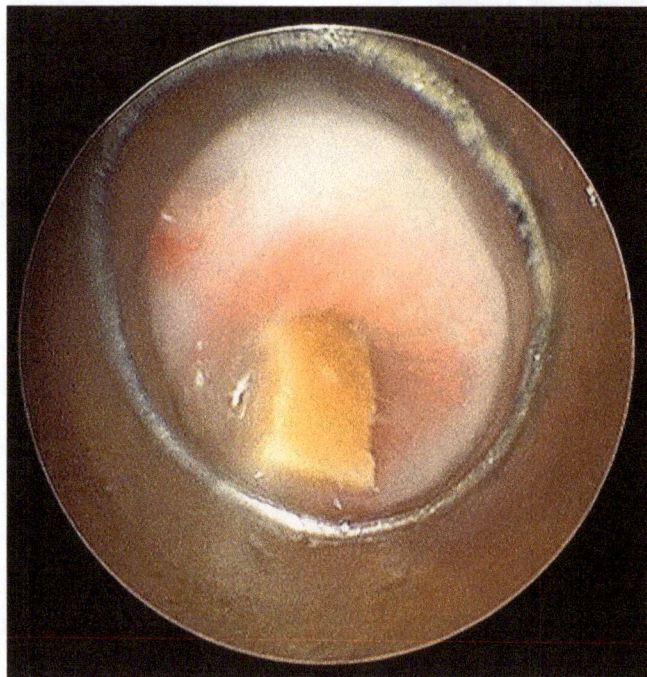

Figure 13. A 2-year-old boy was given peanuts by an older sibling, choked, was in severe respiratory distress, found to have several fragments in the lower airways. These were removed with optical graspers through the rigid bronchoscope.

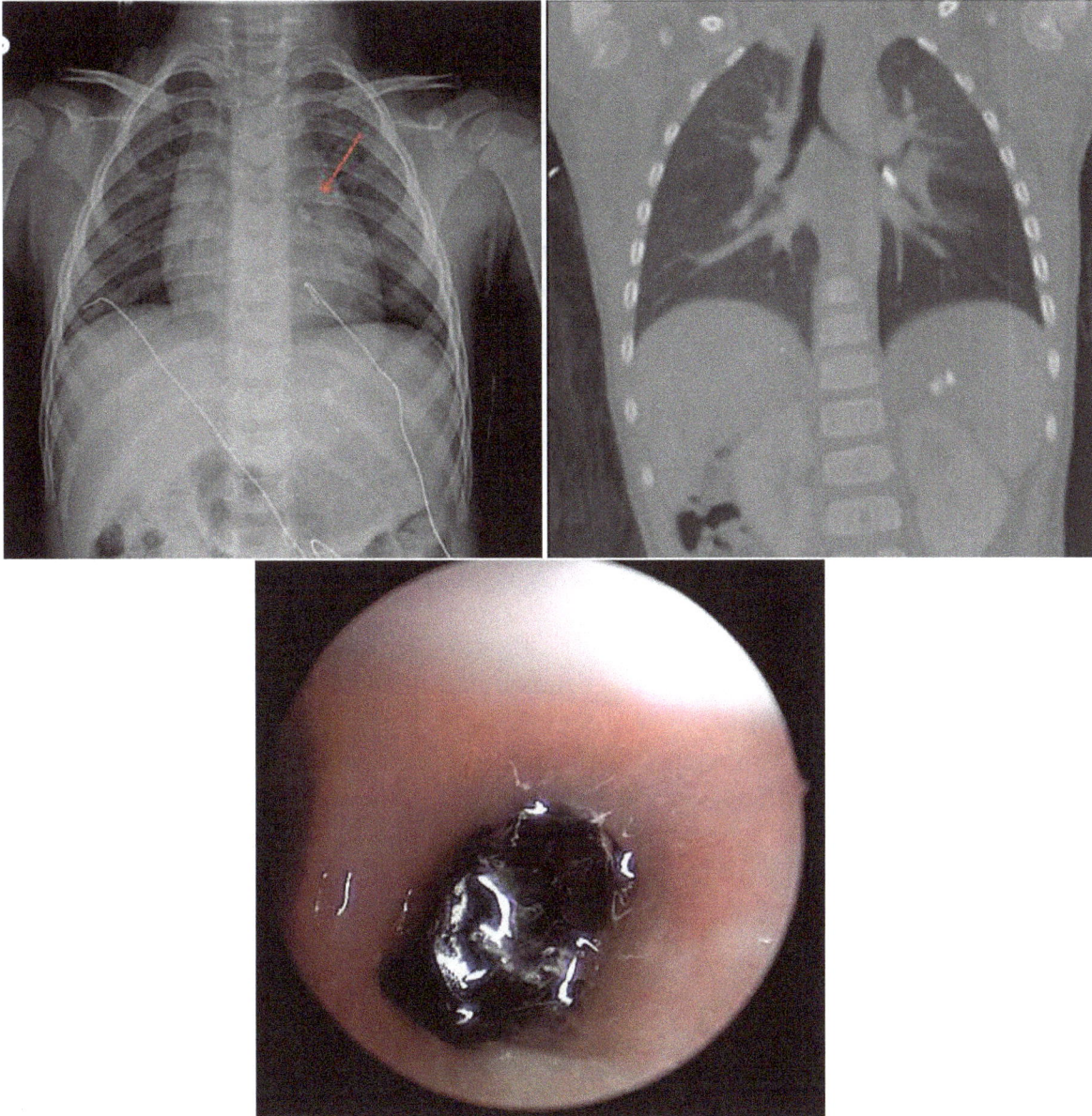

Figure 14. A 2-year-old patient presented to the Emergency Department with multiple facial lacerations following a motor vehicle accident during which she was ejected through the passenger side window. She had no respiratory symptoms as presentation. As part of her trauma workup, she underwent both plain film and CT imaging of the chest, both showed a possible left-sided airway foreign body. Direct laryngoscopy with bronchoscopy confirmed the diagnosis, and the object was endoscopically removed without difficulty.

6. Pediatric Esophageal Foreign Bodies

6.1. Epidemiology

Foreign body ingestion is a relatively common occurrence, with an estimated 100, 000 cases per year in the United States alone. Like airway foreign bodies, the majority of cases occur in children aged between 6 months and 3 years [33]. For the majority of esophageal foreign bodies, a child's caregiver either witnesses or suspects that their child has ingested a foreign body [34]. While the majority of ingested foreign bodies will pass on their own, there is still a real risk of significant morbidity and mortality. Of all patients with esophageal foreign bodies seeking medical attention, 80%–90% pass the foreign body without any intervention, 10%--20% require endoscopic removal, and only 1% require surgical removal [33]. It has been estimated that 1, 500 deaths occur annually in the United States alone due to foreign body ingestion [35].

Recently, there has been a sharp rise in the use of button-battery powered hand-held electronic equipment. This has coincided with a rise in the incidence of button battery--related emergency department visits [36].

6.2. Clinical presentation

As with airway foreign bodies, a thorough history and physical exam are critical in the workup of the pediatric patient with a suspected esophageal foreign body. As previously stated, frequently, a caregiver has witnessed the ingestion and can positively identify the object, which may have implications regarding urgent intervention, such as in the case of an ingested button battery or magnet.

Many esophageal foreign body ingestions go unwitnessed and a large proportion of these pass without incident or development of symptoms [37]. When children do have symptoms, they tend to be nonspecific and can lead to a missed or delayed diagnosis. In a retrospective review by Arana et al. of 325 pediatric patients presenting with esophageal foreign bodies, only 54% of patients had transient symptoms at the time of ingestion [38]. When patients are symptomatic, they primarily present with nonspecific gastrointestinal or pulmonary complaints, including coughing, choking, gagging, drooling, odynophagia, and/or dysphagia. Patients may also present with stridor or wheezing due to inflammation of adjacent tracheobronchial mucosa.

In their retrospective study of 248 cases of patients undergoing esophagogastroduodenoscopy (EGD) for foreign body removal, Denney et al. assessed the incidence of esophageal injury as it related to presenting symptoms. In their series, 59 children (30%) were found to have mucosal ulceration. They found that a presenting complaint of substernal pain correlated with mucosal ulceration, whereas symptoms of vomiting, respiratory distress, and drooling did not. The vast majority of foreign bodies in their series were coins (81%) and 8 cases of batteries were reported. They did not comment on any injuries from batteries [34].

6.3. Radiographic evaluation

The patient's clinical presentation should be corroborated with imaging to ensure that a foreign body requiring urgent removal is not misdiagnosed [35]. Imaging for esophageal foreign body workup should typically include the chest and abdomen in both AP and lateral planes (Figure 15). It should be noted, however, that about 1/3 of foreign bodies are radiolucent [38].

Jatana et al. reported on the utility of plain film radiography in distinguishing esophageal coins from button batteries [39]. They described the "double ring" or "halo" sign created by a button

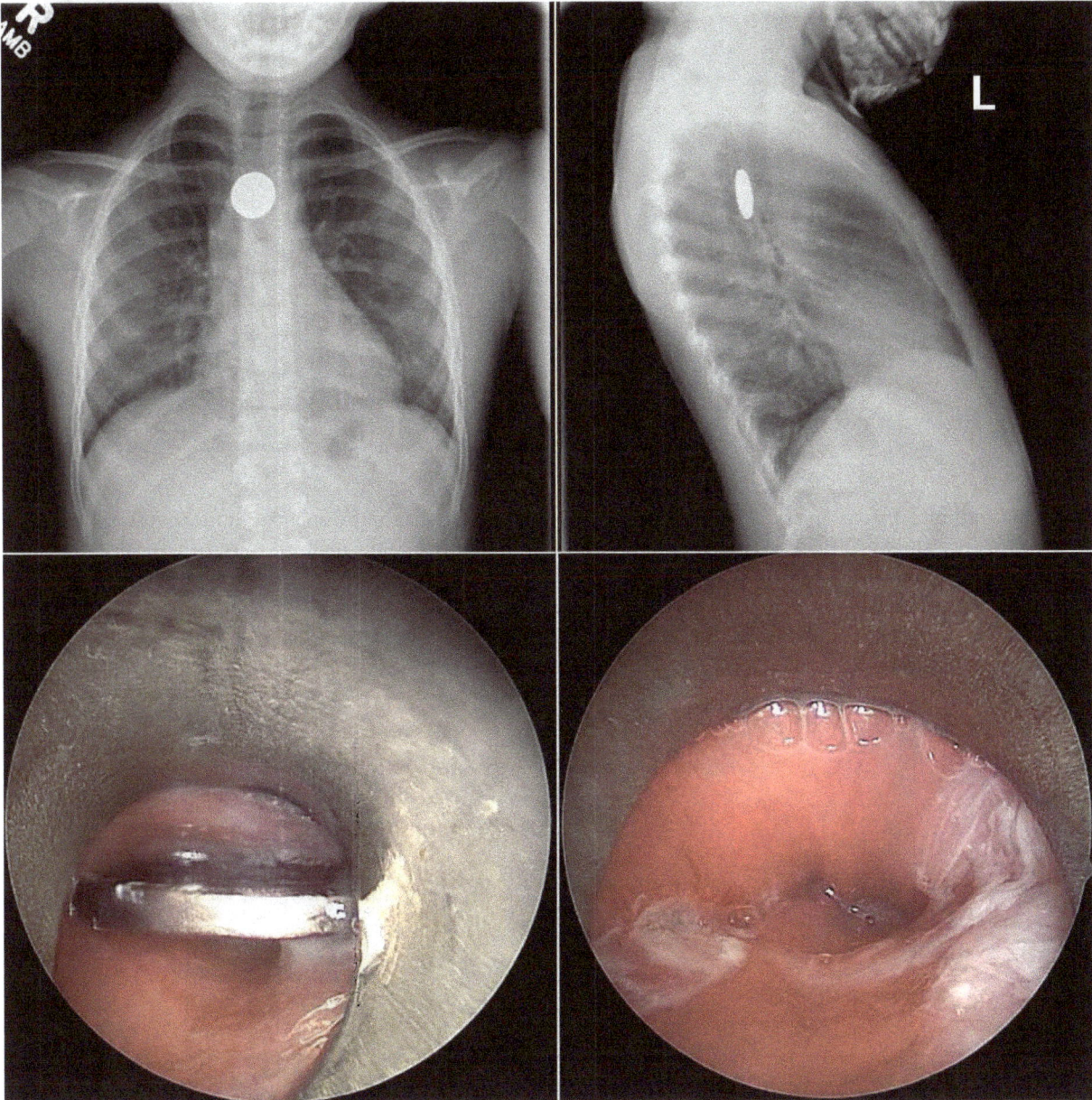

Figure 15. A 5-year old presented to the Emergency Department with several episodes of emesis. She admitted to swallowing a penny while at day care earlier that day. A-P and lateral plain films confirmed the diagnosis of an esophageal foreign body. A penny was identified and removed via rigid esophagoscopy. Minimal esophageal mucosal irritation was noted.

battery on an A-P plain film (Figure 16). The 20mm 3 volt lithium batteries consistently demonstrate this finding. They also demonstrated the "step-off" that can be seen on lateral plain films of button batteries, though they caution that some new thinner button batteries will not demonstrate this finding. Clinicians must not rely on lateral x-rays alone.

Many experts argue against the use of contrast studies for diagnosing esophageal foreign bodies given the increased risk of aspiration with a foreign body obstructing the esophagus. The presence of contrast could compromise the ability of the endoscopist to find the foreign body during retrieval and may also limit mucosal assessment [41]. In addition, the contrast

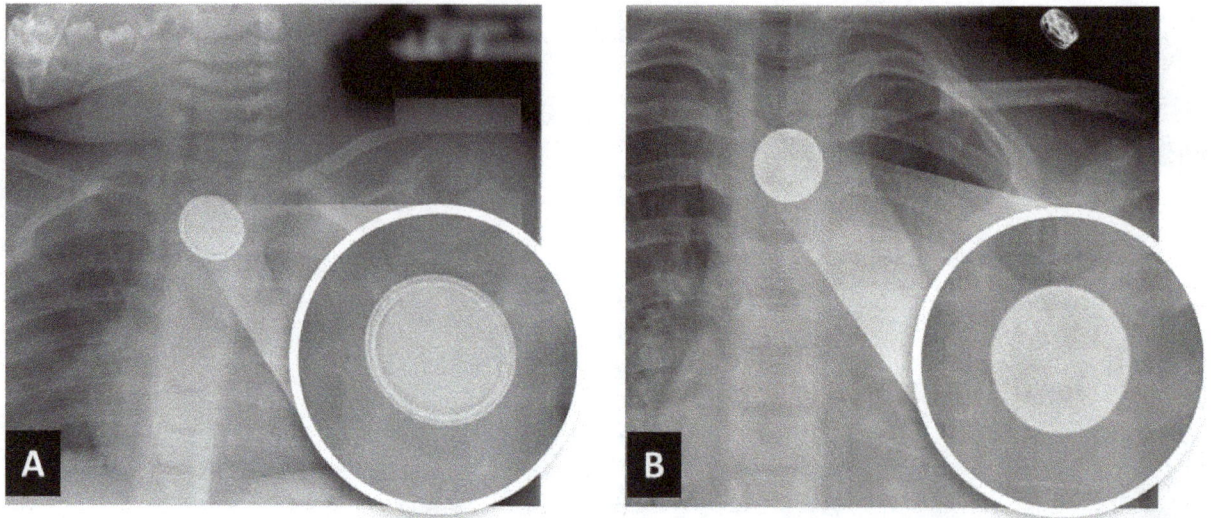

Figure 16. A) Button battery in upper esophagus. B) Coin in upper esophagus. By zooming into the foreign body, the "double ring or halo sign" can be clearly seen for the battery. Zooming into the image is most helpful for differentiation. Reproduced with permission, Jatana [40].

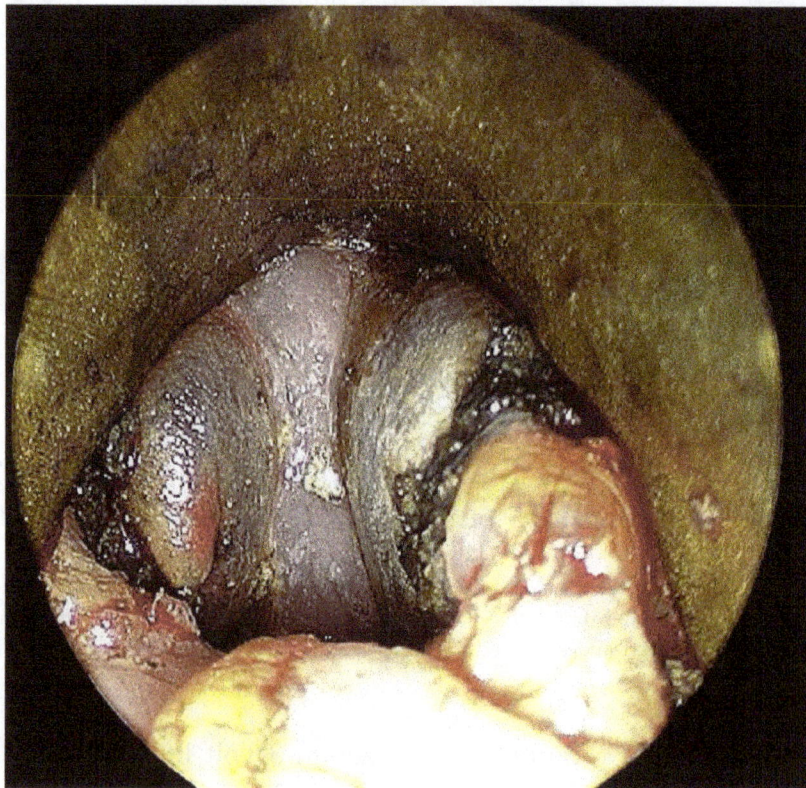

Figure 17. Esophageal injury secondary to a button battery in a 4-year old. The injury involves the muscular layer of the esophagus. Reproduced with permission, Jatana [40].

typically pushes back general anesthesia 8 h, and delays operative intervention. Esophagram does have a role in assessing for esophageal perforation or stricture due to foreign bodies, but generally only after operative removal of the foreign body.

Several authors have described the utility of hand-held metal detectors in the management of patients with suspected coin ingestion. Younger et al. performed a 2-year prospective study of patients presenting for evaluation of esophageal foreign bodies. With a hand-held metal detector, they were able to positively identify the presence and location of esophageal coins in all 26 patients who had positive plain films [42]. Lee et al. performed a systematic review of 11 studies and found that the sensitivity and specificity of identifying the presence of coins was 99.4% and 100%, respectively, when compared to plain films. They do note however, that non-coin metal objects were not detected as frequently as coins in one study reviewed. The authors point out the benefit of avoiding ionizing radiation when using a hand-held metal detector [43].

Repeat imaging has a role in the management of esophageal foreign bodies that are managed expectantly. An x-ray can ensure that an esophageal foreign body has passed into the stomach. In addition, should the object not be found in the stools over time, repeat abdominal x-ray can confirm that there is no retained opaque foreign body in the lower gastrointestinal tract.

6.4. Esophageal foreign body removal

Management of esophageal foreign bodies varies considerably based on several factors, including anatomic location, type of foreign body, patient presenting symptoms, and existing complications. A button battery lodged in the esophagus is an emergency. The current generated around the battery causes hydroxide ion to form at the negative pole, causing rapid injury. Serious injury can occur in only 2 h. The 20 mm diameter, 3 volt lithium batteries cause the most severe injury as they combine high power, with large enough size to get stuck; these are frequently used in many household electronics [39]. A common misconception is that the leaking battery acid is the major source of mucosal injury, rather than the generated electrical current. In addition, "dead" batteries, meaning those that no longer have enough charge to power their intended electronics, can still have enough residual electrical current to cause mucosal injury (Figure 17).

Coins lodged in the esophagus can be managed with an initial period of observation, and if they fail to pass into the stomach, can be removed endoscopically.

Rigid esophagoscopy allows for the scope to be placed under constant direct visualization for removal of the foreign body using endoscopic optical graspers that are most suited for the object. In general, a second-look esophagoscopy can not only confirm the absence of any additional non-opaque foreign bodies, but also assess any injury to the esophageal wall. If a perforation is suspected, keeping the patient with nothing by mouth and obtaining an esophagram is best. When probable perforation or known severe circumferential injury exists, consideration of placing a nasogastric tube under direct visualization through the rigid scope can serve as temporary means of nutrition and keep the region stented open to avoid complete stricture. It should also be kept in mind that when severe injury exists, advancing the esophagoscope past the site of injury can potentially lead to greater injury.

7. Complications of pediatric airway foreign bodies

The most feared acute complication of airway foreign bodies is complete airway obstruction with cardiopulmonary arrest and death. Wheezing is very common after the procedure and close monitoring in the hospital setting is required until symptoms have stabilized. Pneumonia is common due to lower airway obstruction and should be appropriately treated with antibiotics. Intraoperative cultures can be taken to help guide treatment. Given that injury can occur to the tracheobronchial tree, pneumomediastinum and pneumothorax can occur. When the airway is severely inflamed, bleeding and granulation tissue can limit visualization, and the decision to do a planned second-look bronchoscopy must be made to ensure no retained foreign body is present. Laryngeal injury when removing an airway foreign body can occur.

8. Complications of pediatric esophageal foreign bodies

Children who develop a fever after removal of any esophageal foreign body should be assessed for an esophageal perforation by esophagram. Other potential complications include: bleeding or major arterial fistula, mediastinitis, mediastinal abscess, respiratory distress (secondary tracheomalacia/compression), tracheoesophageal fistula, vocal cord paresis/paralysis, esophageal stricture, and death. Repeat endoscopy to follow healing of significant esophageal injury is an alternative to follow-up esophagram, and has the advantage of allowing for debridement or dilation of early stricture formation.

9. Conclusions

The management of pediatric airway and esophageal foreign bodies carries the potential for morbidity and mortality, and can be challenging to diagnose if an unwitnessed aspiration or ingestion occurs in a young child. The symptoms can be somewhat nonspecific, not easily differentiated from common viral illnesses in children. Clinical decision making based on thorough history and physical examination is critical. Centers with airway surgeons and endoscopists trained in foreign body management, and with pediatric ICU care are best equipped to manage the most complex cases in the children.

Author details

Phillip L. Chaffin, Jonathan M. Grischkan, Prashant S. Malhotra and Kris R. Jatana[*]

*Address all correspondence to: Kris.Jatana@nationwidechildrens.org

Department of Otolaryngology-Head and Neck Surgery, Nationwide Children's Hospital and Wexner Medical Center at Ohio State University, Columbus, Ohio, USA

References

[1] Gross SD, Samuel D. A practical treatise on foreign bodies in the air-passages (Internet). Philadelphia, Blanchard and Lea; 1854 (cited 2015 Jan 4). p. 498. Available from: http://archive.org/details/practicaltreagros

[2] Bush RB, Leonhardt H, Bush IM, Landes RR. Dr. Bozzini's Lichtleiter: A translation of his original article (1806). Urology. 1974 Jan;3(1):119–23.

[3] Desormeaux AJ, Antonin J, Hunt RP. The endoscope, and its application to the diagnosis and treatment of affections of the genito-urinary passages: lessons given at Necker Hospital (Internet). Chicago: Robert Fergus' Sons, printers; 1867 (cited 2015 Jan 4). Available from: http://archive.org/details/65910730R.nlm.nih.gov

[4] Moore I. Peroral Endoscopy: An historical survey from its origin to the present day. J Laryngol Otol. 1926 Jun;41(06):361–82.

[5] Marsh BR. Historic development of bronchoesophagology. Otolaryngol Head Neck Surg. 1996 Jun;114(6):689–716.

[6] Thorner MM. A Utoscopy of the larynx and of the trachea. J Am Med Assoc. 1896 Feb 8;XXVI(6):265–7.

[7] Zöllner F. Gustav Killian, father of bronchoscopy. Arch Otolaryngol Chic Ill 1960. 1965 Dec;82(6):656–9.

[8] Hartnick CJ, Hansen MC, Gallagher TQ, editors. Pediatric Airway Surgery (Internet). S. Karger AG; 2012 (cited 2015 Jan 4). Available from: https://www.karger.com/Book/Home/255642

[9] Jackson C. Bronchoscopy and esophagoscopy. WB Saunders; 1922.

[10] Kenna MA, Bluestone CD. Foreign Bodies in the Air and Food Passages. Pediatr Rev. 1988 Jul 1;10(1):25–31.

[11] Nonfatal choking-related episodes among children--United States, 2001. MMWR Morb Mortal Wkly Rep. 2002 Oct 25;51(42):945–8.

[12] Gregori D, Salerni L, Scarinzi C, Morra B, Berchialla P, Snidero S, et al. Foreign bodies in the upper airways causing complications and requiring hospitalization in children aged 0-14 years: results from the ESFBI study. Eur Arch Oto-Rhino-Laryngol Off J Eur Fed Oto-Rhino-Laryngol Soc EUFOS Affil Ger Soc Oto-Rhino-Laryngol - Head Neck Surg. 2008 Aug;265(8):971–8.

[13] Tan HKK, Brown K, McGill T, Kenna MA, Lund DP, Healy GB. Airway foreign bodies (FB): a 10-year review. Int J Pediatr Otorhinolaryngol. 2000 Dec 1;56(2):91–9.

[14] Shubha AM, Das K. Tracheobronchial foreign bodies in infants. Int J Pediatr Otorhinolaryngol. 2009 Oct;73(10):1385–9.

[15] Skoulakis CE, Doxas PG, Papadakis CE, Proimos E, Christodoulou P, Bizakis JG, et al. Bronchoscopy for foreign body removal in children. A review and analysis of 210 cases. Int J Pediatr Otorhinolaryngol. 2000 Jun 30;53(2):143–8.

[16] Chapin MM, Rochette LM, Annest JL, Haileyesus T, Conner KA, Smith GA. Nonfatal choking on food among children 14 years or younger in the United States, 2001-2009. Pediatrics. 2013 Aug;132(2):275–81.

[17] Trachea Foreign Bodies. 2013 Jul 9 (cited 2015 Jan 5); Available from: http://emedicine.medscape.com/article/764615-overview

[18] Chinski A, Foltran F, Gregori D, Ballali S, Passali D, Bellussi L. Foreign bodies in children: A comparison between Argentina and Europe. Int J Pediatr Otorhinolaryngol. 2012 May 14;76, Supplement 1:S76–9.

[19] Claudet I, Salanne S, Debuisson C, Maréchal C, Rekhroukh H, Grouteau E. Corps étranger nasal chez l'enfant. Arch Pédiatrie. 2009 Sep;16(9):1245–51.

[20] François M, Hamrioui R, Narcy P. Nasal foreign bodies in children. Eur Arch Otorhinolaryngol. 1998;255(3):132–4.

[21] Gregori D, Salerni L, Scarinzi C, Morra B, Berchialla P, Snidero S, et al. Foreign bodies in the nose causing complications and requiring hospitalization in children 0-14 age: results from the European survey of foreign bodies injuries study. Rhinology. 2008 Mar;46(1):28–33.

[22] Rodríguez H, Passali GC, Gregori D, Chinski A, Tiscornia C, Botto H, et al. Management of foreign bodies in the airway and oesophagus. Int J Pediatr Otorhinolaryngol. 2012 May 14;76, Supplement 1:S84–91.

[23] Assefa D, Amin N, Stringel G, Dozor AJ. Use of decubitus radiographs in the diagnosis of foreign body aspiration in young children. Pediatr Emerg Care. 2007 Mar;23(3): 154–7.

[24] Silva AB, Muntz HR, Clary R. Utility of conventional radiography in the diagnosis and management of pediatric airway foreign bodies. Ann Otol Rhinol Laryngol. 1998 Oct;107(10 Pt 1):834–8.

[25] Zerella JT, Dimler M, McGill LC, Pippus KJ. Foreign body aspiration in children: Value of radiography and complications of bronchoscopy. J Pediatr Surg. 1998 Nov; 33(11):1651–4.

[26] Brown JC, Chapman T, Klein EJ, Chisholm SL, Phillips GS, Osincup D, et al. The utility of adding expiratory or decubitus chest radiographs to the radiographic evaluation of suspected pediatric airway foreign bodies. Ann Emerg Med. 2013 Jan;61(1): 19–26.

[27] Kocaoglu M, Bulakbasi N, Soylu K, Demirbag S, Tayfun C, Somuncu I. Thin-section axial multidetector computed tomography and multiplanar reformatted imaging of

children with suspected foreign-body aspiration: Is virtual bronchoscopy overemphasized? Acta Radiol Stockh Swed 1987. 2006 Sep;47(7):746–51.

[28] Haliloglu M, Ciftci AO, Oto A, Gumus B, Tanyel FC, Senocak ME, et al. CT virtual bronchoscopy in the evaluation of children with suspected foreign body aspiration. Eur J Radiol. 2003 Nov;48(2):188–92.

[29] Zur KB, Litman RS. Pediatric airway foreign body retrieval: surgical and anesthetic perspectives. Paediatr Anaesth. 2009 Jul;19, Suppl 1:109–17.

[30] Fidkowski CW, Zheng H, Firth PG. The anesthetic considerations of tracheobronchial foreign bodies in children: a literature review of 12, 979 cases. Anesth Analg. 2010 Oct;111(4):1016–25.

[31] Park AH, Tunkel DE, Park E, Barnhart D, Liu E, Lee J, et al. Management of complicated airway foreign body aspiration using extracorporeal membrane oxygenation (ECMO). Int J Pediatr Otorhinolaryngol (Internet). 2014 Oct (cited 2015 Jan 7); Available from: http://linkinghub.elsevier.com/retrieve/pii/S016558761400576X

[32] Ulkü R, Onen A, Onat S, Özçelik C. The value of open surgical approaches for aspirated pen caps. J Pediatr Surg. 2005 Nov;40(11):1780–3.

[33] Wyllie R. Foreign bodies in the gastrointestinal tract. Curr Opin Pediatr. 2006;18(5): 563–4.

[34] Denney W, Ahmad N, Dillard B, Nowicki MJ. Children will eat the strangest things: a 10-year retrospective analysis of foreign body and caustic ingestions from a single academic center. Pediatr Emerg Care. 2012;28(8):731–4.

[35] Uyemura MC. Foreign body ingestion in children. Am Fam Physician. 2005 Jul 15;72(2):287–91.

[36] Sharpe SJ, Rochette LM, Smith GA. Pediatric battery-related emergency department visits in the United States, 1990-2009. Pediatrics. 2012 Jun;129(6):1111–7.

[37] Dahshan A. Management of ingested foreign bodies in children. J Okla State Med Assoc. 2001 Jun;94(6):183–6.

[38] Arana A, Hauser B, Hachimi-Idrissi S, Vandenplas Y. Management of ingested foreign bodies in childhood and review of the literature. Eur J Pediatr. 2001;160(8):468–72.

[39] Jatana KR, Litovitz T, Reilly JS, Koltai PJ, Rider G, Jacobs IN. Pediatric button battery injuries: 2013 task force update. Int J Pediatr Otorhinolaryngol. 2013 Sep;77(9):1392–9.

[40] Jatana K. Button Battery Injuries in Children: A Growing Risk. Everything Matters in Patient Care. Nationwide Children's Hospital, Columbus, OH; 2013.

[41] Eisen GM, Baron TH, Dominitz JA, Faigel DO, Goldstein JL, Johanson JF, et al. Guideline for the management of ingested foreign bodies. Gastrointest Endosc. 2002 Jun;55(7):802–6.

[42] Younger RM, Darrow DH. Handheld metal detector confirmation of radiopaque foreign bodies in the esophagus. Arch Otolaryngol Neck Surg. 2001 Nov 1;127(11):1371–4.

[43] Lee J, Ahmad S, Gale C. Detection of coins ingested by children using a handheld metal detector: a systematic review. Emerg Med J EMJ. 2005 Dec;22(12):839–44.

6

Anesthesia Innovations for Endoscopy of Gastrointestinal Tract

Somchai Amornyotin

Abstract

Gastrointestinal endoscopy (GIE) is a procedure for diagnosis and treatment of gastrointestinal tract abnormalities. This procedure requires some forms of anesthesia. The goal of procedural anesthesia is safe, effective control of pain and anxiety, as well as an appropriate degree of memory loss or reduced awareness. Generally, the majority of GIE procedures are performed by using topical anesthesia and intravenous sedation. General anesthesia is carried out in long and invasive procedures such as endoscopic retrograde cholangiopancreatography, endoscopic ultrasound, and small bowel enteroscopy, as well in patients with history of failed sedation or drug and substance abuse, uncooperative or pediatric patients, and patients with cardiorespiratory system instabilities. The appropriate anesthetic agents for GIE procedures could be short acting, rapid onset with little adverse effects and also improved safety profiles. To date, the new anesthetic drugs and monitoring equipments for safety and efficacy are available. The present review focuses on pre-anesthetic assessment, anesthetic drugs used, monitoring practices, and post-anesthesia care for anesthesia innovations in GIE procedures.

Keywords: Anesthesia, Innovation, Gastrointestinal endoscopy, Safety, Efficacy

1. Introduction

Anesthesia is one of the important components of gastrointestinal endoscopic (GIE) procedures. The aim of anesthesia for these procedures is to improve patient's comfort and endoscopic practice as well as patient and endoscopist satisfaction. The requirement for anesthesia is dependent on the type and duration of endoscopy, experience of endoscopist, and patient's physical status. The anesthetic regimens for GIE procedures are quite different. Several guidelines from American Society of Anesthesiologists (ASA) [1] and American Academy of Pediatrics [2] are established. Appropriate pre-anesthetic assessment, anesthetic drugs used, monitoring practices and post-anesthesia care for anesthesia in GIE procedures are essential.

1.1. Pre-procedure assessment

All patients scheduled to receive anesthesia/sedation should have a history and appropriate physical examination. Several risk factors including history of obstructive sleep apnea, alcohol or drug abuse, and history of adverse reaction to previous anesthesia/sedation are investigated. The patient physical status should be classified according to the ASA. The pregnancy test is recommended in women of childbearing age [3]. Consequently, written consent should be obtained. An anesthesia consultation should be done in high-risk patients including patients with respiratory or hemodynamic instability, obstructive sleep apnea, and high-risk airway management, as well as patients with ASA physical status >III and history of anesthesia-related adverse events.

2. Monitoring

Cardiorespiratory-related adverse events are a leading cause of morbidity and mortality associated with GIE procedures. Continuous monitoring of anesthetized patients is very important for safety. The physicians need to monitor the patients' status throughout the procedure. Clinical observations including pattern of respiration, skin or mucosa color, and level or depth of anesthesia are continuously observed.

2.1. Pulse oximetry

Pulse oximetry is a noninvasive device for continuous measurement of arterial oxygen saturation. Because clinical observation alone is inaccurate in the detection of hypoxemia, pulse oximetry has become a standard of care during GIE procedures. Oxygen saturation levels under 90% must be treated. However, pulse oximetry and oxygen supplementation do not diminish the severity or incidence of cardiorespiratory complications. In addition, oxygen desaturation is relatively a late sign [4].

2.2. Capnography

Moreover, pulse oximetry and clinical observation cannot detect the development of hypercapnea. Capnography has been utilized to permit the safe titration of propofol by a qualified gastroenterologist during invasive procedures such as endoscopic retrograde cholangiopancreatography (ERCP) and endoscopic ultrasonography (EUS).

2.3. Noninvasive blood pressure

Blood pressure and heart rate are important parameters of cardiovascular monitoring. The alterations of blood pressure are mediated by the depressive effects of anesthetic agents. Baseline hemodynamic parameters also provide useful information of the effects of various medical conditions. Generally, blood pressure and heart rate will be documented before anesthesia, and at least 5 min for deep sedation and general anesthesia, as well as every 15 min for mild and moderate sedation. Blood pressure is more likely to predict increasing and decreasing doses of anesthetic drugs.

2.4. Electrocardiography

The use of electrocardiography (ECG) was aimed to detect cardiac arrhythmias in high-risk patients undergoing anesthesia. However, the use of ECG during GIE procedure remains controversial [6]. American Society for Gastrointestinal Endoscopy (ASGE) and ASA practice guidelines recommend the use of ECG during GIE anesthesia in patients with significant cardiovascular diseases or arrhythmias. However, ECG is not recommended for routine use of ECG in patients with ASA physical status I or II [1, 4, 7].

2.5. Other monitors

Other monitors such as invasive arterial blood pressure, central venous pressure (CVP), and pulmonary arterial catheterization (PAC) are infrequently used during GIE anesthesia. However, these invasive monitors should be used in some high-risk patients including patients with severe hemodynamic instabilities and patients with shock.

2.6. Bispectral index monitoring

The depth of anesthesia cannot be reliably judged by clinical assessments alone. Currently, the Bispectral (BIS) index has been reported to be more accurate in measurement of the depth of anesthesia. The BIS scale ranges from 0 to 100 (0, no cortical activity or coma; 40-60, unconscious; 70-90, varying levels of conscious sedation; 100, fully awake). In the past, BIS monitor was used to assess the patient consciousness during general anesthesia [4, 8]. To date, its use has subsequently expanded into the procedural sedation technique. However, the use of BIS during GIE procedures remains a controversial issue.

The usefulness of BIS monitoring for GIE procedure was confirmed by the study of Bower and colleagues. This study showed the correlation of BIS index and the Observer's Assessment of Alertness/Sedation (OAA/S) scale for sedation during GIE procedures. It also suggested that a bispectral index near 82 corresponded with acceptable sedation level for GIE procedure [9]. Al-Sammak and coworkers compared BIS with clinical assessment for sedation during ERCP procedure in pediatric patients. The duration of sedation, recovery period, patient satisfaction, and total dose of sedative agents in the BIS group were better than in the clinical assessment group. This study demonstrated that BIS might be a valuable monitor for safe level of sedation and endoscopist's satisfaction during ERCP [10]. Another study also showed that BIS monitoring guided to a decrease in the propofol dose for sedation in ERCP procedures. Mean BIS values throughout the procedure and during the maintenance period of sedation were 61.68 ± 7.5 and 53.73 ± 8.67, respectively [11].

In contrast, several reports demonstrated that BIS index had low accuracy for detecting deep sedation and it was not helpful for titrating propofol to an adequate depth of sedation level. For example, Chen and Rex evaluated the utility of BIS as a monitoring device for nurse-administered propofol sedation (NAPS) during colonoscopic procedure. The study showed the mean time required to accomplish BIS values ≤60 was significantly longer than the mean time required to achieve an Observer's Assessment of Alertness/Sedation score of 1 (deep sedation). Additionally, there was also a lag time between the time required from the last dose of propofol and the time returned to baseline. The authors concluded that BIS index was not a useful device in titrating propofol to an adequate depth of sedation level [12].

Drake and coworkers also confirmed that BIS did not lead to the reduction in mean propofol dose or recovery time when used for sedation in colonoscopy [13]. Moreover, an observational study also showed that BIS index had a low accuracy for detecting deep sedation because of an overlap of scores across the sedation levels. Further improvements in BIS are needed to differentiate deep from moderate sedation for GIE procedures [14].

2.7. Narcotrend™

Narcotrend™ accomplishes a computerized analysis of the raw EEG. A statistical algorithm is used for analysis, resulting in a six-stage classification from A (awake) to F (general anesthesia/coma) and 14 substages [4, 15]. Wehrmann and colleagues evaluated 80 patients who underwent ERCP procedures by using EEG monitoring and clinical assessment for sedation. Their study demonstrated that mean propofol dose, decrease in blood pressure, and recovery time in the EEG monitoring group were significantly lower than in the clinical assessment group. The authors confirmed that EEG monitoring permitted more effective titration of propofol dosage for sedation during ERCP procedures and was associated with more rapidly patient recovery [16].

My previous study used the Narcotrend™ to guide the depth of sedation for ERCP procedure. Narcotrend™ monitoring was an effective tool for maintenance of the depth of sedation level in this procedure [17]. The other study compared the clinical efficacy of Narcotrend™ monitoring and clinical assessment used to provide deep sedation in patients who underwent ERCP procedure. In the study, Modified Observer's Assessment of Alertness/Sedation scale 1 or 2 and the Narcotrend™ index 47-56 to 57-64 were maintained during the procedure. All endoscopies were completed successfully. Both Narcotrend™ and clinical-assessment-guided propofol deep sedation were equally safe and effective as well as demonstrated comparable propofol dose and recovery time. However, the Narcotrend™-guided sedation showed lower hemodynamic changes and fewer complications compared with the clinical-assessment-guided sedation [18].

3. Anesthetic technique

3.1. Topical anesthesia

Esophagogastroduodenoscopy (EGD) is commonly performed by using topical pharyngeal anesthesia. Topical lidocaine is normally used as pretreatment for pharyngeal anesthesia. My previous study evaluated the clinical efficacy of topical viscous lidocaine solution and lidocaine spray when each was used as a single agent for unsedated EGD [19]. All patients were randomized into the viscous lidocaine (V) group (n = 930) or the lidocaine spray (S) group (n = 934). The results showed the procedure was successfully completed in 868 patients from group V and 931 patients from group S. Patient's and endoscopist's satisfaction, pain score, patient tolerance, and ease of intubation in group S were significantly better than those in group V. Additionally, adverse events in group S also occurred significantly lower than group V. This study demonstrated that the use of topical lidocaine spray was shown to be a better form of pharyngeal anesthesia than viscous lidocaine solution in unsedated EGD procedure [19].

Consequently, the use of posterior lingual lidocaine swab can apply for EGD procedure. Soweid and colleagues evaluated the effect of posterior lingual lidocaine swab in 80 patients who underwent diagnostic EGD procedures on patient tolerance, the ease of performance of EGD procedure, and to determine if such use would decrease the need for intravenous sedation [20]. The result of their study demonstrated that patients in the lidocaine swab group tolerated the procedure better than those in the lidocaine spray group. The procedural difficulty and the need of intravenous sedation in the lidocaine swab group were lower than in the lidocaine spray group. Additionally, the patients and the endoscopists in the lidocaine swab group were more satisfied than in the lidocaine spray group. They suggested the use of posterior lingual lidocaine swab for EGD procedure because of patient comfort and tolerance, endoscopist satisfaction, and reduction of the need for intravenous sedation.

Ramirez and coworkers also compared the effect of glossopharyngeal nerve block and topical anesthetic agent for EGD procedure [21]. The aim of the study was to evaluate the sedation, tolerance to the procedure, hemodynamic stability, and the adverse events. They performed a clinical trial in a total of 100 patients who underwent EGD procedures. All patients in both arms also received intravenous midazolam. The procedures were reported without discomfort in 48 patients (88%) in the glossopharyngeal nerve block group and 32 patients (64%) in the topical anesthetic group. There were no significant differences in the incidence of nausea and retching in both groups. The study confirmed that the use of glossopharyngeal nerve block provided greater patient comfort and tolerance as well as also diminished the need for sedation in EGD patients [21].

3.2. Intravenous sedation

Sedation for GIE procedure can be safely and effectively performed with a multidrug regimen utilizing anesthesiologist or nonanesthetic personnel with appropriate monitoring. Currently, sedation practices for GIE procedures vary widely. The need for sedation is decided by the type of endoscopy, duration of procedure, degree of endoscopic difficulty, patient physical status, and physician's preferences. However, the sedation regimen for GIE procedures is still varied. Benzodiazepines and opioids are commonly used by nonanesthetic personnel. In contrast, propofol in combination with opioids and/or benzodiazepines is usually used by anesthetic personnel.

3.3. General anesthesia

The choice of anesthetic technique for GIE procedure depends on the patient and the type of procedure. General anesthesia is commonly utilized in patients with ASA physical status >III and patients with cardiorespiratory instability, as well as in long duration and complicated procedures. Traditionally, tracheal intubation is also performed when general anesthesia is used. An anesthesiologist usually uses balanced anesthesia technique including opioid, inhalation agent, and neuromuscular blocking drug. The majority of these anesthetic agents have short-acting and short-duration properties.

4. Anesthesia innovative techniques

4.1. Target-controlled infusion

Target-controlled infusion (TCI) is a computer-controlled open-loop administration of anesthetic drugs. A continuous infusion technique uses a pharmacokinetic model to predict the patient plasma and effect site concentrations from the infusion design and allows the anesthesiologist to target a selected concentration. The device computes the appropriate infusion system to accomplish this concentration [22]. The TCI rapidly attains and maintains a predefined plasma or effect site concentration of the anesthetic drug. An appropriate target concentration for achieving the desired clinical endpoint is selected. The TCI delivery system performs better than the manual system. Presently, TCI devices for propofol administration are approved in several countries.

Mazanikov and colleagues compared TCI (initial targeted effect-site concentration 2 mcg/mL) with patient-controlled sedation (PCS) (single bolus 1 mL, lockout time set at zero) in 82 patients who underwent elective ERCP procedures. Alfentanil was supplemented if needed. All procedures were performed successfully. Mean consumption of propofol and the recovery time in the TCI group was significantly greater than in the PCS group. However, mean consumption of alfentanil in both groups was comparable. The authors concluded that there were no benefits of TCI over PCS for propofol administration in ERCP procedures [23].

4.2. Patient-controlled sedation

Because of interindividual variability, new techniques of administration for sedation have been developed. Patient-controlled sedation (PCS) devices deliver a predefined bolus of intravenous drug during a defined time with or without a lockout interval. A prospective, randomized, controlled study compared the use of PCS with propofol and remifentanil and the anesthesiologist-administered propofol sedation for 80 elective ERCP patients. Sedation level was assessed every 5 min by using Ramsay and Gillham sedation scores. All ERCP patients were completely successful except two patients in the PCS group. Mean level of sedation and total propofol consumption in the PCS group were significantly lower than in the anesthesiologist-administered propofol group. However, patient and endoscopist satisfaction were equally high in both groups. The study confirmed that PCS with propofol and remifentanil was a safe and well-accepted sedation technique for ERCP patients [24].

Moreover, the use of PCS with propofol and remifentanil has been compared with fentanyl and midazolam for sedation in patients who underwent colonoscopy by Mandel and colleagues [25]. Their study demonstrated that time to sedation and the recovery time in the PCS with the propofol and remifentanil group were significantly shorter than in the PCS with the fentanyl and midazolam group. However, the perceptions of patients, nurses and endoscopists were comparable between the two groups.

Procedural sedation in cirrhotic patients is challenged. Titration of sedative and analgesic drugs is needed for an optimal sedation level. The use of PCS for sedation in these patients is an alternative technique. Although, dexmedetomidine is suggested for procedural sedation and reported effective for alcohol withdrawal, the efficacy of dexmedetomidine as a sole anesthetic agent is controversial. Mazanikov and coworkers evaluated 50 patients with chronic alcoholism scheduled for elective ERCP procedures. All patients in the PCS with propofol and alfentanil group were successfully sedated, and in 19 of 25 (76%) patients in the dexmedetomidine group. They also suggested that a loading dose of dexmedetomidine 1 mcg/kg over 10 min, followed by continuous intravenous infusion 0.7 mcg/kg/h was insufficient for the ERCP procedure. In addition, dexmedetomidine was also related with prolonged recovery [26].

4.3. Computer-assisted personalized sedation system

The use of propofol for sedation in GIE procedures may allow for better quality of sedation and faster recovery. Computer-assisted personalized sedation system (CAPS) is based on the patient response to stimulation and physiologic profiles. It presents an attractive means of delivering safe and effective doses of propofol. The closed-loop target-controlled system or continuous EEG recordings are used to assess the degree of sedation. Patient-controlled platforms may also be used. These devices may help physicians titrating propofol administration and controlling the physiological functions [27].

The SEDASYS System is a CAPS integrating propofol delivery with patient monitoring to allow physicians to safely administer propofol. The efficacy and safety of this system for sedation during GIE procedures was evaluated and compared with the combination of benzodiazepine and opioid in 1000 adult patients with ASA physical status class I-III. All patients were sedated in mild to moderate depth of sedation level. The study demonstrated that SEDASYS system was safe and effective for sedation during EGD and colonoscopic procedures. Additionally, patient and physician satisfaction as well as recovery time in the SEDASYS group were significantly better than patients in the combination of benzodiazepine and opioid group [28].

The use of inadequate sedative agents results in over and under depth of sedation. The use of CAPS for administration of propofol by nonanesthetic personnel achieving mild to moderate sedation in patients who underwent GIE procedures was evaluated by Pambianco and coworkers [29]. This study showed that propofol administration in mild or moderate sedation level by nonanesthetic personnel used with CAPS system in patients who underwent EGD and colonoscopic procedures was safe and effective. Moreover, low propofol dosage and short recovery time were noted.

4.4. Closed-loop administration of anesthesia

Closed-loop administration of anesthesia systems can provide anesthesia automatically and its effect feedback controlled. This system contains a central system, a target control device such as syringe pump, vaporizer, and other drug delivery systems [30]. Currently, there are several closed-loop administration systems for neuromuscular blockade, depth of anesthesia, and pain control during decreased levels of consciousness. In addition, McSleepy is also a closed-loop control system that displays the patient's depth of consciousness, muscular movement during surgery, and the level of pain [30].

4.5. Teleanesthesia

Teleanesthesia is the use of telemedicine technology in anesthetic management including preoperative assessment at distance, video consultation, and performing anesthesia in remote locations where experienced anesthesiologists are not always present [30, 31]. The impact of telemedicine pre-anesthesia evaluation on periprocedural processes was confirmed by Applegate II and colleagues. Their study demonstrated that telemedicine pre-anesthesia evaluation offered patients time- and cost-saving benefits without more surgical delay. Moreover, telemedicine and in-person assessments were comparable, with high patient and physician satisfaction [32].

5. Anesthetic agents

5.1. Local anesthetic agents

Generally, lidocaine is the most common local anesthetic agent used for GIE procedure. The viscous lidocaine solution and lidocaine spray are usually performed for upper GIE procedure. In addition, lidocaine gel or jelly is frequently employed for lower GIE procedure. Recently, lidocaine lozenge has been tried to use for EGD procedure. Mogensen and colleagues evaluated the effect and acceptance of a lidocaine lozenge compared with a lidocaine viscous oral solution as pharyngeal anesthesia before EGD [33]. The 110 adult patients were randomized to receive either 100 mg lidocaine as a lozenge or 5 mL lidocaine viscous solution 2%. Supplemental intravenous midazolam was administered if needed. They concluded that the lozenge could reduce gag reflex and patients' discomfort, and improved patients' acceptance during the procedure. In addition, the lozenge form had also a good taste [33]. Another study of the lidocaine lozenge used for pharyngeal anesthesia in EGD procedure has been reported by

Tumminakatte and Nagaraj [34]. The authors compared the efficacy, safety, and patient comfort for the lidocaine lozenge and lidocaine viscous as a single agent before EGD procedure. This study showed that lidocaine lozenge was effective and safe for pharyngeal anesthesia before EGD procedure. It was relatively better than lidocaine viscous in terms of lesser discomfort and procedural difficulty as well as increased tolerability of the EGD procedure [34].

Moreover, topical bupivacaine could be used as pretreatment for pharyngeal anesthesia in unsedated EGD. The effect of a bupivacaine lozenge as pharyngeal anesthesia and a lidocaine spray before EGD was assessed by Salale and coworkers [35]. Ninety-nine adult patients were randomized to receive either a bupivacaine lozenge or lidocaine spray. Patient discomfort and the acceptance of gag reflex during EGD procedures were evaluated. The results showed that patient discomfort and gag reflex during procedure in the bupivacaine lozenge group were significantly lower than the lidocaine spray group. The authors also suggested that bupivacaine lozenge for topical pharyngeal anesthesia before an unsedated EGD procedure verified to be a superior option as compared with lidocaine spray [35].

Chan and colleagues studied the effectiveness of 10% lidocaine pump spray plus plain Strepsils and Strepsils anesthetic lozenge plus distilled water spray for EGD procedure in terms of patient tolerance, taste of anesthetic agent, intensity of numbness, amount of cough or gag, and the degree of discomfort at esophageal intubation. They concluded that topical lidocaine spray was superior to the flavored anesthetic lozenge as a topical pharyngeal anesthesia in unsedated EGD procedure [36]. Furthermore, the safety and efficacy of a lidocaine lollipop as single-agent anesthesia for EGD has been evaluated by Ayoub and coworkers [37]. The main outcome variables of the study were the success rate and safety of local anesthesia by using lidocaine lollipop in addition to the need for intravenous sedation. Their study showed that lidocaine lollipop, a favorable form of pharyngeal anesthesia, was safe and well tolerated for EGD procedure.

5.2. Benzodiazepines

5.2.1. Midazolam

Midazolam is one of the most common drugs used for sedation during GIE procedures. It is a rapid-onset, short duration of action, and water-soluble benzodiazepine with anxiolytic, amnesic, sedative, muscle relaxant, and anticonvulsant properties. These actions are due to the effect of binding to gamma-amino butyric acid receptors in the central nervous system. Midazolam has few adverse effects. Respiratory depression is the most important adverse effect and is synergistic when used in combination with opioids. The standard dose in adult patients is 0.015-0.06 mg/kg [38].

5.3. Opioids

5.3.1. Fentanyl

Fentanyl is a potent synthetic opioid and also commonly used for GIE procedures. It has a rapid onset, short duration of action, and lack of direct myocardial depressant effects. The onset of action is 30–60 s, and the duration of action is 30–45 min. Generally, the dose for GIE procedure is usually 1–2 mcg/kg, with a maximum dose of 100–150 mcg in adult healthy patients. Because of its analgesic effect, fentanyl is commonly used for therapeutic GIE procedures. Of late, the combination of fentanyl and midazolam is an accepted regimen with a safety profile [39-41]. However, fentanyl can cause respiratory depression including apnea as well as nausea and vomiting. It can reduce the heart rate.

5.3.2. Remifentanil

Remifentanil is a fentanyl analog with a methyl ester group and is hydrolyzed by plasma and tissue esterases. Its metabolism is not affected by genetics, age, hepatic failure, and renal failure. Its action is rapid. The use of remifentanil for sedation in GIE procedures is not entirely recognized. Remifentanil is generally performed by using the continuous infusion technique. The TCI of remifentanil is another preference. The combination of propofol and remifentanil for sedation in GIE procedures is usually used. The study of Abu-Shahwan and Mack demonstrated the efficacy and safety of a combination of propofol and remifentanil for deep sedation in children who underwent GIE procedures [42]. In their study, anesthesia was induced with sevoflurane and nitrous oxide in oxygen, and was maintained with infusion of propofol and remifentanil. All GIE procedures were successfully completed with no complications. However, this combination of propofol and remifentanil demonstrated the reduction of heart rate, blood pressure, and respiratory rate.

Remifentanil in TCI appears to be a satisfactory drug for sedation in GIE procedures. However, propofol in TCI for GIE procedures demonstrates better sedation than remifentanil in TCI. This issue was confirmed by Munoz and colleagues [43]. They compared remifentanil and propofol in TCI for sedation in 69 patients during GIE procedures. The authors concluded that propofol in TCI for sedation in patients who underwent GIE procedures seemed to be an adequate agent. Additionally, propofol in TCI created less adverse effects and higher patient satisfaction than remifentanil in TCI.

5.4. Remimazolam

Remimazolam is a rapidly acting intravenous sedative drug. It combines the properties of midazolam and remifentanil. Additionally, its tendency to cause apnea is very low. Remimazolam has potential to be used as a sedative drug in the intensive care unit and as a novel agent for procedural sedation [44, 45]. Recently, remimazolam was evaluated for sedation in patients who underwent upper GIE procedures by Rogers and McDowell. This clinical trial demonstrated that the time to recovery from sedation of remimazolam was faster and more reliable than midazolam [46]. Moreover, Worthington and colleagues assessed the feasibility of remimazolam for sedation during colonoscopy and reversing the sedative effects of remimazolam with flumazenil in 15 healthy volunteers. The sedation for colonoscopy was successfully completed in more than 70% of subjects. In addition, all subjects rapidly reversed with flumazenil and also rapidly recovered within 10 min. No serious adverse events were observed [47].

5.5. Propofol

Propofol has sedative, hypnotic, and anesthetic properties. However, it does not have analgesic effects. Propofol rapidly crosses the blood–brain barrier. The onset of action is 30–60 s. Dose reduction is needed in patients with cardiac dysfunction and in elderly patients. However, the dose reduction of propofol in patients with moderately severe liver disease or renal failure is not required. Propofol potentiates the effects of analgesic and sedative drugs. The advantage of propofol has been demonstrated for therapeutic GIE procedures and not for diagnostic GIE procedures.

Propofol in combination with opioid or benzodiazepine can cause significant cardiovascular depression and may result in a deeper than expected depth of sedation because of its narrow therapeutic window. Pain at the injection site is the most frequent local complication. Several methods for propofol delivery have been used for GIE procedures. Generally, propofol is administered intravenously as a repeated bolus injection, continuous infusion, or a mixture of both. Currently, the nonanesthesiologist-administered propofol is a controversial issue and also varies among countries.

5.5.1. Propofol for GIE procedures

Generally, propofol is usually used for various GIE procedures. A previous study confirmed that sedation with propofol alone or propofol combined with fentanyl or midazolam in children was safe and effective. However, the use of propofol alone provides lesser sedation and ease of endoscopy than the use of propofol in combination with fentanyl or midazolam [48]. In Siriraj GI Endoscopy Center, the combination of propofol, fentanyl, and/or midazolam was usually used for GIE procedures even in pediatric patients. Moreover, our previous studies also demonstrated the clinical effectiveness of an anesthesiologist-administered sedation outside of the operating room for pediatric GIE procedures. Although, all sedation-related complications were relatively high, all of these complications were transient and easily treated [39, 40, 49, 50]. In terms of procedure-related complications, propofol-based sedation does not increase the rate of colonoscopic perforation [51].

For invasive GIE procedures, propofol-based sedation for ERCP and percutaneous endoscopic gastrostomy procedures in sick and elderly patients by anesthetic personnel with appropriate monitoring was also safe and effective without any serious complications [52-54]. The safety of propofol sedation for EUS with fine needle aspiration procedure was confirmed by Pagano and coworkers [55]. The complication rates for propofol deep sedation and meperidine/midazolam administered for moderate sedation were not significantly different. Furthermore, propofol combined with fentanyl and midazolam is frequently used for GIE procedures including EUS and small bowel enteroscopy [56-60].

5.5.2. Nurse-administered propofol

Several guidelines do not recommend the use of propofol for routine GIE procedures. The safety and efficacy of propofol administered by registered nurses has been reported in a case series including 2000 patients undergoing elective EGD and/or colonoscopy [61]. Another study demonstrated that trained nurse-administered propofol for GIE sedation in patients with ASA class I, II, and III was safe and effective. The anesthetic support was assisted in 11 patients (0.4%) [62].

5.5.3. Gastroenterologist-administered propofol

Similar to qualified nurses, the gastroenterologist can administer propofol effectively. Several guidelines recommend that gastroenterologist-administered propofol should be used to sedate patients only at mild or moderate sedation levels. Additionally, the patients must have ASA physical status not more than III. The study of Vargo and colleagues confirmed that gastro-enterologist-administered propofol for elective ERCP and EUS procedures resulted in the reduction of propofol dosage and the improvement of recovery activity as well as the rapid detection of respiratory depression. This study also demonstrated that gastroenterologist-administered propofol should be a cost-effective sedation technique [63].

5.5.4. Anesthesiologist-administered propofol

Propofol is commonly used by anesthesiologists for anesthesia in GIE procedures. To date, the use of propofol is still controversial. Propofol can be used by well-trained registered nurses or physicians in some countries. However, in developing countries, propofol-based sedation is performed by anesthesiologists or anesthetic nurses. Berzin and coworkers accomplished a cohort study of sedation-related adverse events, patient- and procedure-related risk factors associated with sedation, as well as endoscopist and patient satisfaction with anesthesiologist-administered sedation in 528 patients who underwent ERCP procedures. The study confirmed that anesthesiologist-administered sedation for ERCP patients was safe and effective. Cardi-orespiratory-related adverse events were generally minimal [64].

5.6. Fospropofol

Fospropofol is a water-soluble prodrug of propofol that is currently approved for sedation for diagnostic and therapeutic procedures. It is characterized by a smooth and predictable rise and decline rapidly observed following intravenous administration. It does not cause pain on intravenous injection, but it has been associated with paresthesia in the perineal and perianal area. However, fospropofol causes dose-dependent hypotension, respiratory depression, and apnea. Generally, a standard of fospropofol sedation is 6.5 mg/kg. In high-risk and elderly patients, a lower dose should be administered. Bergese and coworkers compared the efficacy and safety of fospropofol in a dose of 4.875 mg/kg and 6.5 mg/kg for sedation in high-risk elderly patients who underwent colonoscopy. This study showed that fospropofol in a dose of 4.875 mg/kg for sedation in high-risk elderly patients who underwent colonoscopy was not a clinically significant advantage. Fospropofol in a dose of 6.5 mg/kg was recommended in the elderly, obese, and high-risk patients when used for moderate sedation [65].

5.7. Ketofol

Ketofol is the combination of ketamine and propofol in various concentrations. It isan agent of choice for a variety of GIE procedures. Ketamine, a neuroleptic anesthetic agent, works on thalamocortical and limbic N-methyl-D-aspartate receptors. Ketamine stimulates the cardiorespiratory system. A direct effect increases cardiac output, arterial blood pressure, heart rate, and central venous pressures [66]. In contrast, propofol has antiemetic, anxiolytic, hypnotic, and anesthetic properties. Additionally, propofol has a short recovery time without an increase of cardiorespiratory side effects. As a result, the combination of these two drugs has several benefits because of hemodynamic stability, lack of respiratory depression, good recovery and post-procedural analgesia. The safety and efficacy of ketofol as a sedoanalgesic agent are dependent on the dose and the ratio of the mixture [67].

Ketofol is also commonly used for sedation during GIE procedures. My previous study evaluated the clinical efficacy of the ketofol and propofol alone when each regimen is used as sedative agents for colonoscopic procedure. A 194 patients were randomized into two groups; 97 patients in group PK received propofol and ketamine and 97 patients in group P received propofol and normal saline for sedation. All patients were premedicated with 0.02–0.03 mg/kg of midazolam. All colonoscopic procedures were completely successful. There were no significant differences in patient tolerance, hemodynamic parameters, recovery activity, patient and endoscopist satisfaction, as well as the sedation-related adverse events between the two groups. In addition, these adverse events were transient and mild in degree [68].

5.8. Dexmedetomidine

Dexmedetomidine is a specific central alpha-2 adrenoreceptor agonist with sedative and analgesic properties. Dexmedetomidine has no effect at the GABA receptor, and is not associated with significant respiratory depression. The patients can be sedated but are able to be awakened to full consciousness easily. It induces a biphasic blood pressure response: high doses cause hypertension, and lower doses cause hypotension and bradycardia. The other disadvantages of dexmedetomidine include a slow onset and longer duration of action [42].

To date, the role of dexmedetomidine for GIE procedures is not entirely established and remains a controversial issue. Samson and colleagues compared the sedation efficacy and the hemodynamic effects of dexmedetomidine, midazolam, and propofol in 90 patients with ASA physical status I or II, who underwent elective diagnostic upper GIE procedures. The results demonstrated that endoscopist satisfaction level, recovery, and the hemodynamic stability in the dexmedetomidine group were significantly better than in the midazolam and the propofol groups [69]. However, dexmedetomidine alone is less effective than the combination of propofol and fentanyl for moderate sedation during ERCP procedure [70]. Most of the patients needed supplementary analgesic and sedative drugs to accomplish the depth of sedation level. However, these findings do not allow us to conclude that propofol alone is better than dexmedetomidine alone, because the conclusion was established for propofol combined with fentanyl. Moreover, dexmedetomidine was associated with higher hemodynamic instability and a prolonged recovery phase [70].

5.9. Ketodex

Ketamine is a dissociative anesthetic agent and works on thalamocortical and limbic N-methyl-D-aspartate (NMDA) receptors. Its actions are described by catalepsy in which eyes remain open and there is slow nystagmic gaze while corneal and light reflexes remain intact. Direct effects increase cardiac output, blood pressure, heart rate as well as pulmonary arterial and central venous pressures, which stimulates the cardiorespiratory system. However, ketamine produces unpleasant psychological effects including hallucinations, nightmares, and emergence reactions. Dexmedetomidine is a specific central alpha-2 adrenergic agonist that decreases central presynaptic catecholamine release. It has no effect at the GABA receptor, and is not associated with significant respiratory depression. Its properties of sedation, anxiolysis, and analgesia together with its beneficial pharmacokinetics make it a valuable adjunct for procedural and intensive care sedation [66].

The use of ketodex for GIE procedures was reported by Goyal and colleagues [71]. They used a bolus dose of ketamine 2 mg/kg and dexmedetomidine 1 mcg/kg for upper GIE procedures in pediatric patients. The results of the study showed that blood pressure, heart rate, and oxygen saturation did not change significantly from the baseline. The airway interventions were not used. In addition, there were also no laryngospasm and postprocedural shivering. The delirium score was lower than 4 in all patients except for two cases. This case series supported the use of ketodex was safe and clinically effective for upper GIE procedure in pediatric patients [71].

5.10. Muscle relaxants

5.10.1. Cisatracurium

Cisatracurium, an isomer of atracurium, is about three times more potent than atracurium and less tendency to release histamine than atracurium. It experiences spontaneous degradation at physiological pH and temperature by Hofmann elimination. Liver disease does not appear to have an effect on cisatracurium. Pharmacokinetics and pharmacodynamics of cisatracurium in normal adult and liver transplant patients do not show clinically significant differences in the recovery profiles [72]. Because of its beneficial properties, cisatracurium is a muscle relaxant drug of choice for tracheal intubation and maintenance during general anesthesia in GIE procedures [50, 59].

5.10.2. Rocuronium

Rocuronium is a steroidal nondepolarizing neuromuscular blocking drug and has a rapid onset of action. It is a muscle relaxant drug of choice for tracheal intubation and maintenance during general anesthesia in GIE procedures [50, 59, 73]. Rocuronium has emerged as an alternative to succinylcholine for facilitating rapid tracheal intubation in full stomach patients. It is predominantly useful as a relaxant agent for tracheal intubation in patients at risk of hyperkalemia and patients with known or suspected increased intracranial or intraocular pressure. However, rocuronium may be used cautiously in patients with impaired liver function [74].

5.11. Reversal drugs

5.11.1. Naloxone

Naloxone is a pure mu-opioid antagonist with a high affinity for the receptor. It can reverse both the analgesic and respiratory effects of opioids [4, 42]. The standard dosage of intravenous naloxone is 1–2 mcg/kg with a maximum dose of 0.1 mg/kg and up to 2 mg. However, naloxone has a short duration of action and one dose typically only lasts for 30–45 min. Patients should be monitored for at least 2 h after the last dose of naloxone. The adverse reactions of naloxone include reversal of opioid withdrawal, nausea/vomiting, hypertension, tachycardia, pulmonary edema, and cardiac dysrhythmias.

5.11.2. Flumazenil

Flumazenil is a benzodiazepine antagonist. It is a highly specific benzodiazepine receptor antagonist and can safely reverse the sedative and respiratory effects caused by benzodiazepines. The adult dose is 0.01 mg/kg and up to 1 mg. Its duration of action is just about 1 h. However, this effect is reversible. Importantly, the patients should be observed for at least 2 h after the administration of flumazenil [4, 42]. The adverse reactions of flumazenil consist of sweating, flushing, nausea/vomiting, hiccup, agitation, abnormal vision, paresthesia, and seizure.

5.12. Sugammadex

Sugammadex is a selective relaxant binding drug that quickly reverses the effects of aminosteroid neuromuscular blocking agents such as rocuronium and vecuronium. It was successfully used to reverse rocuronium-induced neuromuscular block in patients where neostigmine was insufficient. Dogan and colleagues investigated the efficacy of sugammadex after unsatisfactory decurarization following neostigmine administration. This study was performed on 14 patients who experienced inadequate decurarization (TOF < 0.9) with neostigmine after general anesthesia. A dose of 2 mg/kg of sugammadex was used. The result confirmed that sugammadex was successfully performed to reverse rocuronium-induced neuromuscular block in patients where neostigmine was insufficient [75]. The capability to reverse a rocuronium-induced neuromuscular block at any stage and possibly to improve patients' safety might make sugammadex a very attractive drug for the use in day-case anesthesia.

Another study compared the efficacy of sugammadex and neostigmine for the reversal of vecuronium-induced neuromuscular blockade in elective surgical patients [76]. All patients, ASA physical status I-III obtained a dose of 0.1 mg/kg vecuronium for tracheal intubation and maintenance dose of 0.02–0.03 mg/kg if needed. Neuromuscular blockade was monitored by using acceleromyography. At the end of surgery, patients were randomized to receive either sugammadex 2 mg/kg or neostigmine 50 mcg/kg and glycopyrrolate 10 mcg/kg. The study showed that mean recovery times to a TOF ratio of 0.8 and 0.7 in the sugammadex group were significantly shorter than in the neostigmine group. No serious adverse events were noted.

The authors concluded that sugammadex presented significantly quicker reversal of vecuronium-induced neuromuscular blockade compared with neostigmine [76].

5.13. Inhalation agents

5.13.1. Sevoflurane

Sevoflurane is an inhalation agent with ideal properties for deep sedation during GIE procedures in pediatric patients. In addition, it is commonly used for balanced general anesthesia. A retrospective study reviewed data from children receiving sevoflurane inhalation administered by an anesthesiologist via laryngeal insufflation to attain deep sedation for outpatient GIE procedures. All patients were adequately sedated with sevoflurane, and no intravenous line was needed. Time to awakening, discharge, and complication rate in the sevoflurane group were significantly lower than in the combination of midazolam, fentanyl, and ketamine, as well as in the propofol alone groups. This report suggested that deep sedation with sevoflurane insufflation for pediatric outpatient GIE procedure is as safe as conventional sedation techniques [77].

Consequently, Meretoja and colleagues compared anesthesia with sevoflurane or halothane for bronchoscopy or gastroscopy, or both in 120 infants and children. All pediatric patients were assigned to receive either 7% sevoflurane or 3% halothane in 66% nitrous oxide in oxygen for induction of anesthesia. Induction time and psychomotor recovery as well as the incidence of nausea/vomiting and cardiac arrhythmia in the sevoflurane group were significantly lower than in the halothane group. This study confirmed that the use of sevoflurane was better than the use of halothane for bronchoscopy and gastroscopy procedures in pediatric patients [78].

5.13.2. Desflurane

Desflurane is an ether inhalational anesthetic agent. It offers the advantage of precise control over depth of anesthesia along with a rapid, predictable, and clear-headed recovery with minimal postoperative adverse events. It also has advantages when used in extremes of age and in obese patients. Desflurane is generally used for the maintenance of balanced general anesthesia because of its rapid recovery. Currently, the use of desflurane may increase the direct costs of anesthetic care [79]. However, no significant differences were demonstrated between desflurane and sevoflurane in the late recovery period.

6. Post-anesthesia care

Blood pressure, heart rate, respiratory rate, oxygen saturation, and level of consciousness are monitored and documented at least every 15 min or less, for a minimum of 30 min after the last dose of sedation drug. These parameters should be monitored and noted in the recovery period. Moreover, the patients should be monitored for at least 2 h after the last dose of a reversal drug. All patients will be discharged from the recovery room once the discharge criteria are completed. Generally, the majority of sedated patients would complete an acceptable score on or before 1 h after GIE procedure. Most delays after satisfactory scores were due to nonmedical causes [80]. In ambulatory cases, the presence of an escort must be confirmed, and the patients should not drive for at least 24 h.

7. Conclusion

GIE procedure requires some forms of anesthesia. To date, sedation for GIE procedure can be effectively and safely performed by anesthesiologist or nonanesthetic personnel with appropriate patient selection and monitoring. The new anesthetic drugs and monitoring equipments for safety and efficacy are available. However, pre-anesthetic evaluation and preparation, anesthetic drugs used, monitoring practices and post-anesthesia management are still essential for the anesthesia innovations in GIE procedures.

Author details

Somchai Amornyotin

Address all correspondence to: somchai.amo@mahidol.ac.th

Department of Anesthesiology and Siriraj GI Endoscopy Center, Faculty of Medicine Siriraj Hospital, Mahidol University, Bangkok, Thailand

References

[1] American Society of Anesthesiologists Task Force on Sedation and Analgesia by Non Anesthesiologists. Practice guidelines for sedation and analgesia by non-anesthesiologists. *Anesthesiology* 2002; 96: 1004-17

[2] Cote CJ, Wilson S. Guidelines for monitoring and management of pediatric patients during and after sedation for diagnostic and therapeutic procedures: an update. *Pediatrics* 2006; 118: 2587-602

[3] Muller M, Wehrmann T. How best to approach endoscopic sedation? *Nat Rev Gastroenterol Hepatol* 2011; 8: 481-90

[4] Amornyotin S. Sedation and monitoring for gastrointestinal endoscopy. *World J Gastrointest Endosc* 2013; 5: 47-55

[5] Cacho G, Perez-Calle JL, Barbado A, et al. Capnography is superior to pulse oximetry for the detection of respiratory depression during colonoscopy. *Rev Esp Enferm Dig* 2010; 102: 86-9

[6]   Cohen LB. Patient monitoring during gastrointestinal endoscopy: why, when, and how? *Gastrointest Endosc Clin N Am* 2008; 18: 651-63

[7]   Lichtenstein DR, Jagannath S, Baron TH, et al. Sedation and anesthesia in GI endoscopy. *Gastrointest Endosc* 2008; 68: 815-26

[8]   Amornyotin S. Monitoring for depth of anesthesia: a review. *J Biomed Graph Comput* 2012; 2: 119-27

[9]   Bower AL, Ripepi A, Dilger J, et al. Bispectral index monitoring of sedation during endoscopy. *Gastrointest Endosc* 2000; 52: 192-6

[10] Al-Sammak Z, Al-Falaki MM, Gamal HM. Predictor of sedation during endoscopic retrograde cholangiopancreatography-bispectral index vs clinical assessment. *Middle East J Anesthesiol* 2005; 18: 141-8

[11] Paspatis GA, Chainaki I, Manolaraki MM, et al. Efficacy of bispectral index monitoring as an adjunct to propofol deep sedation for ERCP: a randomized controlled trial. *Endoscopy* 2009; 41: 1046-51

[12] Chen SC, Rex DK. An initial investigation of bispectral monitoring as an adjunct to nurse-administered propofol sedation for colonoscopy. *Am J Gastroenterol* 2004; 99: 1081-6

[13] Drake LM, Chen SC, Rex DK. Efficacy of bispectral monitoring as an adjunct to nurse-administered propofol sedation for colonoscopy: a randomized controlled trial. *Am J Gastroenterol* 2006; 101: 2003-7

[14] Qadeer MA, Vargo JJ, Patel S, et al. Bispectral index monitoring of conscious sedation with the combination of meperidine and midazolam during endoscopy. *Clin Gastroenterol Hepatol* 2008; 6: 102-8

[15] Kreuer S, Biedler A, Larsen R, Altmann S, Wilhelm W. Narcotrend monitoring allows faster emergence and a reduction of drug consumption in propofol-remifentanil anesthesia. *Anesthesiology* 2003; 99: 34-41

[16] Wehmann T, Grotkamp J, Stergiou N, et al. Electroencephalogram monitoring facilitates sedation with propofol for routine ERCP: a randomized, controlled trial. *Gastrointest Endosc* 2002; 56: 817-24

[17] Amornyotin S, Srikureja W, Chalayonnawin W, Kongphlay S. Dose requirement and complication of diluted and undiluted propofol for deep sedation for endoscopic retrograde cholangiopancreatography. *Hepatobiliary Pancreat Dis Int* 2011; 10: 313-8

[18] Amornyotin S, Chalayonnawin W, Kongphlay S. Deep sedation for endoscopic retrograde cholangiopancreatography: a comparison between clinical assessment and Narcotrend™ monitoring. *Med Devices* (Auckl) 2011; 4: 43-9

[19] Amornyotin S, Srikureja W, Chalayonnavin W, Kongphlay S, Chatchawankitkul S. Topical viscous lidocaine solution versus lidocaine spray for pharyngeal anesthesia in unsedated esophagogastroduodenoscopy. *Endoscopy* 2009; 41: 581-6

[20] Soweid AM, Yaghi SR, Jamali FR, et al. Posterior lingual lidocaine: a novel method to improve tolerance in upper gastrointestinal endoscopy. *World J Gastroenterol* 2011; 17: 5191-6

[21] Ramirez MO, Segovia BL, Cuevas MAG, et al. Glossopharyngeal nerve block versus lidocaine spray to improve tolerance in upper gastrointestinal endoscopy. *Gastroenterol Res Pract* 2013; Article ID 264509, 4 pages, http://dx.doi.org/10.1155/2013/264509

[22] Guarracino F, Lapolla F, Cariello C, et al. Target controlled infusion: TCI. *Minerva Anestesiol* 2005; 71: 335-7

[23] Mazanikov M, Udd M, Kylanpaa L, et al. A randomized comparison of target-controlled propofol infusion and patient-controlled sedation during ERCP. *Endoscopy* 2013; 45: 915-9

[24] Mazanikov M, Udd M, Kylanpaa L, et al. Patient-controlled sedation with propofol and remifentanil for ERCP: a randomized, controlled study. *Gastrointest Endosc* 2011; 73: 260-6

[25] Mandel JE, Tanner JW, Lichtenstein GR, et al. A randomized, controlled, double-blind trial of patient-controlled sedation with propofol/remifentanil versus midazolam/fentanyl for colonoscopy. *Anesth Analg* 2008; 106: 434-9

[26] Mazanikov M, Udd M, Kylanpaa L, et al. Dexmedetomidine impairs success of patient-controlled sedation in alcoholics during ERCP: a randomized, double-blind, placebo-controlled study. *Surg Endosc* 2013; 27: 2163-8

[27] O'Connor JPA, O'Morain CA, Vargo JJ. Computer-assisted propofol administration. *Digestion* 2010; 82: 124-6

[28] Pambianco DJ, Vargo JJ, Pruitt RE, Hardi R, Martin JF. Computer-assisted personalized sedation for upper endoscopy and colonoscopy: a comparative, multicenter randomized study. *Gastrointest Endosc* 2011; 73: 765-72

[29] Pambianco DJ, Whitten CJ, Moerman A, Struys MM, Martin JF. An assessment of computer-assisted personalized sedation: a sedation delivery system to administer propofol for gastrointestinal endoscopy. *Gastrointest Endosc* 2008; 68: 542-7

[30] Hemmerling TM. Automated anesthesia. *Curr Opin Anesthesiol* 2009; 22: 757-63

[31] Hemmerling TM, Terrasini N. Robotic anesthesia: not the realm of science fiction any more. *Curr Opin Anesthesiol* 2012; 25:736-42

[32] Applegate II RL, Gildea B, Patchin R, et al. Telemedicine pre-anesthesia evaluation: a randomized pilot trial. Telemed e-Health 2013; 19: 211-6

[33] Mogensen S, Treldal C, Feldager E, et al. New lidocaine lozenge as topical anesthesia compared to lidocaine viscous oral solution before upper gastrointestinal endoscopy. *Local Reg Anesth* 2012; 5: 17-22

[34] Tumminakatte ZU, Nagaraj P. Double blinded randomized controlled trial comparing lidocaine viscous and lidocaine lozenges prior to upper gastrointestinal endoscopy. *Indian J Public Health Res Develop* 2013; 4: 256-60

[35] Salale N, Treldal C, Mogensen S, et al. Bupivacaine lozenge compared with lidocaine spray as topical pharyngeal anesthetic before unsedated upper gastrointestinal endoscopy: a randomized, controlled trial. *Clin Med Insights: Gastroenterol* 2014; 7: 55-9

[36] Chan CKO, Fok KL, Poon CM. Flavored anesthetic lozenge versus Xylocaine spray used as topical pharyngeal anesthesia for unsedated esophagogastroduodenoscopy: a randomized placebo-controlled trial. *Surg Endosc* 2010; 24: 897-901

[37] Ayoub C, Skoury A, Abdul-Baki H, et al. Lidocaine lollipop as single-agent anesthesia in upper GI endoscopy. *Gastrointest Endosc* 2007; 66: 786-93

[38] Hausman LM, Reich DL. Providing safe sedation/analgesia: an anesthesiologist's perspective. *Gastrointest Endosc Clin N Am* 2008; 18: 707-16

[39] Amornyotin S, Srikureja W, Pausawasdi N, Prakanrattana U, Kachintorn U. Intravenous sedation for gastrointestinal endoscopy in very elderly patients of Thailand. *Asian Biomed* 2011; 5: 485-91

[40] Amornyotin S, Aanpreung P, Prakarnrattana U, et al. Experience of intravenous sedation for pediatric gastrointestinal endoscopy in a large tertiary referral center in a developing country. *Pediatr Anesth* 2009; 19: 784-91

[41] Amornyotin S, Prakanrattana U, Chalayonnavin W, Kongphlay S. Intravenous sedation for endoscopic ultrasonography in Siriraj Hospital. *Thai J Anesthesiol* 2009; 35: 181-90

[42] Amornyotin S. Sedative and analgesic drugs for gastrointestinal endoscopic procedure. *J Gastroenterol Hepatol Res* 2014; 3: 1133-44

[43] Abu-Shahwan I, Mack D. Propofol and remifentanil for deep sedation in children undergoing gastrointestinal endoscopy. *Pediatr Anesth* 2007; 17: 460-3

[44] Munoz L, Arevalo JJ, Reyesc LE, et al. Remifentanil vs. propofol controlled infusion for sedation of patients undergoing gastrointestinal endoscopic procedures: a clinical randomized controlled clinical trial. *Rev Colomb Anestesiol* 2013; 41: 114-9

[45] Goudra BG, Singh PM. Remimazolam: the future of its sedative potential. *Saudi J Anesth* 2014; 8: 388-91

[46] Rogers WK, McDowell TS. Remimazolam, a short-acting GABA (A) receptor agonist for intravenous sedation and/or anesthesia in day-case surgical and non-surgical procedures. *IDrugs* 2010; 13: 929-37

[47]   Worthington MT, Antonik LJ, Goldwater DR, et al. A phase Ib, dose-finding study of multiple doses of remimazolam (CNS 7056) in volunteers undergoing colonoscopy. *Anesth Analg* 2013; 117: 1093-100

[48]   Disma N, Astuto M, Rizzo G, et al. Propofol sedation with fentanyl or midazolam during esophagogastroduodenoscopy in children. *Eur J Anesthesiol* 2005; 22: 848-52

[49]   Amornyotin S, Aanpreung P. Clinical effectiveness of an anesthesiologist-administered intravenous sedation outside of the main operating room for pediatric upper gastrointestinal endoscopy in Thailand. *Int J Pediatr* 2010; 2010 [DOI: 10.1155/2010/748564]

[50]   Amornyotin S, Prakanrattana U, Chalayonnavin W, Kongphlay S, Chantakard S. Anesthesia for pediatric gastrointestinal endoscopy in a tertiary care teaching hospital. *Thai J Anesthesiol* 2008; 34: 265-72

[51]   Amornyotin S, Prakanrattana U, Kachintorn U, Chalayonnavin W, Kongphlay S. Propofol-based sedation does not increase rate of perforation during colonoscopic procedure. *Gastroenterol Insights* 2010; 2: e4

[52]   Amornyotin S, Kachintorn U, Chalayonnawin W, Kongphlay S. Propofol-based deep sedation for endoscopic retrograde cholangiopancreatography procedure in sick elderly patients in a developing country. *Ther Clin Risk Manage* 2011; 7: 251-5

[53]   Amornyotin S, Prakanrattana U, Chalayonnavin W, Kongphlay S, Kongmueng B. Anesthesia for percutaneous endoscopic gastrostomy in Siriraj Hospital. *Thai J Anesthesiol* 2009; 35: 39-47

[54]   Amornyotin S, Chalayonnavin W, Kongphlay S. Propofol-based sedation does not increase rate of complication during percutaneous endoscopic gastrostomy procedure. *Gastroenterol Res Pract* 2011; 2011 [DOI: 10.1155/2011/134819]

[55]   Pagano N, Arosio M, Romeo F, et al. Balanced propofol sedation in patients undergoing EUS-FNA: a pilot study to assess feasibility and safety. *Diagn Ther Endosc* 2011; 2011: 542159

[56]   Amornyotin S. Sedation for colonoscopy in children. *J Gastroenterol Hepatol Res* 2013; 2: 555-60

[57]   Amornyotin S, Songarj P, Kongphlay S. Deep sedation with propofol and pethidine versus moderate sedation with midazolam and fentanyl in colonoscopic procedure. *J Gastroenterol Hepatol Res* 2013; 2: 885-90

[58]   Amornyotin S, Kongphlay S. Esophagogastroduodenoscopy procedure in sick pediatric patients: a comparison between deep sedation and general anesthesia technique. *J Anesth Clin Res* 2012; 3: 1000185

[59] Amornyotin S, Kachintorn U, Kongphlay S. Anesthetic management for small bowel enteroscopy in a World Gastroenterology Organizing Endoscopy Training Center. *World J Gastrointest Endosc* 2012; 4: 189-93

[60] Amornyotin S, Kongphlay S. Anesthetic trainee-administered propofol deep sedation for small bowel enteroscopy procedure in elderly patients. *J Gastroenterol Hepatol Res* 2014; 3: 1117-29

[61] Rex DK, Overley C, Kinser K, et al. Safety of propofol administered by registered nurses with gastroenterologist supervision in 2000 endoscopic cases. *Am J Gastroenterol* 2002; 97: 1159-63

[62] Slagelse C, Vilmann P, Hornslet P, Hammering A, Mantoni T. Nurse-administered propofol sedation for gastrointestinal endoscopic procedures: first Nordic results from implementation of a structured training program. Scand J Gastroenterol 2011; 46: 1503-9

[63] Vargo JJ, Zuccaro G, Dumot JA, et al. Gastroenterologist administered propofol versus meperidine and midazolam for advanced upper endoscopy: a prospective, randomized trial. *Gastroenterology* 2002; 123: 8-16

[64] Berzin TM, Sanaka S, Barnett SR, et al. A prospective assessment of sedation-related adverse events and patient and endoscopist satisfaction in ERCP with anesthesiologist-administered sedation. *Gastrointest Endosc* 2011; 73: 710-7

[65] Bergese SD, Dalal P, Vandse R, et al. A double-blind, randomized, multicenter, dose-ranging study to evaluate the safety and efficacy of fospropofol disodium as an intravenous sedative for colonoscopy in high-risk populations. *Am J Ther* 2013; 20: 163-71

[66] Amornyotin S. Ketamine: pharmacology revisited. *Int J Anesthesiol Res* 2014; 2: 42-4 [DOI: 10.14205/2310-9394.2014.02.02.4]

[67] Amornyotin S. Ketofol: a combination of ketamine and propofol. *J Anesth Crit Care Open Access* 2014; 1: 00031 [DOI:10.15406/jaccoa.2014.01.00031]

[68] Amornyotin S, Chalayonnawin W, Kongphlay S. Clinical efficacy of the combination of propofol and ketamine (ketofol) for deep sedation for colonoscopy. Gut 2012; 61 (Suppl 2): A339-40

[69] Samson S, George SK, Vinoth B, Khan MS, Akila B. Comparison of dexmedetomidine, midazolam, and propofol as an optimal sedative for upper gastrointestinal endoscopy: a randomized controlled trial. *J Dig Endosc* 2014; 5: 51-7

[70] Muller S, Borowics SM, Fortis EAF, et al. Clinical efficacy of dexmedetomidine alone is less than propofol for conscious sedation during ERCP. *Gastrointest Endosc* 2008; 67: 651-9

[71]   Goyal R, Singh S, Shukla RN, Patra AK, Bhargava DV. Ketodex, a combination of dexmedetomidine and ketamine for upper gastrointestinal endoscopy in children: a preliminary report. *J Anesth* 2013; 27: 461-3

[72]   De Wolf AM, Freeman JA, Scott VL, et al. Pharmacokinetics and pharmacodynamics of cisatracurium in patients with end-stage liver disease undergoing liver transplantation. *Br J Anesth* 1996; 76: 624-8

[73]   Amornyotin S, Pranootnarabhal T, Chalayonnavin W, Kongphlay S. Anesthesia for gastrointestinal endoscopy from 2005-2006 in Siriraj Hospital: a prospective study. *Thai J Anesthesiol* 2007; 33: 93-101

[74]   Magorian T, Wood P, Caldwell J, et al. The pharmacokinetics and neuromuscular effects of rocuronium bromide in patients with liver disease. *Anesth Analg* 1995; 80: 754-9

[75]   Dogan E, Akdemir MS, Guzel A, et al. A miracle that accelerates operating room functionality: sugammadex. *Bio Med Res Int* 2014 (2014), Article ID 945310, 4 pages [10.1155/2014/945310]

[76]   Khuenl-Brady K, Wattwil M, Vanacker BF, et al. Sugammadex provides faster reversal of vecuronium-induced neuromuscular blockade compared with neostigmine: a multicenter, randomized, controlled trial. *Anesth Analg* 2010; 110: 64-73

[77]   Montes RG, Bohn RA. Deep sedation with inhaled sevoflurane for pediatric outpatient gastrointestinal endoscopy. *J Pediatr Gastroenterol Nutr* 2000; 31: 41-6

[78]   Meretoja OA, Taivainen T, Raiha L, Korpela R, Wirtavuori K. Sevoflurane-nitrous oxide or halothane-nitrous oxide for pediatric bronchoscopy and gastroscopy. *Br J Anesth* 1996; 76: 767-71

[79]   Kapoor MC, Vakamudi M. Desflurane-revisited. *J Anesthesiol Clin Pharmacol* 2012; 28: 92-100

[80]   Amornyotin S, Chalayonnavin W, Kongphlay S. Recovery pattern and home-readiness after ambulatory gastrointestinal endoscopy. J Med Assoc Thai 2007; 90: 2352-8

7

Endoscopy for Skull Base Surgery

Boonsam Roongpuvapaht,

Kangsadarn Tanjararak and Ake Hansasuta

Abstract

The endonasal approaches for skull base surgery have evolved in the recent decade. There are many publications of this technical safety and good outcomes, comparable with conventional procedure and have less morbidities. In this chapter, the authors describe the approach and surgical technique for each area of the skull base.

Keywords: Endoscopy, Skull base

1. Introduction

Lesions of paranasal sinuses, as well as those within skull base region, have long been challenging to rhinologists and neurosurgeons for several decades. Historically, the only available surgical approaches for these pathologies have traditionally been extensive and, often, invasive open procedures. Despite ample corridor created by open surgery, its major drawbacks during the surgery have been the poor visualization due to suboptimal illumination and magnification of the surgical fields. This fact could become more significant in those with pathologies in deep, narrow or complex anatomical areas. In some cases, en bloc tumor resection can be more easily performed through an open technique while in deep and difficult lesion may not possible to obtain the precise and free surgical margin due to poor visualization. In addition to the limited visualization by open surgery, these massive maneuvers can result in significant blood loss, morbidity or mortality.

Based on important principles, any evolution of surgical equipment and techniques has the same crucial concepts. First, it needs to minimize the associated surgical morbidity/mortality.

Second, it should maintain the patients' functional outcomes, parallel to the high success rate of surgery, i.e., for neoplasms, to achieve oncological control.

Later, development of surgical technique utilizing microscopy has been applied to the operative management of intracranial pathologies. Microsurgery had proven better patients' outcome compared to the historic open procedures, likely from the improved visualization and magnification of the operative field. Consequently, smaller skin incision and less amount of bone removal can achieve similar, if not better, overall result of the same lesions. Patients' safety as well as satisfaction has been greater with microscopic surgery. Therefore, microsurgery has been recognized as the standard of care for many neurosurgical and otolaryngological procedures. However, despite the vast usefulness of the microscope in neurosurgery and otolaryngology, it is not perfect. For the fact, shadow from an outside light source, an operating microscope, can hinder clear visualization at corners of the lesions or critical structures. This drawback is very obvious if one performs an operation through a small and narrow passage, i.e., transsphenoidal route either by sublabial or transnasal technique. This may, indeed, result in a subtotal resection.

For the past few decades, innovation of endoscopy has been developed and accepted as a minimally invasive technique. Various endoscopic tools and techniques have been applied to appropriate organs in different surgical fields. Unlike an outside light source from an operating microscope as mentioned above, visualization under endoscope has the superiority, obtaining a panoramic view with minimal or no shadow due to its light coming off the end of an endoscope. This is very factual through the narrow corridor, i.e., transsphenoidal route. In addition, endoscope provides excellent magnification that enhances the critical anatomical view beyond the operating site. Furthermore, the variety of angled lens endoscope allows surgeons to inspect "hidden" areas, especially "around the corners." Hence, some surgeons have been utilizing endoscopy as an assisting tool along with open or microsurgery so that it enhances visualization around the corners to improve resection of the target pathology. It reassures the complete removal of the tumors.

The treatment of the sinonasal tumors by endoscopy has been widely employed after the evolution of the endoscopic application for the paranasal and sinus diseases in the 1980s, which was introduced by Wigand and Messerklinger.[1, 2] Subsequently, the more properly designed endonasal instruments were developed and adapted to the endoscopic methods. This was popularized and spread over the otolaryngologists world by Stammberger and Kennedy.[3, 6] The endoscopic surgery for the intracranial pathology was first described in 1920s. Then, it was mainly applied within the ventricular system for the treatment of hydrocephalus. In 1990s it was, for the first time, reported for the treatment of pituitary lesions via transsphenoidal route as a collaboration between the otolaringologists and the neurosurgeons.[7, 11]

Recently, endoscopy has been employed for surgical treatment of various sinonasal pathologies. With the success of endoscopic sinus surgery, this approach has progressed further to the treatment of intracranial lesions namely in the vicinity of the skull base. In the aspect of skull base area, by accessing the cranial base via the natural anatomical corridors such as the nostrils or the oral cavity, endoscopic procedures can preserve critical and normal structures without leaving patients with cutaneous/visible scar. Moreover, better visualization with little, or no, brain retraction can be obtained. Hence, improvement of oncological control along with minimal functional morbidities has been reported by many authors. To date, there have been several publications that reiterated excellent results of the surgical outcomes to prove the efficacy of this innovative technique. Therefore, in some pathology, endoscopic procedures are considered one of the available standard treatments.

The endoscopic surgery has been expanded for the treatment of the lesions along the skull base, including both the median sagittal and paramedian coronal planes in the fashion of the multidisciplinary team approach.[12, 14] True team work can enhance the most benefit of the surgical techniques. The maintaining of clear visualization simultaneous with the two-hand dissecting technique cannot be accomplished independently. Moreover, the team approach has more efficient potential to manage the inevitable crisis during surgery.

Parallel to the surgical technique advancement, the safety from the new surgical method should be assessed for clinical use. Although, the endoscopic surgery has been known as a minimally invasive technique, it also carries a risk of complications. The incidence of complication has the different degrees of possibility depending on the surgical pathologies and procedures. The death and neurological deficits (transient or permanent) are the definite sequelae of the major complications from the endoscopic skull base surgery that includes the cerebrospinal fluid (CSF) leak, the intracranial infection and the neurovascular injury. The following rhinological symptoms have been considered as the minor complications as they don't cause severe morbidities for the patients: the nasal obstruction, the change of smell and sinusitis.

2. Patient selection

Not all the diseases could manage with endonasal technique. If the disease involves subcutaneous of skin or skin itself, the external approach should be more proper. If the tumor extends lateral to the center of the orbit, the orbit itself will be in the axis of the surgical corridor and block the working space. However, the patient selection depends on surgeon's experience.

3. Instrument

Author recommends using a high-definition camera, 4-mm telescopes in various angles (0, 30, 45, 70 degree), a powered instrument (microdebrider, ultrasonic aspirator, drill), hemostatic materials and devices and material for skull base reconstruction. The image-guided surgery system is highly recommended.

4. Surgical approaches

Surgical approaches for endonasal skull base can be classified into two groups based on anatomical view: sagittal plane (Figure 1) and coronal plane (Table 1).

Sagittal plane	Coronal view
Transfrontal	Anterior cranial fossa
Transcribiform	-Orbital approach
Transplanum	Middle cranial fossa
Transellar	-Pterygomaxillary fossa
Transclival	-Infratemporal fossa
Transodontoid	Posterior cranial fossa
	-Parapharyngeal space

Table 1. Surgical approaches

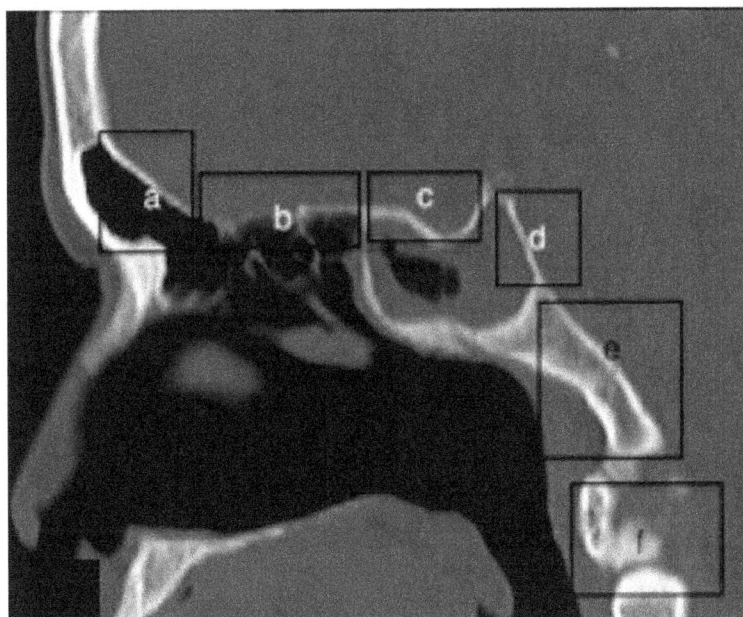

Figure 1. Endonasal approaches to the skull base in sagittal view. a) Transfrontal b) Transcribiform c) Transplanum d) Transsellar e) Transclival f) Transodontoid

4.1. Sagittal view

4.1.1. Transfrontal approach

This approach can be used in chronic frontal sinusitis, frontal fibro-osseous lesion and frontal sinus mucocele. This area can be reached by Draf III procedure or modified Lothrop which has to remove posterior part of nasal septum, remove the bone anterior to frontal sinus and connect both frontal sinus together by removing interfrontal sinus septum (Figures 3 and 4).

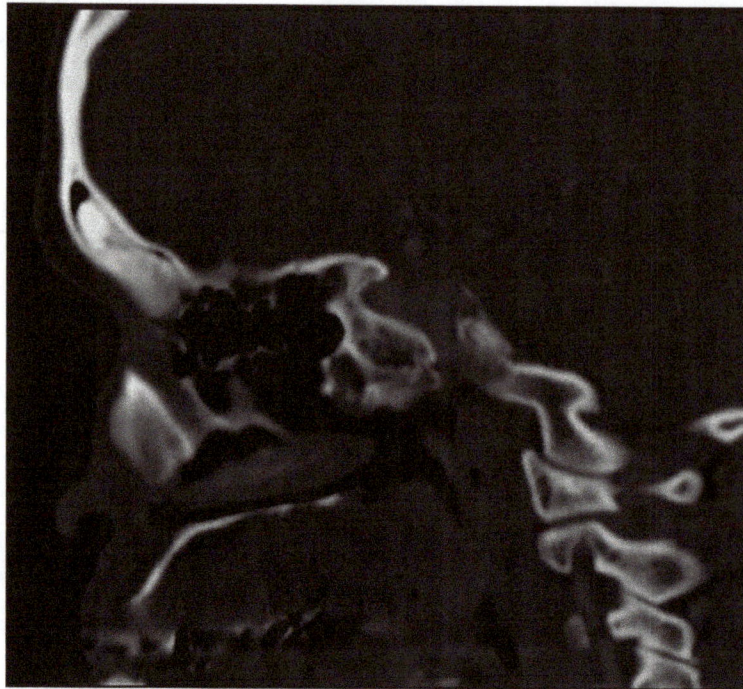

Figure 2. Sagittal view of CT scan shows osteoma in frontal sinus.

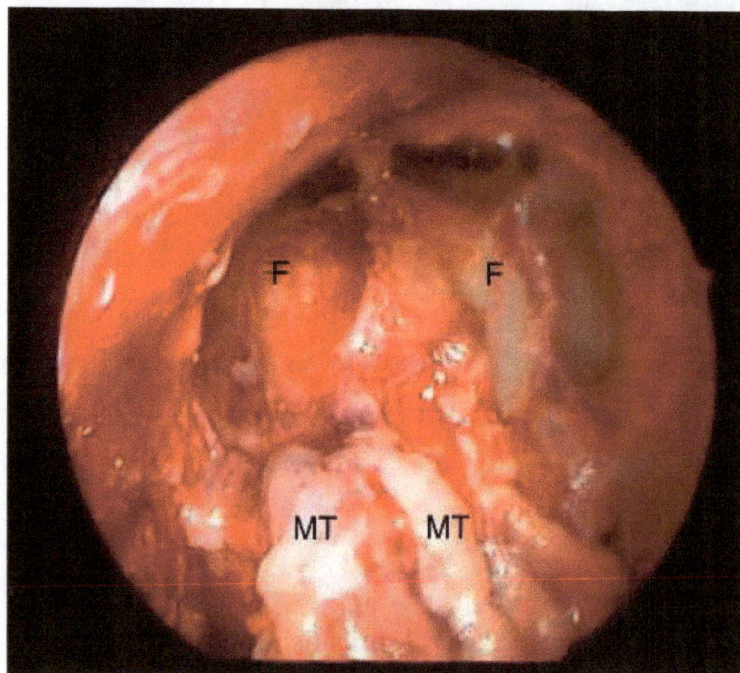

Figure 3. Endonasal view of both frontal sinus after Draf III procedure; F, frontal sinus; MT, middle turbinate.

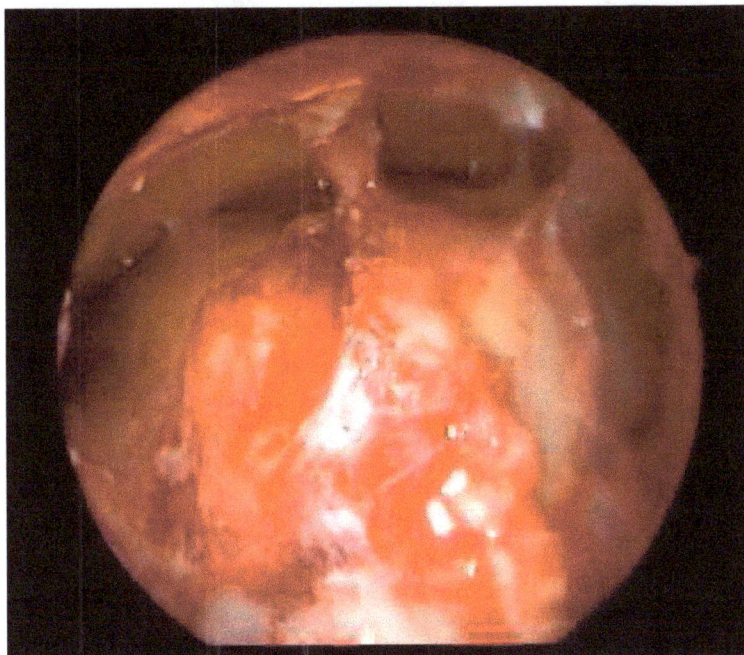

Figure 4. Endonasal view of both frontal sinus after Draf III procedure; F, frontal sinus; MT, middle turbinate.

4.1.2. Transcribiform approach

This approach is commonly utilized for olfactory area tumor such as olfactory neuroblastoma (esthesioneuroblastoma) and olfactory groove meningioma. This approach starts with complete sphenoethmoidectomy and Draf IIa/b or Draf III. The nasal septum removal should start from the crista galli to the sphenoid sinus.The anterior ethmoidal artery and posterior ethmoidal artery should be cauterized and transected to prevent bleeding and decrease the blood supply to the tumor. Cribiform plate should be thinned with diamond burr prior to its removal by bone rongeur so that the dura is clearly seen. The required area of bone exposure usually depends on oncological margin. The maximal bone removal at the cribiform plate can be from posterior wall of frontal sinus to planum sphenoidale in sagittal view and from medial wall of orbit to the other one in coronal view. The crista galli is thinned and removed from from its dural attachment, the falx cerebri. After dural opening, similar microsurgical technique for tumor dissection is employed by two-hand method.

4.1.3. Transplanum approach

Neoplasms at suprasellar area, such as tuberculum meningioma (Figure 9) or craniopharyngioma, typically require this particular approach. Bone removal at the posterior nasal septum and bilateral sphenoidotomy must be done as well as identification of optic nerves and optico-carotid recesses on both sides. Using similar steps as previously mentioned, the bone of skull base should be thinned and removed (Figures 10, 11). After dural opening, awareness of and early identification of critical structures, i.e., optic nerves and chiasm, internal carotid and anterior cerebral arteries and pituitary gland and its stalk (Figures 12, 13, 14), are critically

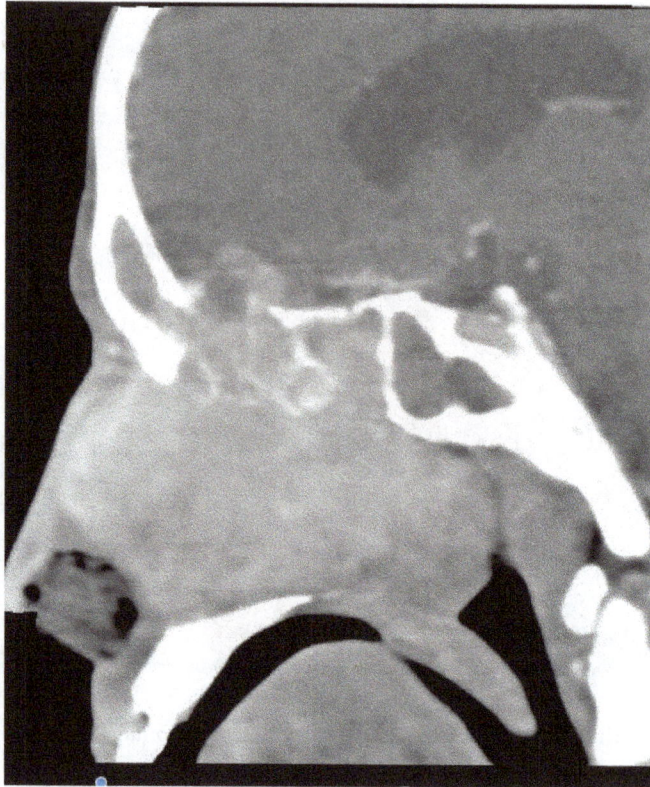

Figure 5. CT of an olfactory neuroblastoma. The tumor fully occupies the sino-nasal cavity and destroys the cribiform plate with intracranial extension.

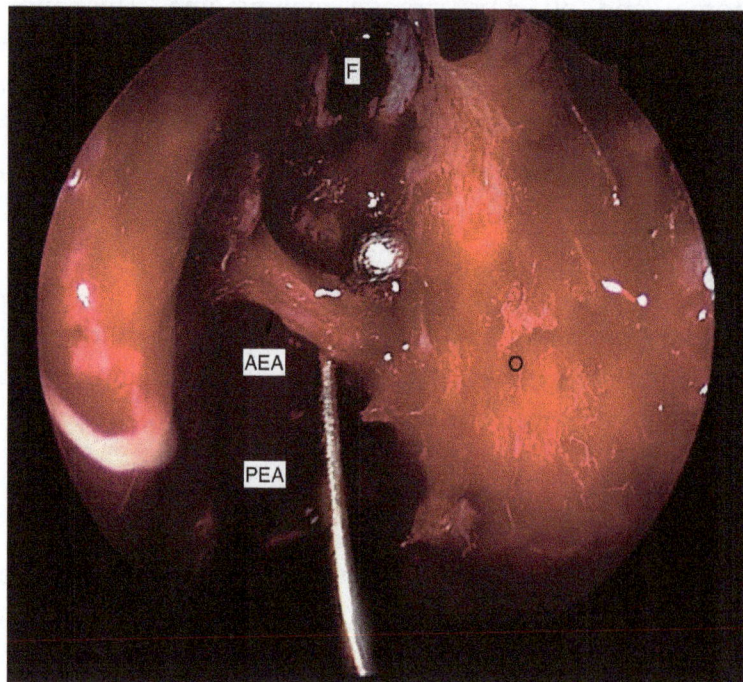

Figure 6. Left endonasal view, after endoscopic sinus surgery. The anterior ethmoidal artery was pulled with sinus seeker. F: frontal sinus O: orbit AEA: anterior ethmoidal artery PEA posterior ethmoidal artery

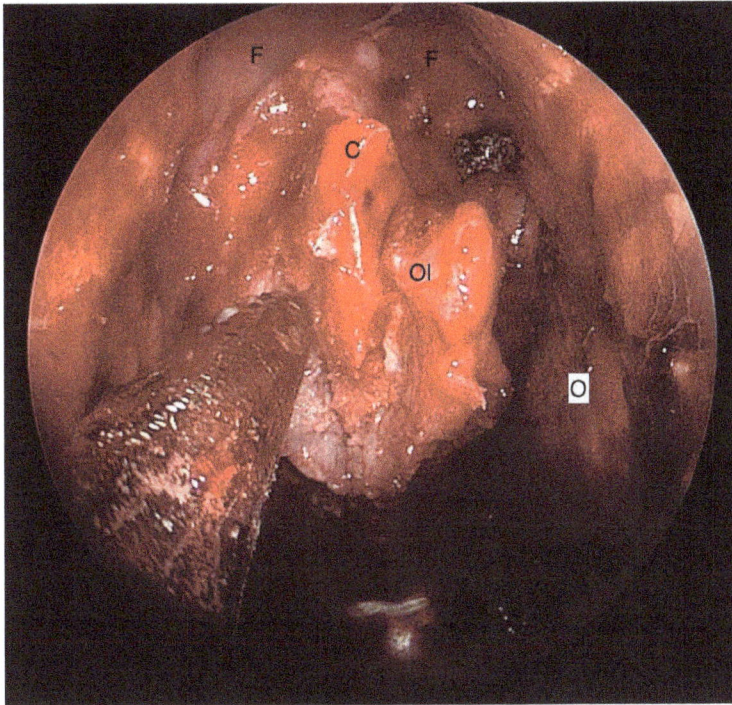

Figure 7. Endoscopic view of Draft III procedure and removal of nasal septum. The crista galli (C) in midline and first branch of olfactory nerve lateral to crista galli both sides are shown. F: frontal sinus C: crista galli Ol: first branch of olfactory nerve O: orbit

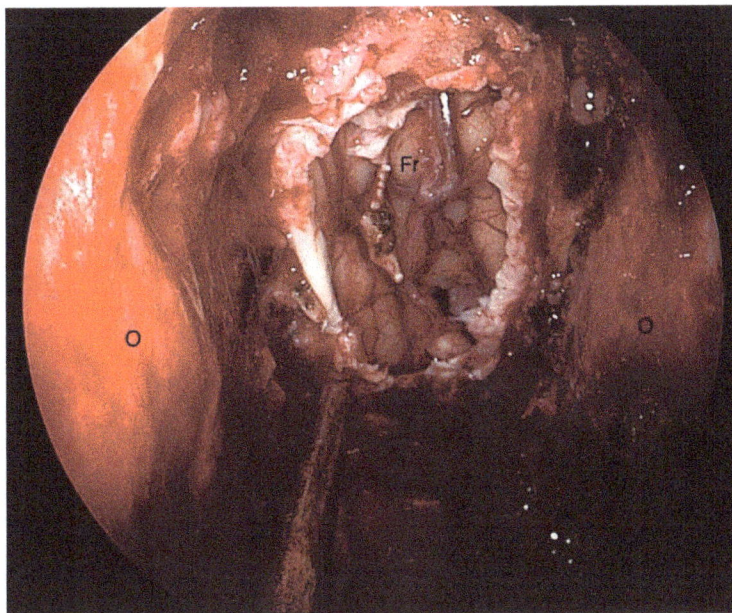

Figure 8. Endoscopic view after removing cribiform plate and dural opening demonstrates frontal lobe and orbit on both sides. O: orbit Fr: frontal lobe

important. Bi-manual technique, using similar microsurgical dissection, should be delicately performed. In some craniopharyngiomas, entry to the third ventricle is necessary for further tumor resection (Figures 15, 16).

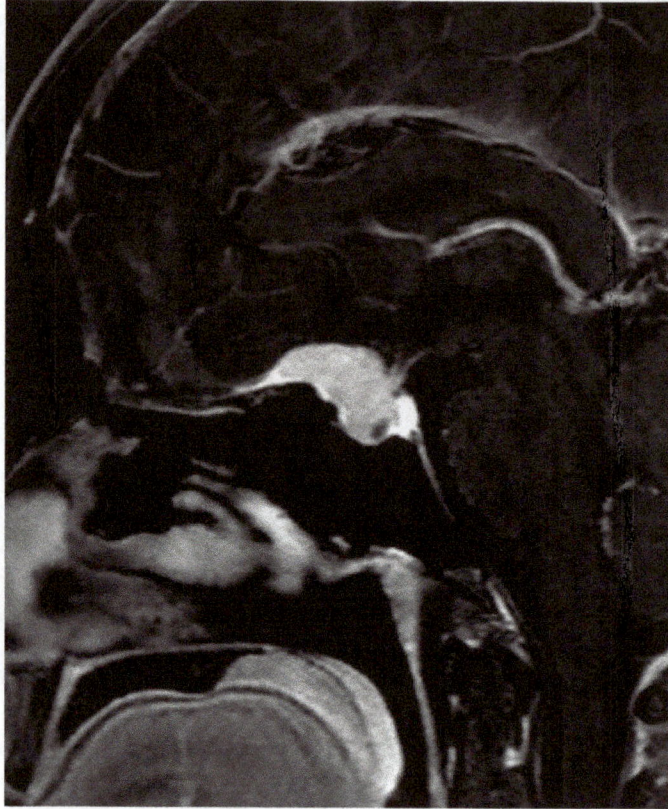

Figure 9. Sagittal MRI shows planum meningioma with compression of optic apparatus. The anterior cerebral artery complex is superior to the tumor.

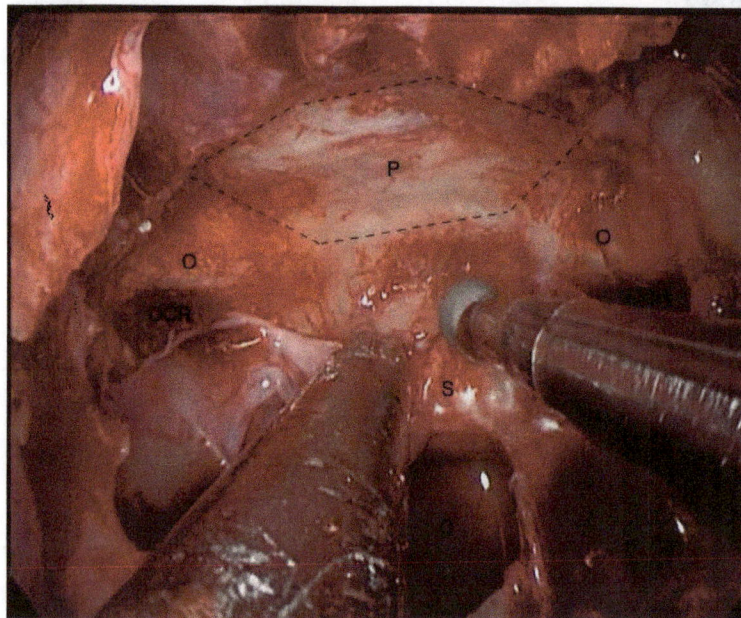

Figure 10. Endonasal view of planum sphenoidale and sella. P: planum sphenoidale (bony area within dashed line needs to be removed) O: optic nerve OCR: optico-carotid recess S: sellar C: clivus

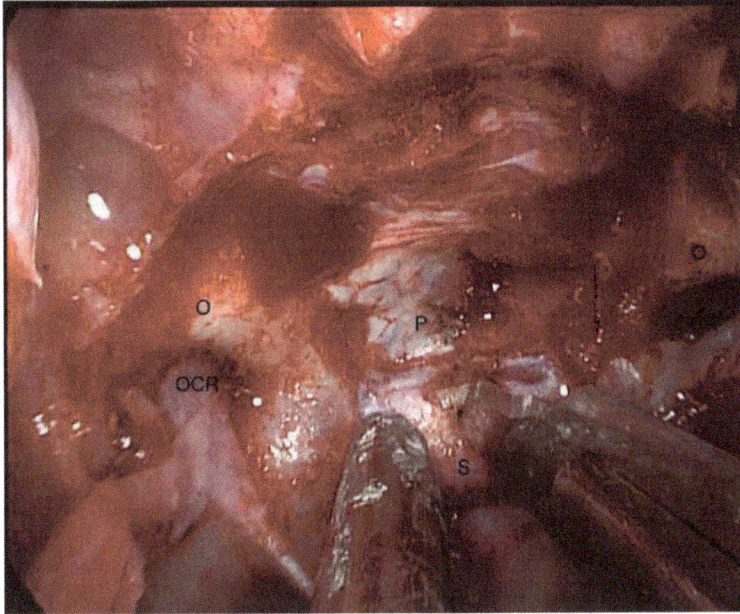

Figure 11. Endoscopic view demonstrates incision of the dura after removal of bony part of skull base. O: optic nerve OCR: optico-carotid recess P: planum sphenoidale S: sellar

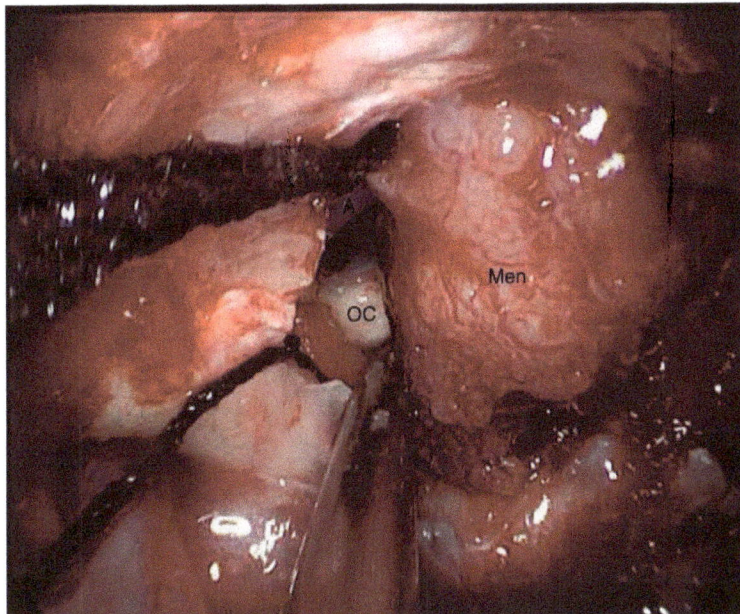

Figure 12. Endoscopic view after partial tumor removal illustrates the meningioma(Men), showing optic chiasm(OC) and anterior cerebral artery(A). Men: meningioma OC: optic chiasm A: anterior cerebral artery (A1 segment)

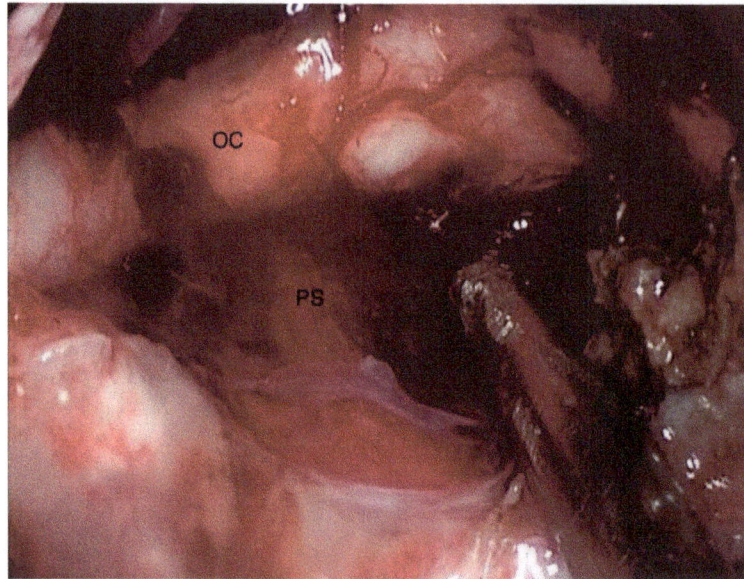

Figure 13. Endoscopic view after complete tumor removal depicts optic chiasm and pituitary stalk. OC: optic chiasm PS: pituitary stalk

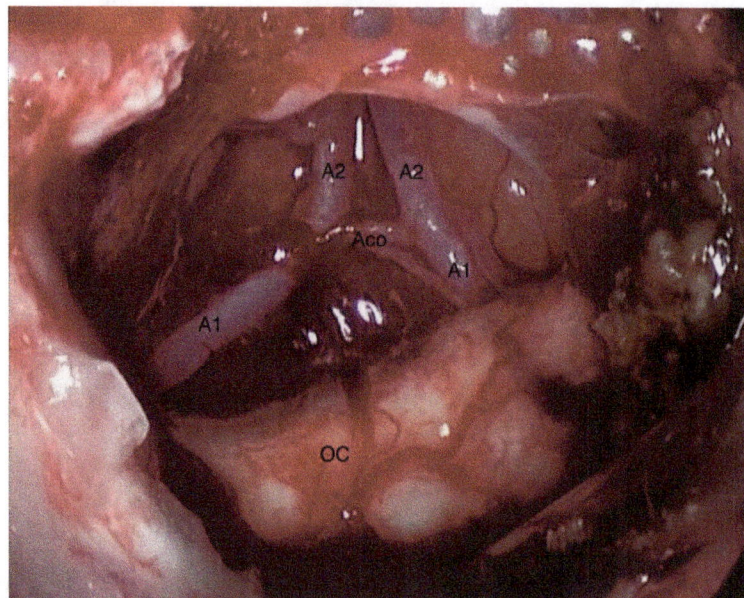

Figure 14. Endoscopic view of 30 degree angle lens, after complete tumor removal, shows more superiorly located structure. OC: optic chiasm A1: left and right anterior cerebral artery (A1 segment) Aco: Anterior communicating artery A2: left and right anterior cerebral artery (A2 segment)

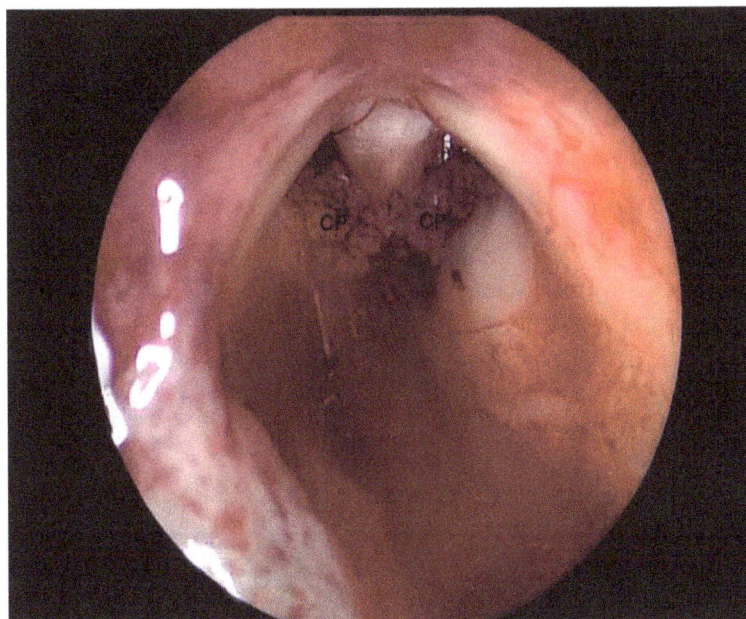

Figure 15. Endoscopic view using 30 degree lens looking upward after removal of craniopharyngioma depictsboth foramen of Monroe. CP: choroid plexus running from both lateral ventricle into the third ventricle

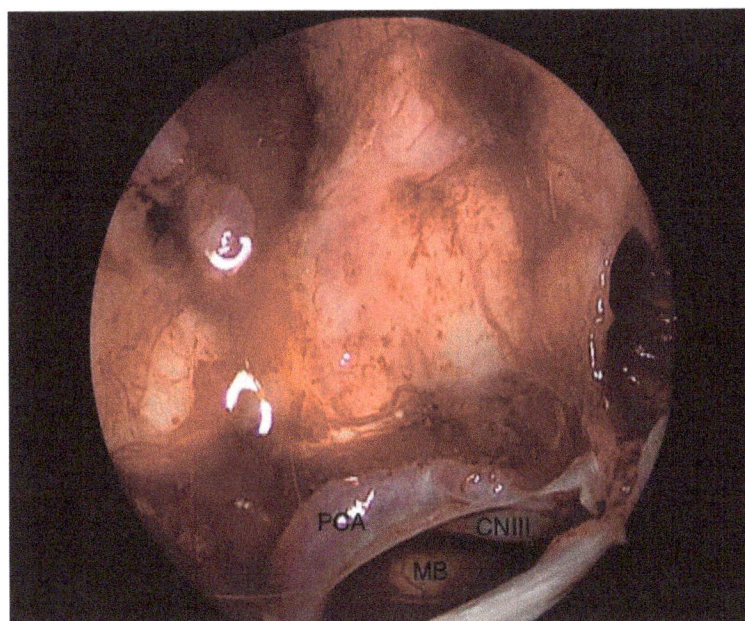

Figure 16. Endoscopic view using 30 degree lens looking downward after removal of craniopharyngioma reveals posterior structures. PCA: posterior cerebral artery CNIII: oculomotor nerve MB: mammillary bod

4.1.4. Transsellar approach

The most common disease for this approach is pituitary adenoma. This is the basic procedure of skull base that a surgeon should start to practice. After posterior nasal septectomy and bilateral sphenoidotomy, the sellar will come into the center of view. All the landmarks structures, e.g., internal carotid artery (ICA), optic nerve, optico-carotid recess, sellar, clivus and planum sphenoidale, should be identified. Sellar bone can be removed with diamond bur and manual instrument to expose the dura. The dura needs to be opened by using bipolar diathermy for hemostasis prior to incision with knife. The pituitary adenoma could be removed in a variety of techniques depending on the consistency of the tumor. The pituitary stalk, superior hypophyseal should be taken care for prevention of long-term endocrine malfunction.

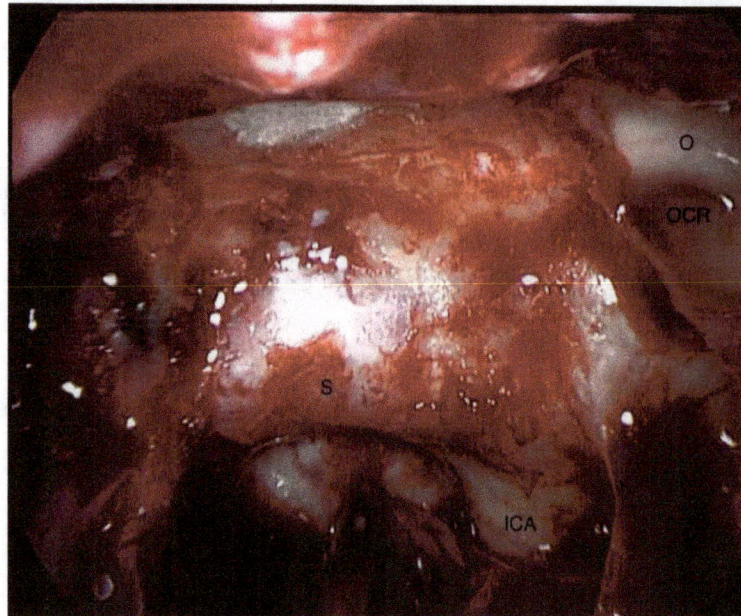

Figure 17. After removal of sellar bone, the sellar dura is exposed. O: optic nerve OCR: optico-carotid recess S: sellar ICA: internal carotid artery

4.1.5. Transclival approach

The clivus extends from sphenoid floor to foramen magnum. The common disease in this area includes meningioma and chordoma. This approach provides direct access to anterior surface of brainstem. The bony part of the clivus has a rich blood supply which surgeon should be cautious. After bony removal with diamond drill, the dura should carefully be incised because the 6th cranial nerve could be injured as it runs more superficially laterally. The vertebrobasillar artery should be carefully dissected and preserved.

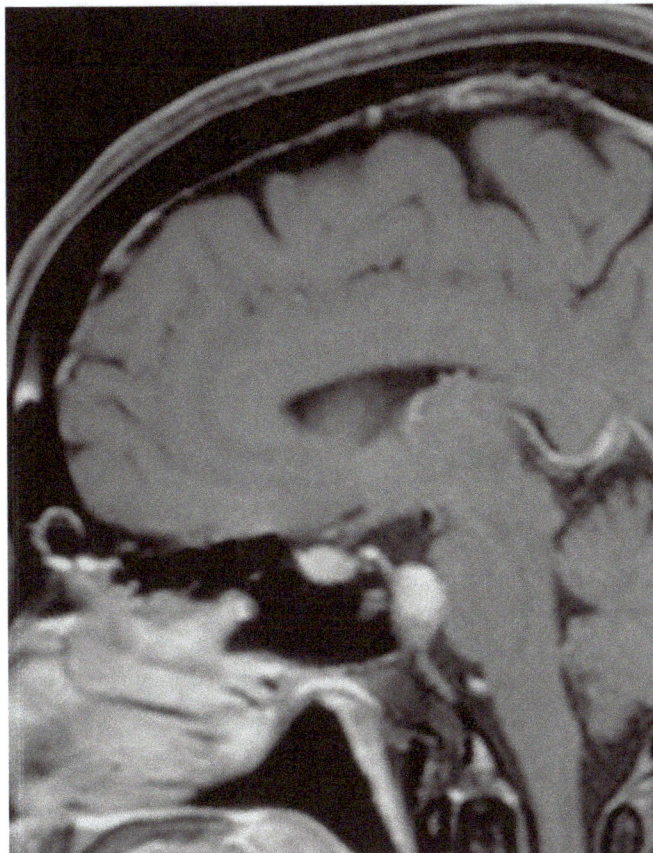

Figure 18. Sagittal MRI shows clivus chordoma pushing on brainstem, patient visit with diplopia from left lateral rectus muscle palsy.

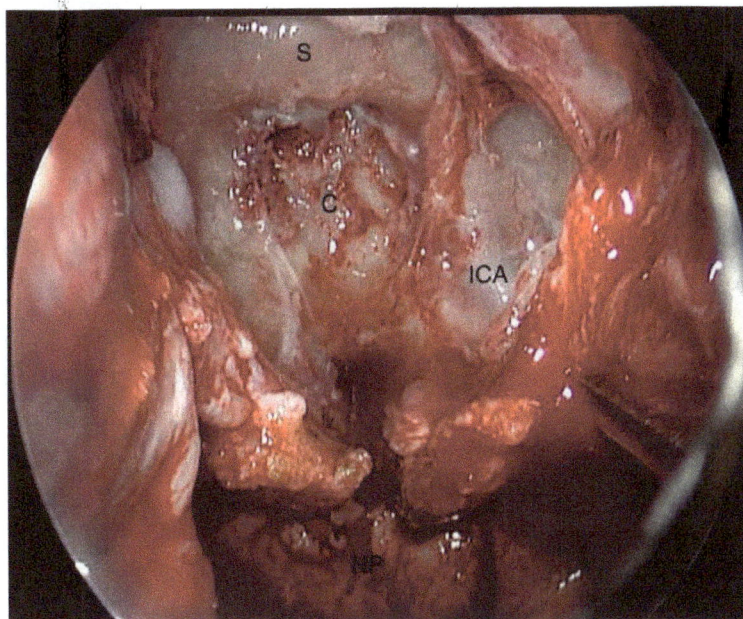

Figure 19. Endonasal view while drilling clivus. S: sellar C: clivus ICA: internal carotid artery NP: nasopharynx

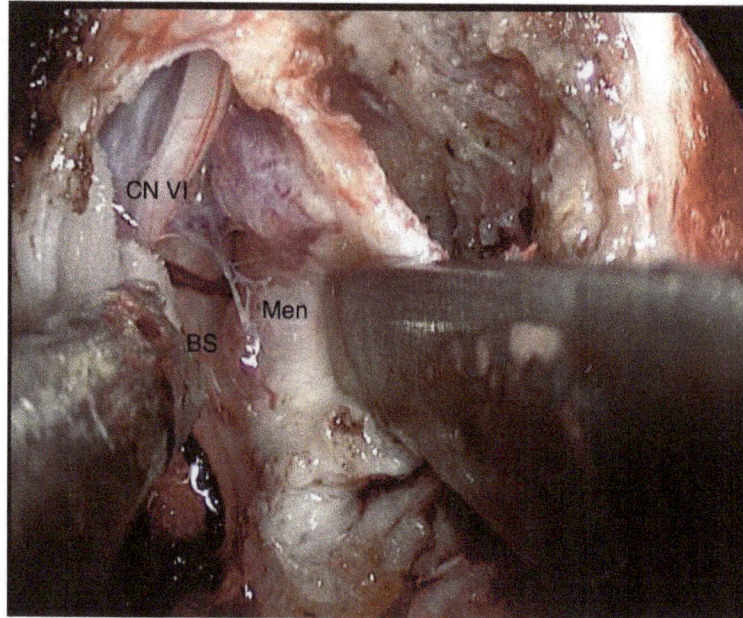

Figure 20. Endoscopic view after removal of bony clivus and incision of dura; meningioma was partially removed and retracted laterally. CN VI: abducens nerve Men: meningioma BS: brainstem

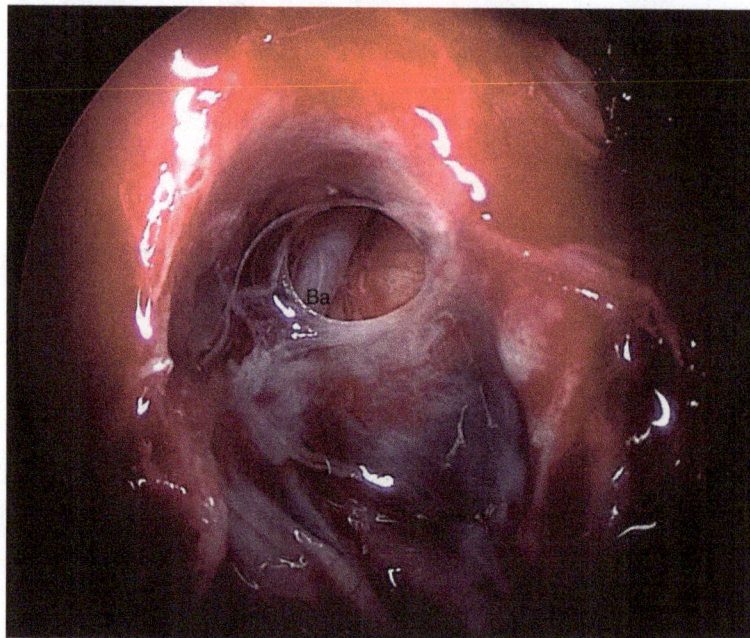

Figure 21. Endoscopic view after complete removal of tumor depicts the basilar artery lies posterior to arachnoid membrane, running vertically in front of the brainstem. Ba: basilar artery

4.1.6. Transodontoid approach

This approach allows access to foramen magnum and upper cervical spine (C1 and C2). Common diseases are pannus formation in rheumatoid arthritis and foramen magnum meningioma. This procedure is identical with transclival approach but necessitates further inferior dissection of nasopharyngeal mucosa and muscular structures. Again, the bone of anterior C1 and C2 should be thinned with high-speed drill before its removal.

4.2. Coronal view

4.2.1. Orbital approach

This approach use for tumor involve orbit, orbital roof. Start with complete endoscopic sinus surgery (middle maxillary antrostomy, complete sphenoethmoidectomy, frontal sinusotomy) and make a wide sinus cavity to ensure the orbital fat after decompression will not occlude to sinonasal drainage pathway. The lamina papyracea is elevated from periorbita like peeling an egg shell. The periorbita can be resected with sharp instrument. If the tumor is intraconal, the surgical corridor should be done between medial and inferior rectus muscle while having medial rectus retraction externally.

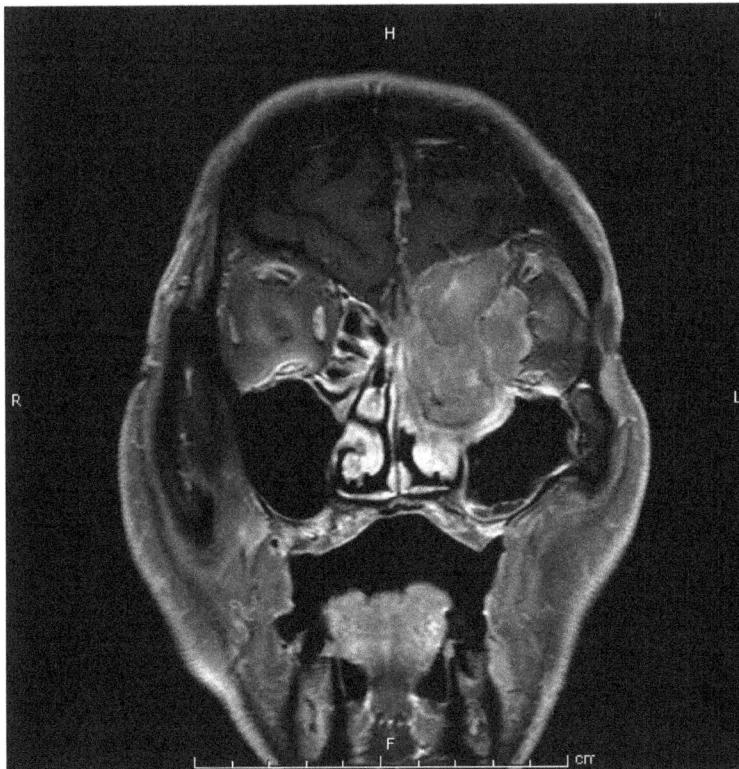

Figure 22. MRI shows tumor in left ethmoid sinus invading the left orbit.

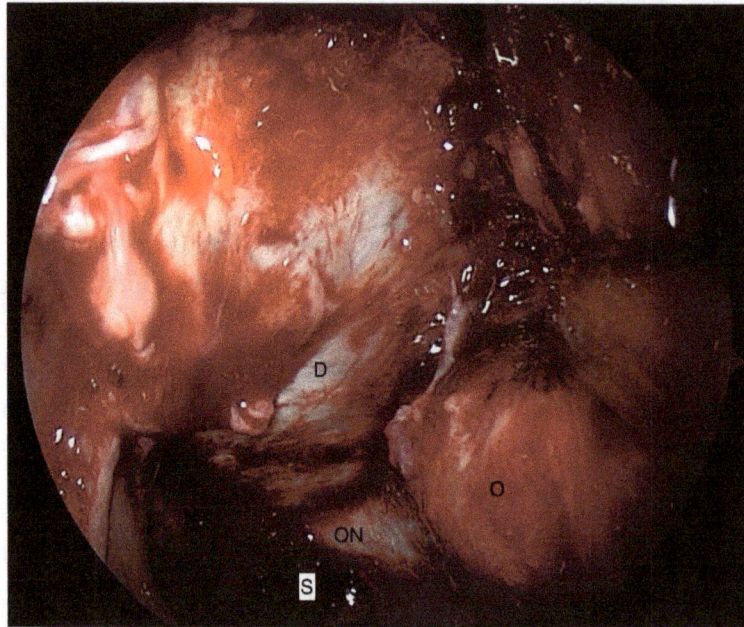

Figure 23. Endoscopic view after removal of the tumor, left cribiform plate, lamina papyracea and decompression of left optic nerve. The medial wall of orbit still bulging from the residual intraconal tumor. O: orbit D: dura ON: optic nerve S: sphenoid sinus (left)

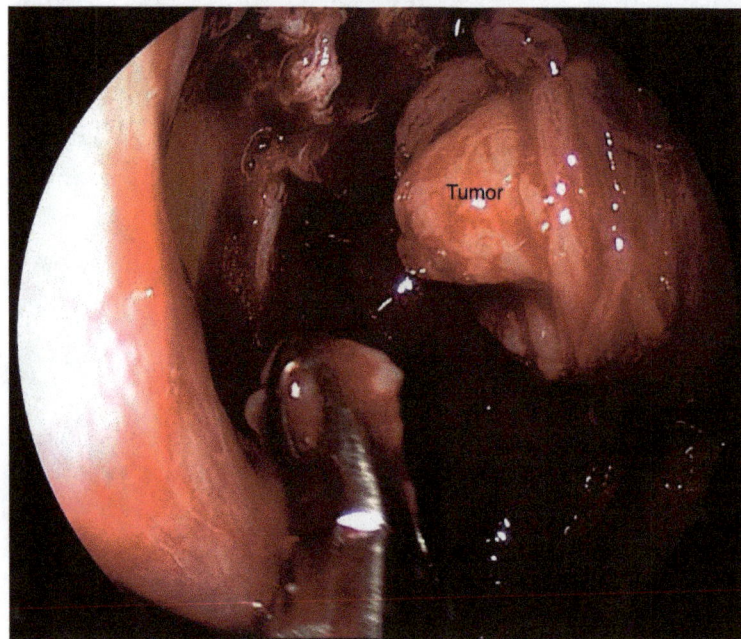

Figure 24. After incision of the periorbita, eye ball was gently compressed by assistant surgeon; the tumor will show up into the surgical field. The tumor could be removed by pushing externally and by intranasal dissection.

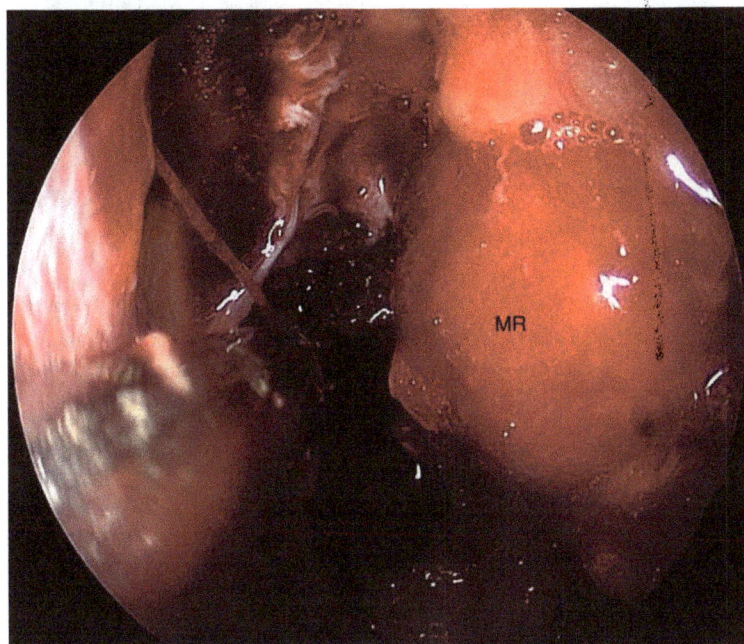

Figure 25. After total removal of the tumor, the medial rectus muscle can be clearly seen. The medial rectus muscle is retracted downward and upward for inspection with angle telescope to confirm that no tumor was left behind. MR: medial rectus muscle

4.2.2. Transpterygoid approach

This approach is utilized for access to middle cranial fossa. By removing the pterygoid bone, it can be used as a margin for tumor in sinus area, e.g., nasopharyngeal carcinoma. Other pathologies require access to the lateral recess of sphenoid such as meningoencephalocele and dural defect repair. This approach starts with maxillary antrostomy (medial maxillectomy is necessary if dissection has to be done at the lower level of inferior turbinate) and complete sphenoethmoidectomy. The sphenopalatine artery, which runs just behind ethmoidal process of palatine bone, should be cauterized or ligated (Figure 26). High-speed drill is typically necessary for removing medial and lateral pterygoid plate. The medial and lateral pterygoid muscles lie beneath the bone plate where there is rich vascular supply; hence, careful hemostasis should be employed prior to performing deeper dissection (Figure 27).

4.2.3. Infratemporal fossa approach

The location of infratemporal space is lateral to the lateral pterygoid plate. This space contains fat, internal maxillary artery, CN V2 (infraorbital nerve) and CN V3(mandibular nerve). The internal maxillary artery should be controlled with vascular clip or electrocautery. Infraorbital nerve is typically identified at the roof of posterior wall of maxillary sinus. For the mandibular nerve, it usually runs laterally to the lateral pterygoid muscle.

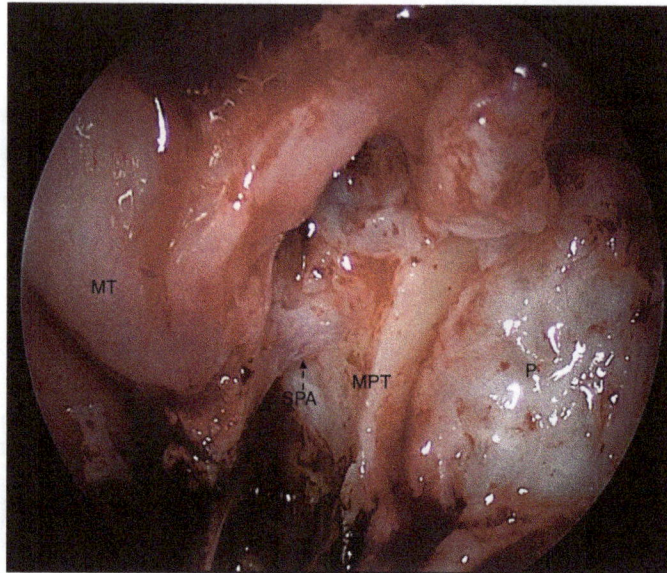

Figure 26. Endoscopic view of left nasal cavity after endoscopic sinus surgery and medial maxillectomy showing sphenopalatine artery running horizontally. MT: middle turbinate SPA: sphenopalatine artery MPT: medial pterygoid plate P: posterior wall of maxillary sinus

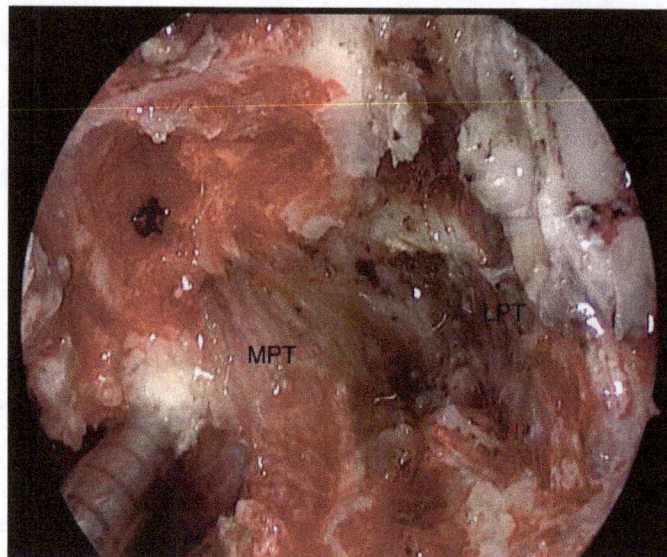

Figure 27. Endoscopic view after sphenopalatine artery is cauterized along with removal of pterygoid plate; the medial pterygoid and lateral pterygoid muscles can be identified. MPT: medial pterygoid muscle LPT: lateral pterygoid muscle

5. Reconstruction of skull base with endonasal technique

In the past, craniotomy for CSF leakage and reconstruction of skull base defect commonly utilized vascularized pericranial or fascial flap harvested from skull. In this new era of endoscopy, with external scar and need for some brain retraction, craniotomy for CSF leak repair has been preserved for those who failed endonasal endoscopic surgery. Upon access from skull base, similar to approaches with violation of dura and arachnoid membranes, CSF leak is one of the most common complications reported by many endoscopic series. However, few studies found that the incidence of CSF leakage from conventional surgery was not less frequent than endoscopic method. Among endoscopic procedures, the probability for CSF leakage is usually higher for the extrasellar lesions than limited pituitary-sellar surgery. The postresection communication between intracranial and nasal cavity must be thoroughly repaired to prevent any possibility of intracranial infection. For small defects, repair is accomplished independently of techniques for reconstruction.[15, 16] Conversely, larger defects, particularly for the high flow CSF leak, need a vascularized mucosal flap reconstruction in addition to a multilayer closure (Figure 28). It has been proven to yield better outcome with the incidence of CSF leakage < 5%.[17, 21] The advent of new technique for the intranasally harvested vascularized mucosal flap has been popularized. It has become well-known as the Hadad-Bassagasteguy flap (HBF).[22] The flap was developed from the mucoperiosteum and mucoperichondrium of the nasal septum that is supplied by the nasoseptal artery (Figures 29, 30, 31, 32, 33, 34). This reconstruction technique has improved the outcome of endonasal endoscopy for the skull base. Although the endoscopic skull base surgery via the endonasal corridor has the potential contamination from the sinonasal tract, the incidence of intracranial infections is still relatively low. The common intracranial infections are meningitis and intracranial abscess that have been reported in various incidences among the endoscopic series from less than 1% up to 10%,[23, 27] while the traditional approaches had the higher incidences from 15–30%.[28, 29] The intracranial infections were associated with the intradural resection, and some studies stated that they were related to the refractory postoperative CSF leak. Perioperative antibiotic prophylaxis is recommended to prevent the intracranial infections.

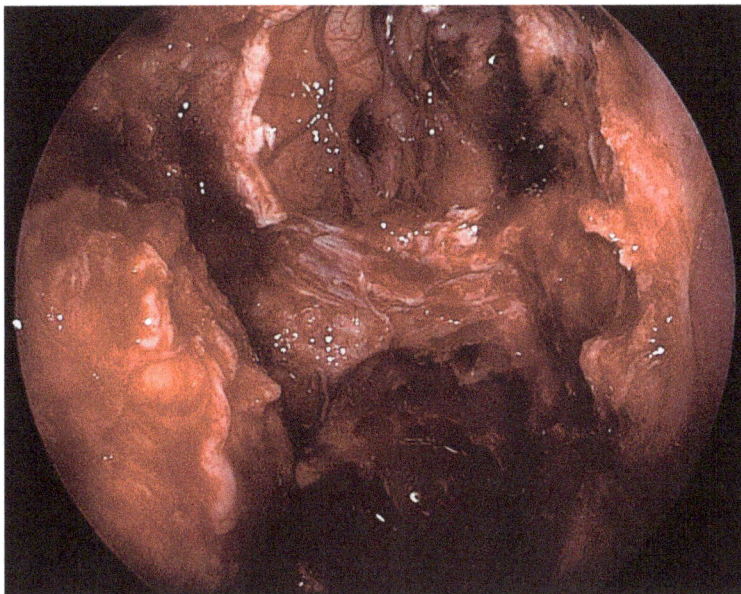

Figure 28. Endoscopic view of cribiform defect in pediatric patient after resection of fibro-osseous lesion.

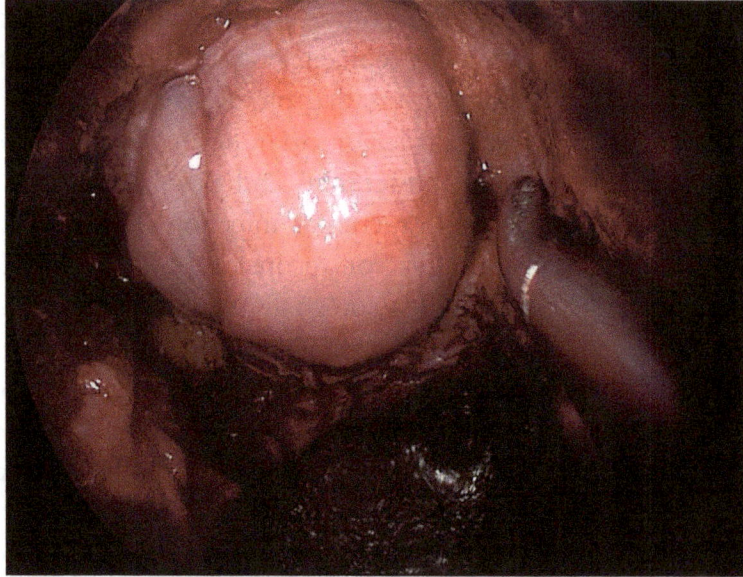

Figure 29. Endoscopic view of the same patient in Figure 28. The defect was reconstructed with multiple layers (fat graft and two layers of fascia lata).

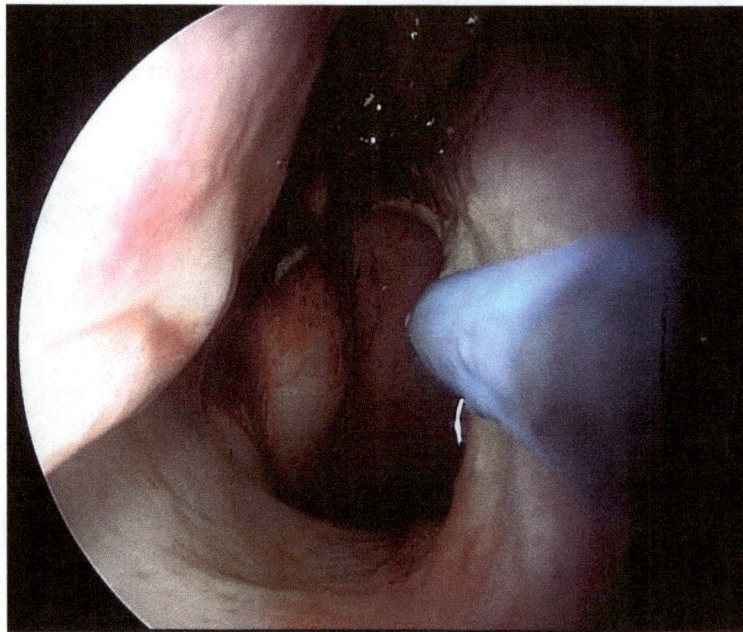

Figure 30. Endoscopic view, inferior incision for creation of nasoseptal flap is illustrated. This inferior incision typically starts at the roof of nasopharynx then advances anteriorly to mucocutaneous junction of nasal septum. Superior incision (not pictured) ideally starts at inferior level of sphenoid natural ostium and moves anteriorly to mucocutaneous junction of nasal septum.

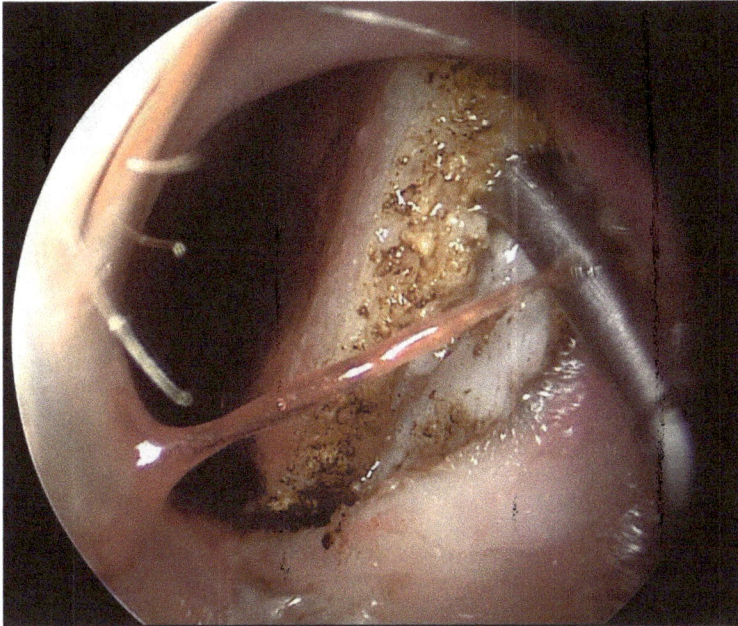

Figure 31. Endoscopic view of same patient in Figure 30. The superior and inferior incision will be connected by a vertical incision at mucocutaneous junction. Submucoperichondrium dissection should proceed from anterior to posterior toward its pedicle at the nasopharynx.

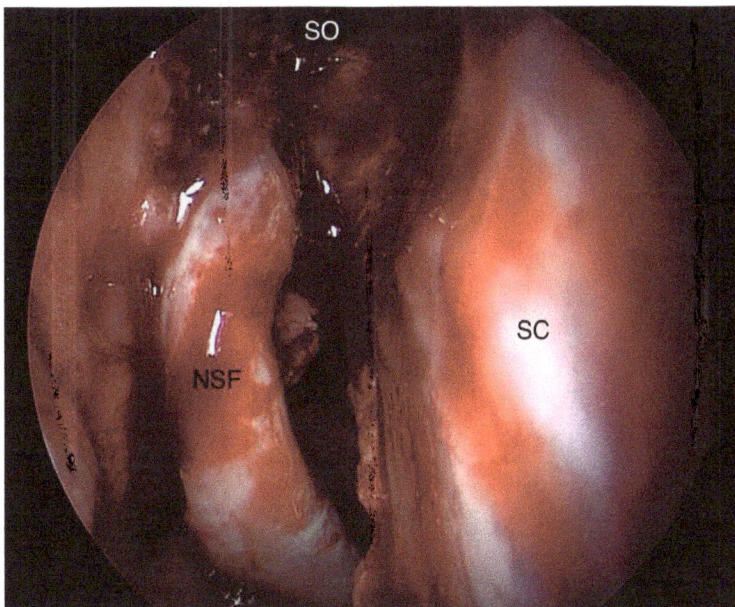

Figure 32. Endoscopic view of same patient in Figure 30. After elevation of nasoseptal flap, the pedicle is protected at posterior to preserve arterial supply by septal branch of sphenopalatine artery. NSF: nasoseptal flap SC: septal cartilage SO: sphenoid ostium

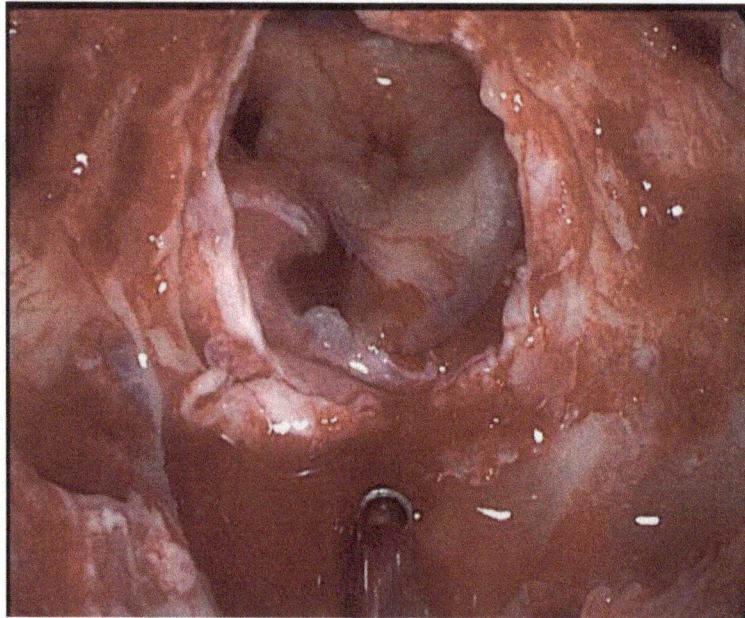

Figure 33. Endoscopic view of same patient in Figure 30 demonstrates the large skull base defect at sellar and planum after craniopharyngioma removal.

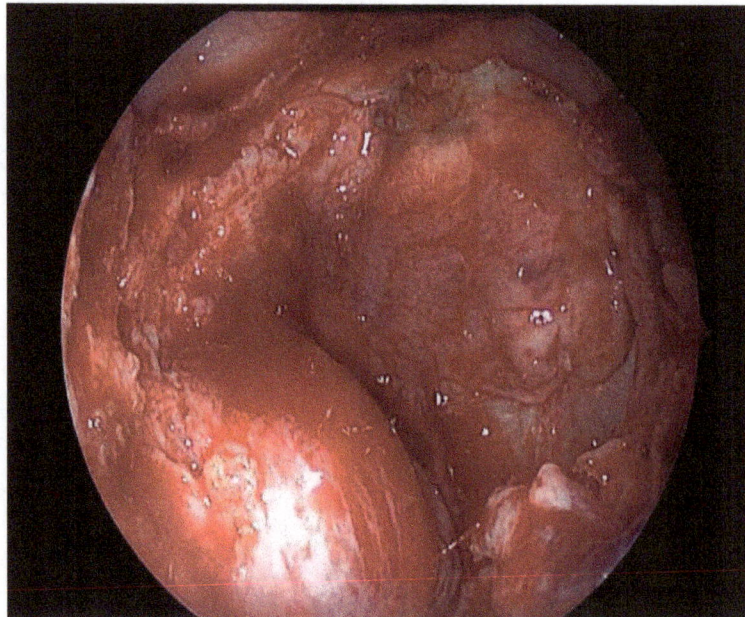

Figure 34. Endoscopic view of same patient in Figure 30. The nasoseptal flap was placed over the defect area after inlay placement of fat.

6. Surgical complications and morbidities

As mentioned earlier, although endoscopic skull base surgery creates direct communication between intracranial and nasal compartment, the incidence of intracranial infections is relatively low. Reports of the postoperative incidence of intracranial infection varied from less than 1% up to 10%.[23, 27]

Vascular injury during endoscopic procedures can be catastrophic, in particular when it involves the ICA. The ventral perspective of ICA that is perceived via endoscopic view is less familiar to surgeons than transcranial procedures. Higher rate of the ICA injury was more commonly associated with paramedian coronal plane dissection. Complete understanding of the ICA pathway and its surgical landmarks together with advanced intraoperative image-guided technology can minimize this feared intraoperative vascular complication. Fortunately, major ICA injury is uncommon with overall incidence of 0.9%. Experienced surgeons with multidisciplinary team approach as well as efficient instruments must be prepared to promptly deal with this critical event.[27] Though the ideal concept for management of an injured artery is to maintain lumen patency of the vessel, it is, unfortunately, extremely difficult to achieve in real situation. Direct repair with suture is close to impossible given the narrow corridor in light of profuse hemorrhage. Although several hemostatic agents or patches have varying success in damage control, at least temporarily, from our experience, crushed muscle has been the best. When all attempts fail, nasal packing is performed. Subsequently, angiographic study of the ICA is necessary. In some, balloon occlusion test is advocated in the preoperative plan in selected patients who carry high risk of vascular complications. Previous surgery or irradiation as well as tumor encasing ICA have been found to be factors predicting arterial injury.

Intraoperative neural injury from endoscopic series has been reported, with lower incidence than the traditional techniques. In addition, its majority was transient. The most commonly injured nerve was the CN VI. This could be related to its poor tolerance for manipulation.[27] Electromyographic cranial nerve monitoring during the surgery can signal surgeons of proximity to cranial nerves while dissecting a lesion. Dissection beyond the lateral limit of given cranial nerves is principally contraindicated for the endoscopic approach. Therefore, combined approaches from traditional craniotomy may occasionally be required for an extensive pathology.

The lower rate of overall complications from endonasal endoscopic approach seems more encouraging than the traditional techniques. Nevertheless, specialized training to gain experiences in this complex anatomical area along with advanced technological equipment is essential to surgeons to overcome obstacles in the course of his/her learning curve. With increased experience after several cases, the incidences of complication should typically approach acceptable reported incidence.

Over the past few decades, many authors have reported the feasibility and safety in the clinical uses of pure endoscopy in treatment of skull base pathologies. Understandably, with shorter follow-up time, endoscopic endonasal surgery cannot perfectly prove its efficacy, namely the long-term oncological control and functional outcome that has been its common target for criticism.

The general principle to achieve the oncological control is the complete resection of the tumor. The malignant pathologies, the surgical margins need to be extended. Via endoscopic approach, the en bloc tumor removal at the invasion site has been considered more fundamental than the en bloc resection of the entire tumor. The intraoperative frozen section is a tool to confirm the surgical margin after the en bloc resection at the tumor invasion site. The tumors arising in the sinonasal cavities usually have some parts situated in the air-filled space. The floating tumors in the cavities can be debulked in order to allow the surgeons comfortably insert the surgical instruments through the limited space and gain access to manage the tumors. At present, there is limited data to evaluate the oncological recurrence and disease-free survival rate. Many authors reported a small number of patients in the series of endonasal endoscopic surgery for skull base lesions for whom the oncological outcomes were favorable and comparable to the open techniques with lesser morbidities.[30, 33]

Although most of the surgeons have been experienced with the excellent functional outcomes and quality of life of the patients who underwent the endonasal endoscopic surgery, the published data has been limited. The obviously favorable outcomes include faster recovery without external scar and that the patients can regain normal or near-normal functions. The endonasal endoscopic skull base surgery has many steps of operation that can affect the patient's life in different ways. The further subanalysis of quality of life in each aspect of the procedure can lead to development of the completed data in the endoscopic surgical field.

7. Conclusion

Endoscopic endonasal surgery is challenging and dynamic. Coupling between the adjustments of the endoscopic lens position to acquire optimal view and the movement of instruments to provide the surgical freedom in the limited space requires tremendous experience and teamwork. It delivers enormous advantages for the various skull base pathologies which surgical corridor provides the most direct access to the ventral cranial base area. Proper selection of patients for endoscopic approach is crucial to achieve good outcome while avoiding untoward events. Comprehensive knowledge in complex skull base anatomy, training in advanced and high-volume institutes, advanced surgical technologies and strong teamwork are the keystones to gain the most benefit from this surgical method.

Author details

Boonsam Roongpuvapaht[1*], Kangsadarn Tanjararak[1] and Ake Hansasuta[2]

*Address all correspondence to: boonsamr@yahoo.com

1 Department of Otolaryngology Head and Neck Surgery, Ramathibodi Hospital, Faculty of Medicine, Mahidol University, Thailand

2 Division of Neurosurgery, Department of Surgery, Ramathibodi Hospital, Faculty of Medicine, Mahidol University, Thailand

References

[1] Messerklinger W: Diagnosis and endoscopic surgery of the nose and its adjoining structures. Acta Otorhinolaryngol Belg 1980;34:170–176.

[2] Wigand ME: Transnasal ethmoidectomy under endoscopical control. Rhinology 1981;19:7–15.

[3] Kennedy DW: Functional endoscopic sinus surgery: technique. Arch Otolaryngol 1985;111:643–649.

[4] Stammberger H: Endoscopic endonasal surgery – concepts in treatment of recurring rhinosinusitis. I. Anatomic and pathophysiologic considerations. Otolaryngol Head Neck Surg 1986;94:143–147.

[5] Stammberger H: Endoscopic endonasal surgery – concepts in treatment of recurring rhinosinusitis. II. Surgical technique. Otolaryngol Head Neck Surg 1986;94:147– 156.

[6] Stammberger H, Posawetz W: Functional endo- scopic sinus surgery: concept, indications and results of the Messerklinger technique. Eur Arch Otorhinolaryngol 1990;247:63–76.

[7] Duffner F, Freudenstein D, Wacker A, Straub Duffner S, Grote EH: 75 years after Dandy, Fay and Mixter – looking back on the history of neuroendoscopy. Zentralbl Neurochir 1998;59:121–128.

[8] Harris LW: Endoscopic techniques in neurosurgery. Microsurgery 1994;15:541–546.

[9] Carrau RL, Jho HD, Ko Y: Transnasal-transsphenoidal endoscopic surgery of the pituitary gland. Laryngoscope 1996;106:914–918.

[10] Jho HD, Carrau RL: Endoscopy assisted transsphenoidal surgery for pituitary adenoma: technical note. Acta Neurochir (Wien) 1996;138:1416–1425.

[11] Jho HD, Carrau RL, Ko Y, Daly MA: Endoscopic pituitary surgery: an early experience. Surg Neurol 1997;47:213–222; discussion 222–223.

[12] Kassam AB, Snyderman CH, Mintz A, Gardner P, Carrau RL: Expanded endonasal approach: the rostrocaudal axis. Part I. Crista galli to the sella turcica. Neurosurg Focus 2005;19:E3.

[13] Kassam AB, Snyderman CH, Mintz A, Gardner P, Carrau RL: Expanded endonasal approach: the rostrocaudal axis. Part II. Posterior clinoids to the foramen magnum. Neurosurg Focus 2005;19(1):E4.

[14] Kassam AB, Gardner P, Snyderman CH, Mintz A, Carrau RL: Expanded endonasal

[15] approach: fully endoscopic, completely transnasal approach to the middle third of

[16] the clivus, petrous bone, middle cranial fossa, and infratenporal fossa. Neurosurg Focus 2005;19(1):E6.

[17] Hegazy HM, Carrau RL, Snyderman CH, Kassam AB, Zweig J: Transnasal endoscopic repair of

[18] cerebrospinal fluid rhinorrhea: a meta-analysis. Laryngoscope 2000;110(7): 1166–1172.

[19] Senior BA, Jafri K, Benninger M: Safety and efficacy of endoscopic repair of CSF leaks and encephaloceles: a survey of the members of the American Rhinologic Society. Am J Rhinol 2001;15(1):21–25.

[20] Kassam AB, Thomas A, Carrau RL, Snyderman CH, Vescan A, Prevedello D, et al.: Endoscopic reconstruction of the cranial base using a pedicled nasoseptal flap. Neurosurgery 2008; 63(1 suppl 1):ONS44–ONS53.

[21] Zanation AM, Carrau RL, Snyderman CH, Germanwala AV, Gardner PA, Prevedello DM, et al.: Nasoseptal flap reconstruction of high flow intraoperative cerebral spinal fluid leaks during endoscopic skull base surgery. American Journal of Rhinology & Allergy 2009;23(5):518–521.

[22] Shah RN, Surowitz JB, Patel MR, Huang BY, Snyderman CH, Carrau RL, et al.: Endoscopic pedicled nasoseptal flap reconstruction for paediatric skull base defects. Laryngoscope 2009;119(6):1067–1075.

[23] El Sayed IH, Roediger FC, Goldberg AN, Parsa AT, McDermott MW: Endoscopic reconstruction of skull base defects with the nasal septal flap. Skull Base: An Interdisciplinary Approach 2008;18(6):385–394.

[24] Harvey RJ, Nogueira JF, Schlosser RJ, Patel SJ, Vellutini E, Stamm AC: Closure of large skull base defects after endoscopic transnasal craniotomy. Clinical article. Journal of Neurosurgery 2009;111(2):371–379.

[25] Hadad G, Bassagasteguy L, Carrau RL, Mataza JC, Kassam A, Snyderman CH, et al.: A novel reconstructive technique after endoscopic expanded endonasal approaches: vascular pedicle nasoseptal flap. Laryngoscope 2006;116:1882–1886.

[26] Cappabianca P, Cavallo LM, Colao A, De Divitiis E: Surgical complications associated with the endoscopic endonasal transsphenoidal approach for pituitary adenomas. J Neuro- surg 2002; 97:293–298.

[27] Dehdashti AR, Ganna A, Karabatsou K, Gentili F: Pure endoscopic endonasal approach for pituitary adenomas: early surgical results in 200 patients and comparison with previous microsurgical series. Neurosurgery 2008; 62:1006–1017.

[28] Frank G, Pasquini E, Doglietto F, Mazzatenta D, Sciarretta V, Farneti G, et al.: The endoscopic extended transsphenoidal approach for craniopharyngiomas. Neurosurgery 2006; 59 (1 Suppl 1):ONS75–ONS83.

[29] Frank G, Sciarretta V, Calbucci F, Farneti G, Mazzatenta D, Pasquini E: The endoscopic transnasal transsphenoidal approach for the treatment of cranial base chordomas and chondrosarcomas. Neurosurgery 2006; 59 (1 Suppl 1): ONS50–ONS57.

[30] Kassam AB, Preveldello DM, Carrau RL, et al.: Endoscopic endonasal skull base surgery: analysis of complications in the authors' initial 800 patients. J Neurosurg

[31] 2011;114:1544–1568.

[32] Sen C, Triana A: Cranial chordomas: results of radical excision. Neurosurg Focus 2001;10(3):E3.

[33] Feiz-ErfanI, Han PP, Spetzler RF, Horn EM, Klopfenstein JD, Porter RW, et al.: The radical transbasal approach for resection of anterior and midline skull base lesions. J Neurosurg 2005;103:485–490.

[34] Stammberger H, Anderhuber W, Walch C, et al.: Possibilities and limitations of endoscopic management of nasal and paranasal sinus malignancies. Acta Otorhinolaryngol Belg 1999;53:199– 205.

[35] Casiano RR, Numa WA, Falquez AM: Endoscopic resection of esthesioneuroblastoma. Am J Rhinol 2001;15:271.

[36] Castelnuovo PG, Delu G, Sberze F, et al.: Esthesioneuroblastoma: Endonasal endoscopic treatment. Skull Base 2006;16:25–230.

[37] Snyderman CH, Carrau RL, Kassam AB, et al.: Endoscopic skull base surgery: principles of endonasal oncological surgery. Journal of Surgical Oncology 2008;97:658–664.

8

New Frontiers in Managing Clival Tumors —
The Extended Endoscopic Endonasal Approach

G. Cossu, R.T. Daniel, M. George, F. Parker,
N. Aghakhani, M. Levivier and M. Messerer

Abstract

Clival lesions still represent a challenge for neurosurgeons. A variety of expansive process, either benign or malignant, may be identified in the clival and paraclival region.

Surgery of this region with classical open approaches is associated with a significant rate of complication, and the treatment is risky despite technological progress. The acceptance and utilization of endoscopic techniques on a regular basis in transsphenoidal surgery have allowed its application to regions far beyond the *sella turcica*, such as to reach the clival and paraclival region.

Long-term follow-up studies show how the extent of oncological resection is related to long-term prognosis for the most common clival malignancies. Gross total removal is therefore mandatory, and the selection of the best surgical approach is essential for the achievement of this goal.

The choice of the surgical approach depends on the location and the extent of the lesion. Through a complete overview of surgical anatomy, we propose a surgical classification with three corridors in the sagittal plane and three zones in the coronal plane. We finally summarize the indications and the limits for the endoscopic technique. In selected cases, endoscopic approaches allow similar oncological outcomes as classical open approaches with a lower rate of complications.

Keywords: Clival tumors, Clival chordoma, Clival chondrosarcoma, Meningioma, Extended endoscopic endonasal approach, Skull base surgery

1. Introduction

The clival region may be involved in a copious number of disorders. The most common clival lesions are chordomas, but meningiomas, chondroma and chondrosarcoma may also occur. Furthermore, the clivus may be secondarily invaded by a variety of metastatic malignancies. A radical excision is related to long-term prognosis and survival and a gross total resection is the *primum movens* of every surgical procedure when judged possible. The deep location and the presence of important neurovascular structures make of the clivus a challenging working area. Surgery of this region through classical open approaches implies neurovascular and cerebral retraction with a significant rate of neurological morbidities. Neurosurgeons have thus progressively searched for innovative ways to reach the clival region and to limit the complication rate.

Endoscopy started to be used as a diagnostic tool [1, 2] and then developed as a therapeutic option for sellar lesions [3, 4]. During the last decades, endoscopic techniques were applied to the skull base with encouraging results in terms of surgical resection and rate of complications [5]. Clear advantages of endoscopic surgery are principally a limited retraction on neurovascular structures with a concomitant wide vision and large exposure. Furthermore, patients have no external marks, and the length of hospitalization is normally shorter than with open procedures.

According to their location and extension, clival tumors may be reached through an anterior approach, as extended subfrontal, Le Fort I, transoral approach or maxillotomy, or through a lateral approach as the transpterygoid or infratemporal craniotomy or as the transpetrosal or far lateral approach. The endoscopic technique may represent a valid alternative to these open approaches, and the aim of this chapter is to expose the expanded endoscopic approach as first-line treatment in well-selected patients.

2. Preoperative evaluation

A satisfying preoperative evaluation implies T1 and T2-weighted MRI sequences, with and without gadolinium administration, to evaluate the extent and the precise localization of the lesion in the axial, coronal and sagittal plane. A high-resolution skull base CT scan with bone windows will help to plane the surgical approach and to evaluate bone invasion and osseous pneumatization. A CT angiography will then help to characterize vessels' characteristics, in particular of the ICA, and their reciprocal relationship with the lesion, thus defining the extent of resection. A 3D-scannographic reconstruction may better help understanding the real surgical anatomy of the ventral skull base, with a particular concern for the location of foramen lacerum and vidian canal. Patients should also have an ENT evaluation with a specialized neuro-otological examination and undergo a preoperative endonasal endoscopy to plan the access for the surgery.

3. Surgical procedure

3.1. Surgical anatomy and classification of the surgical approach

The clivus separates the nasopharynx from the posterior cranial fossa and a natural access is possible through the nasal cavities.

From a purely anatomical point of view, the clivus is traditionally divided into basisphenoid (sphenoid body) and basiocciput (basilar part of the occipital bone) (Figure 1).

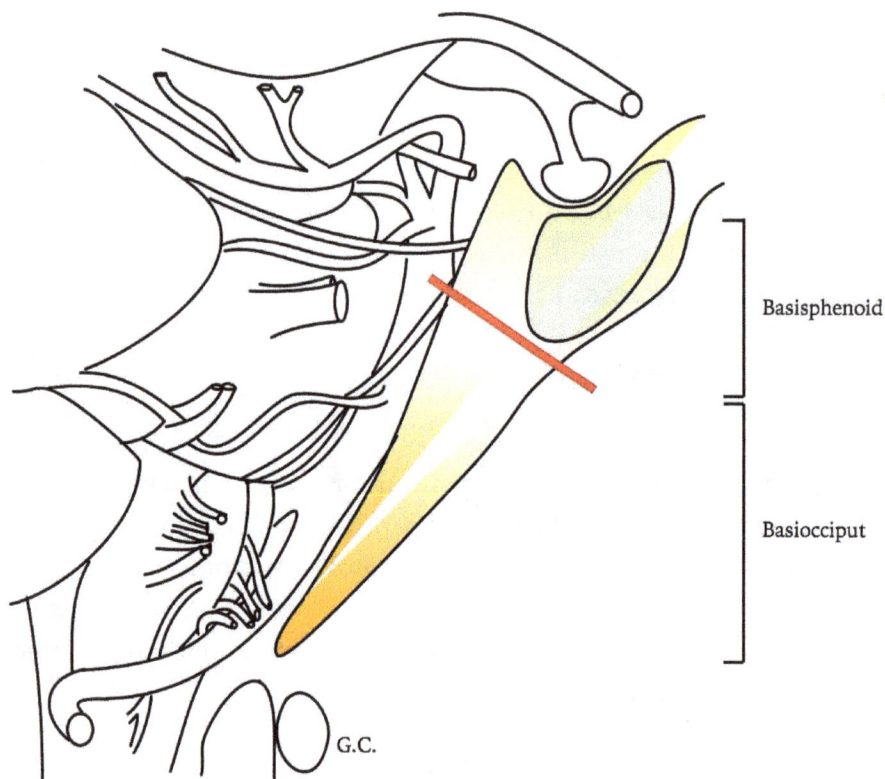

Figure 1. Anatomical classification of the clivus, which is divided into basisphenoid and basiocciput. Classically the sphenoid body forms the basisphenoid while the basiocciput belongs to the occipital bone.

From a surgical point of view, the clivus has classically been divided into [6] (Figure 2):

- an upper clivus extending from the dorsum sellae to the plane of Dorello canal;

- a middle clivus extending from the Dorello canal to the pars nervosa of the jugular foramen;

- a lower clivus extending from the pars nervosa of the jugular foramen to the foramen magnum.

The choice of the surgical approach depends on the location and extension of the lesion, which are the principal determinants for the extent of bone removal. The relationship between the lesion and the pneumatization of the sphenoidal sinus represents the basis of our surgical classification proposed here.

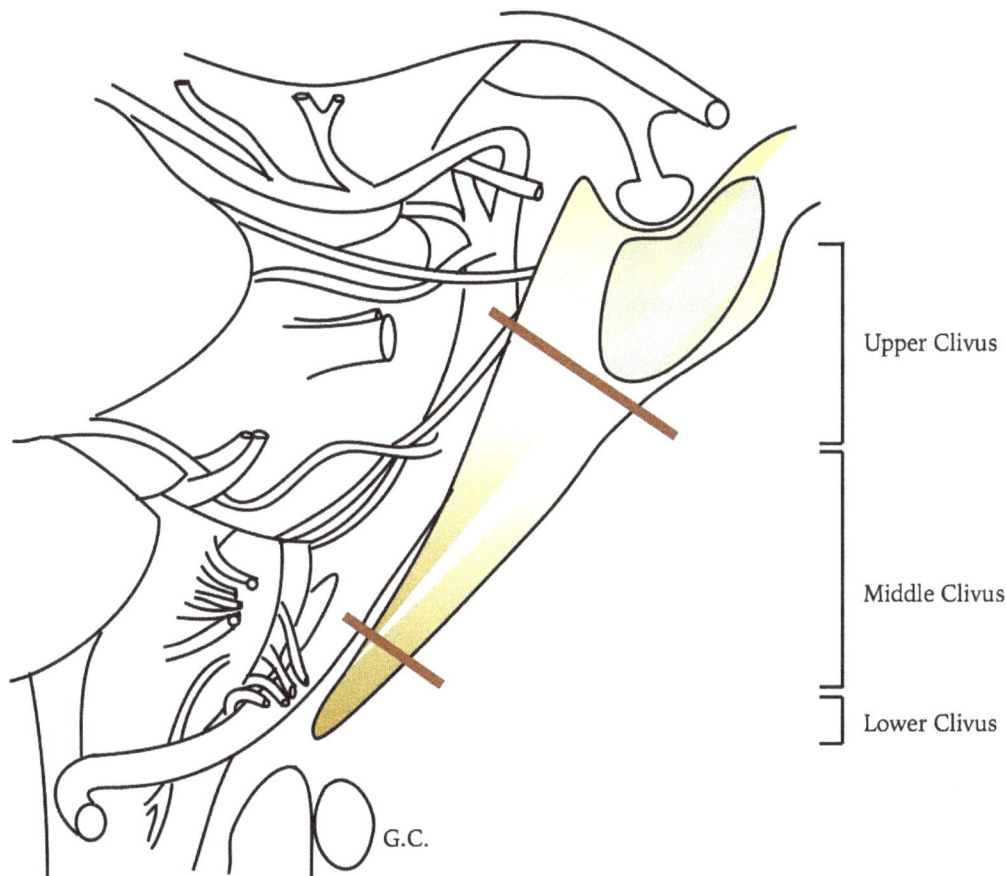

Figure 2. Surgical classification of the clivus. The upper third extends from the dorsum sellae to the Dorello canal. The middle third extends inferiorly till the jugular foramen, while the inferior third extends to the foramen magnum.

Three corridors may be identified in the sagittal plane, separated by two lines (Figure 3). The superior line joins the nostril with the sellar floor, while the inferior line joins the nostril with the inferior wall of the sphenoidal sinus. The superior line separates the trans-sellar corridor, used for lesions of the anterior cranial base and extending till the posterior clinoid process, and the sphenoidal corridor, where the natural pneumatization allows a direct access to the sellar and retrosellar region without the necessity to transpose the pituitary gland as in the trans-sellar corridor [7] (Figure 4). In front of a well-pneumatized sphenoid sinus, the sphenoidal corridor gives an excellent access to mid-clival lesions. The inferior line separates the sphenoidal corridor from the infra-sphenoidal corridor, used to access to the lower part of the clivus after the lateralization of the *longus capitis* and *longus colli* muscles. The identification of the foramen magnum and hypoglossal canals is fundamental to safely use this corridor. A different inclination of the endoscope in the sagittal plane combined with a more or less pronounced flexion or extension of the head of the patient allows direct access to one of the three corridors.

According to our endoscopic conception, three zones are also identified in the coronal plane: the median, paramedian and lateral zone (Figure 5). The medial line, extending from the medial wall of the cavernous sinus to the medial border of the foramen lacerum, separates the median from the paramedian zone. The lateral line, extending from the lateral wall of the

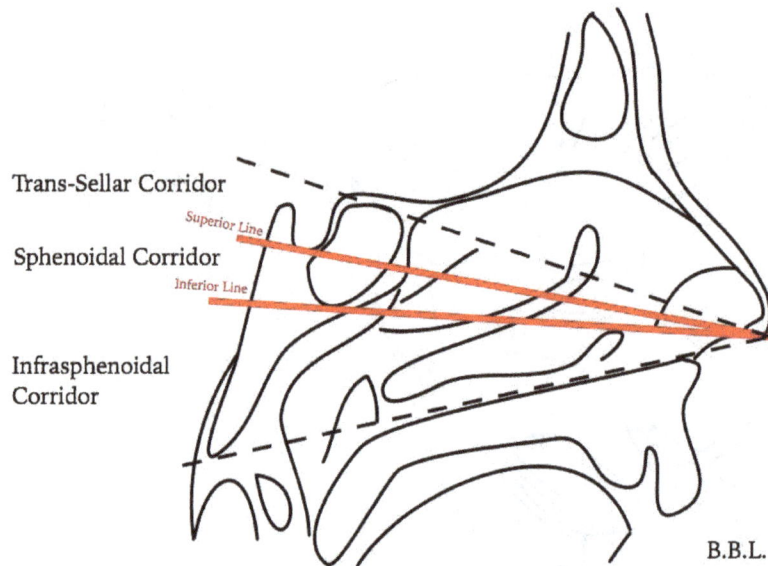

Figure 3. Sagittal view showing the three surgical corridors: the trans-sellar, the sphenoidal and the infra-sphenoidal corridors. The corridor must be chosen on the basis of the location of the lesion. Head flexion and the use of angulated endoscope may help in performing the procedure.

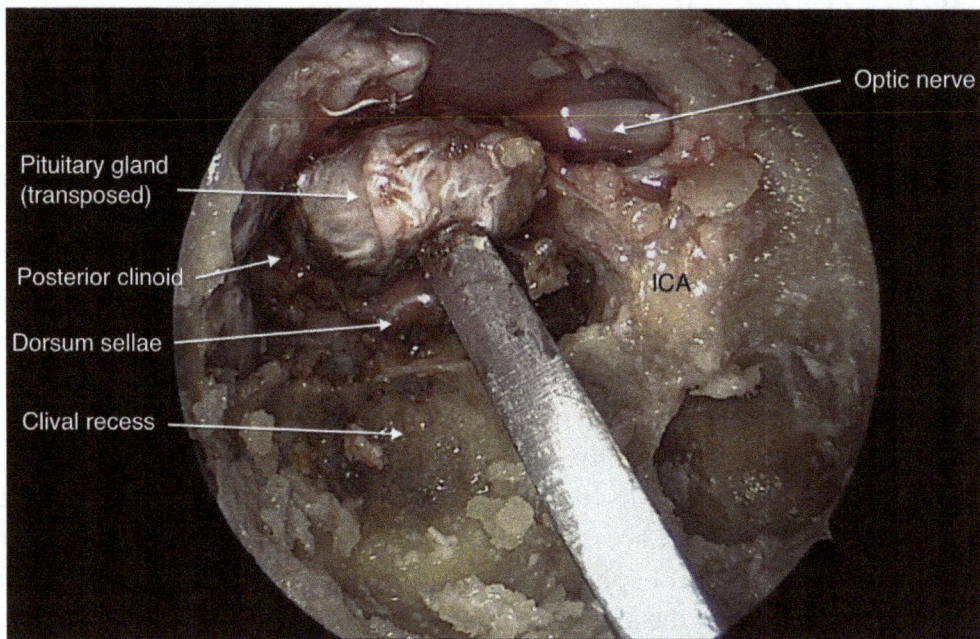

Figure 4. Cadaveric view of a trans-sellar corridor. The pituitary is transposed to drill out the posterior clinoids and the dorsum sellae. The posterior ethmoidal cells are also opened and the left optic nerve is here exposed.

cavernous sinus to the lateral edge of the foramen lacerum, separates the paramedian zone from the lateral zone.

To work safely in the paramedian zone, the identification of the vidian nerve and of the ICA is fundamental [8]. Lesions limited to the median and paramedian zones may be completely excised through an endoscopic approach, while for lesions extending to the lateral zone a pterygoid or infratemporal craniotomy may be preferred or combined with endoscopy.

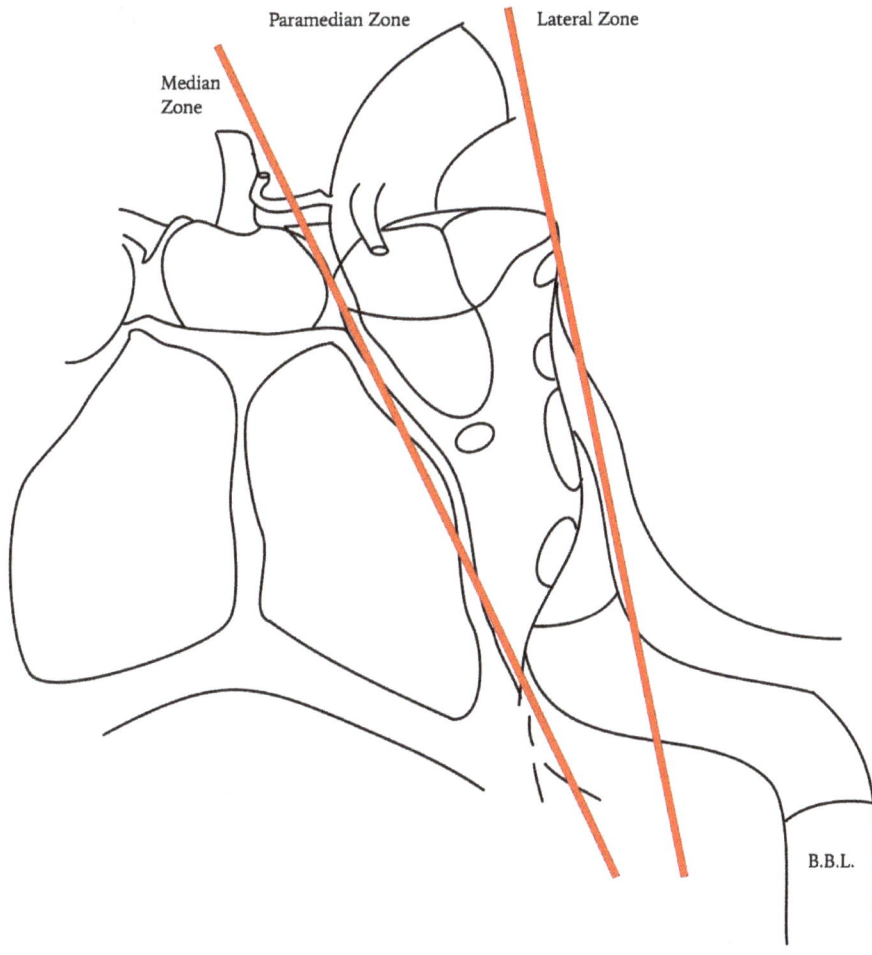

Figure 5. Coronal representation of the three coronal zones. The cavernous sinus and the foramen lacerum represent two important landmarks. A lesion situated solely in the median or paramedian zone may be completely resected through an endoscopic approach. For lesions extending to the lateral zone a combined approach must be considered.

3.2. Operative technique

In most centers, an interdisciplinary team consisting of a neurosurgeon and an otolaryngologist performs the surgery. The patient is positioned supine with the head elevated of 30° and slightly hyperextended. A general anesthesia is performed with an orotracheal intubation. As nerves retraction represent one of the main risk, intraoperative neuromonitoring is performed, allowing direct monitoring of cranial nerve function. Direct stimulation through a monopolar device is commonly used, with a frequency of 1Hz, a monophasic negative 200 μs duration and a 1 to 5 mA intensity stimulation. Eyeball movements are thus monitored through electrodes capturing the displacement of the retina dipole to evaluate the integrity of oculomotor, trochlear and abducens nerves. The frontalis, orbicularis oculi, orbicularis ori and mentalis muscles are evaluated to monitor the functionality of the facial nerve. Electrodes incorporated in the endotracheal tube (Xomed®) are used for glossopharyngeal and vagus nerves while electrodes in trapezius and hypoglossal muscles are used to monitor accessory-spinal and hypoglossal nerves respectively. Somatosensory evoked potentials and brain stem auditory potentials are also used as complement for brainstem function assessment.

Some centers guide their extent of resection with a neuronavigation system and a Doppler ultrasonography to better visualize adjacent vascular structures as the sphenopalatine artery, the ICA and the basilar artery.

A binostral approach is used according to the four-hand technique *(Figure 6)*. The procedure is performed with a hand-held short 0°, 30° or 45° endoscope till the sellar floor opening. The endoscope is classically first introduced from the right nostril unless the preoperative endo-nasal evaluation showed a preferential way in the left nostril. The endoscope is oriented slightly rostrally to better visualize the clivus and normally handled in the nostril contralateral to the lesion during the operative procedure.

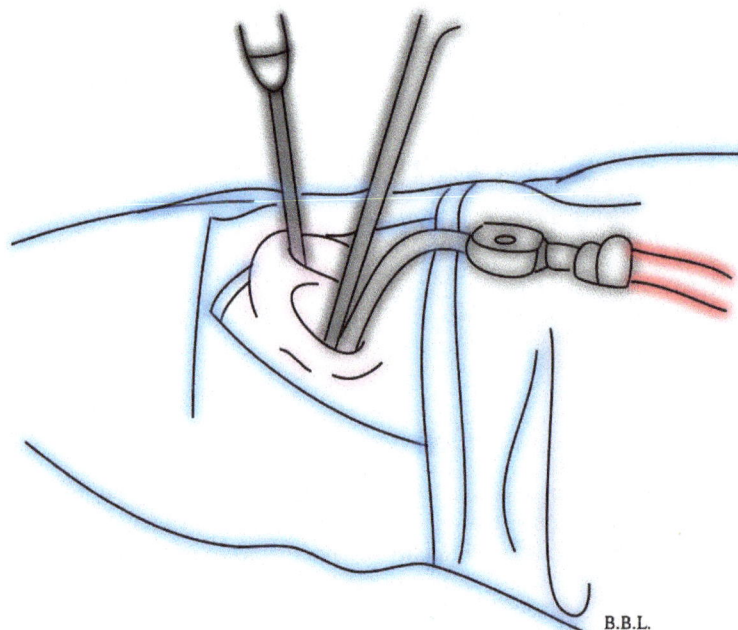

Figure 6. Representation of the *four-hand technique*. The endoscopic is kept by the operative aid in the nostril contrala-teral to the lesion, while the surgeon freely operates with both hands in the other nostril. This technique implies the presence of two well-trained operators and a strong collaboration between the two surgeons.

Through the endonasal approach, the inferior turbinate is encountered first, then the medial and the superior one, which may be resected or just retracted (Figure 7). To obtain a wider surgical corridor, a resection of the middle and superior turbinates is preferred for extended endoscopic approaches [9, 10, 11, 12, 13] (Figure 8 and 9). Turbinectomies allows also a better visualization of branches of the sphenopalatine arteries, important to preserve for the closure stage.

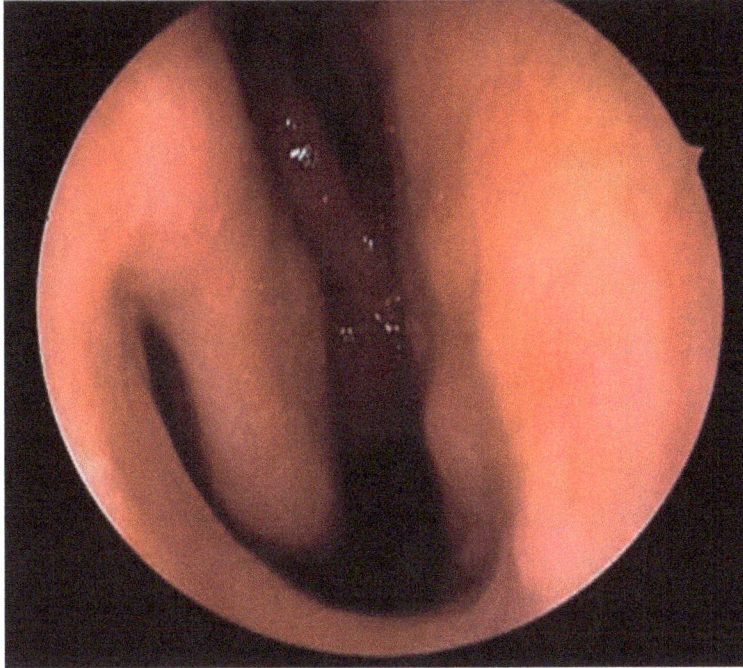

Figure 7. *In vivo* visualisation of the right nasal cavity through a 0° endoscope. At the beginning of the endonasal approach the inferior turbinate is first visualized (left). More deeply the middle turbinate is identified and laterally displaced or resected to gain a wider access to the clival region.

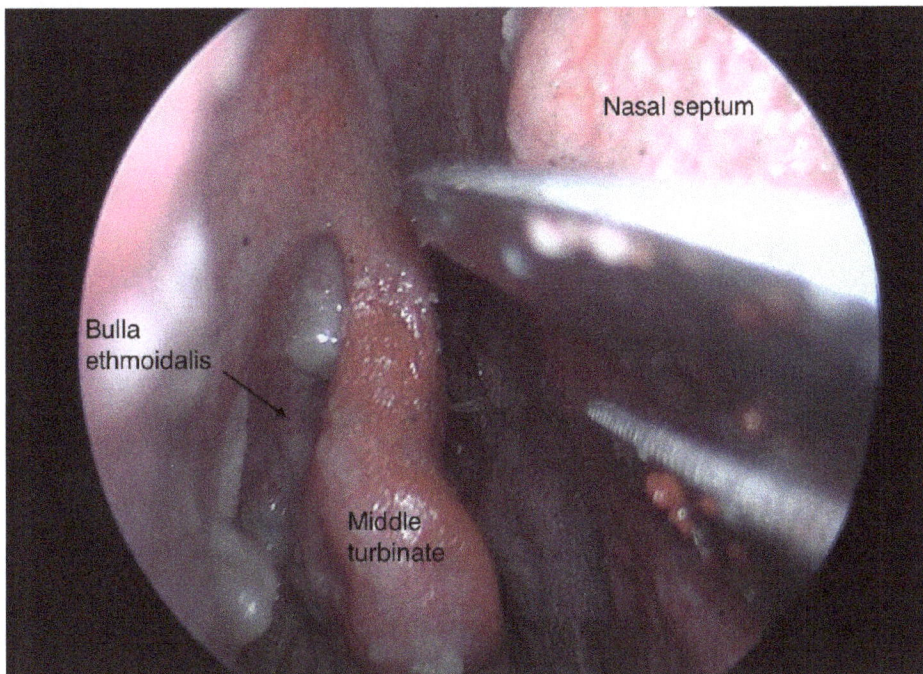

Figure 8. Cadaveric view of the right nasal fossa. The middle turbinate is visualized as well as the bulla ethmoidalis in the lateral wall of the nasal cavity.

The coanes and the inferior wall of the sphenoid sinus are identified.

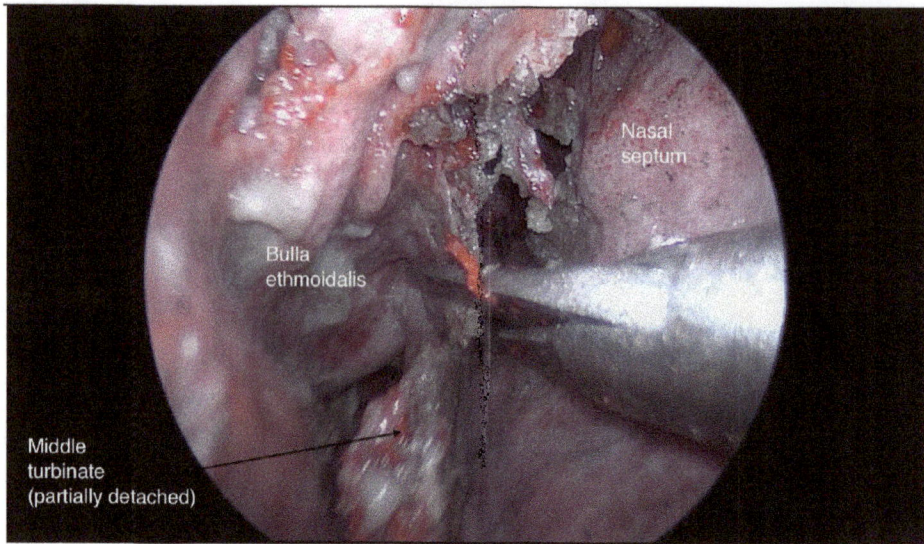

Figure 9. A middle turbinectomy is performed in a cadaveric specimen. A wider endonasal access is thus obtained for more extended approaches. The middle turbinate may then be used during the closure stage.

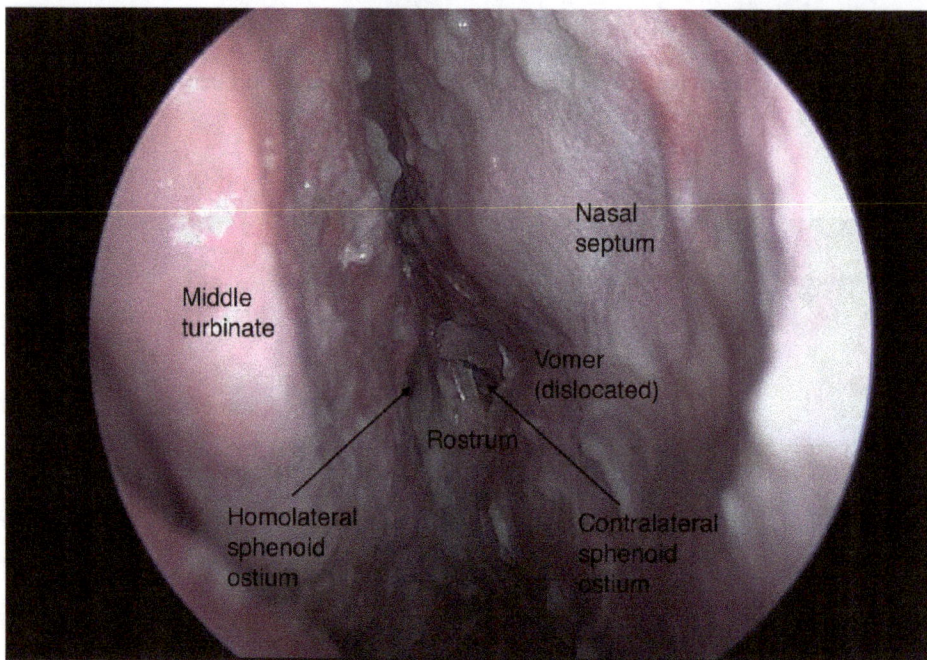

Figure 10. Cadaveric view showing sphenoid rostrum exposition after the septal mucosa is incised and the vomer is dislocated laterally. The two sphenoid ostia are here visualized, giving access to the sphenoid sinus.

The mucosa is incised with an endoscopic knife over the vomer (Figure 10) and retracted laterally until the vidian nerve, which represents the lateral limit for exposure and resection. The vidian nerve conducts in fact to the junction between the horizontal portion of the petrous ICA and the vertical paraclival segment of the ICA at the foramen lacerum.

After vomer subluxation and bilateral wide sphenoidotomies (Figure 11), the following steps of the surgery depend on the location and the extent of surgery (Figure 12). The osseous structure of the clivus is exposed and resected through a diamond burr drill (Figure 13) and secondarily a 1 and 2 mm Kerrison bone punch, according to a cranio-caudal direction from the inferior wall of the sphenoid ostium down to the foramen magnum (Figure 14). The paraclival ICA represents the lateral limit for exposure at this level. If necessary the ICA can be carefully dissected and mobilized in the medio-lateral plane to provide adequate access to the tumor in the paramedian zone.

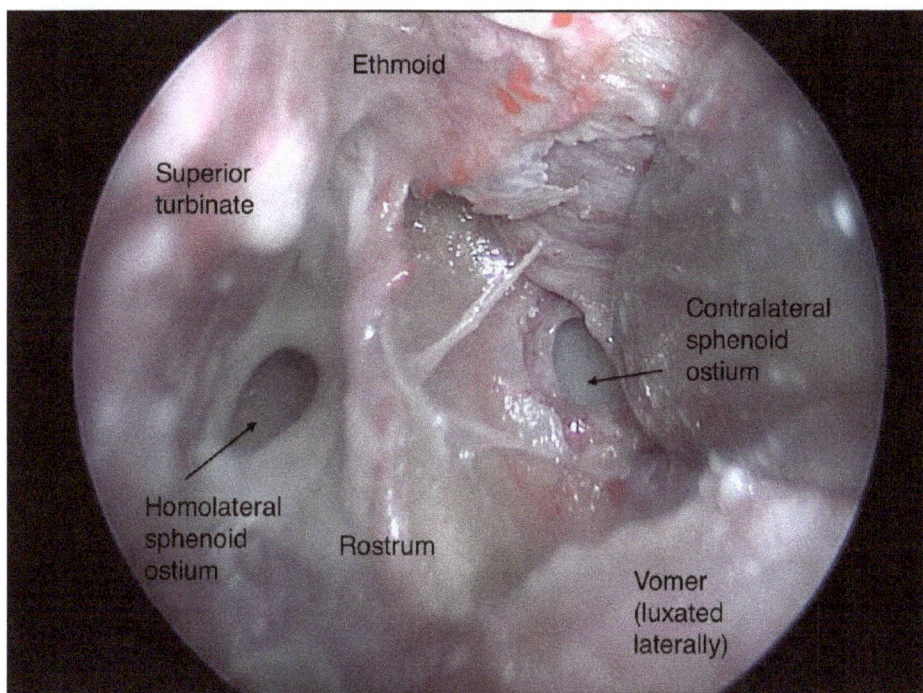

Figure 11. Bilateral exposition of the sphenoid ostia. A bilateral sphenoidotomy is then performed trhough a diamond drill and a small Kerrison bone punch to gain access to the sphenoid sinus.

The lateral extension of bone removal is defined by the pterygoid canal, which is found about 5mm lateral to the vomer-sphenoid junction. The vidian nerve may be followed proximally till the pterygoidcanal. The lateral boundaries limiting bone resection are thus represented in a craniocaudal fashion by the cavernous sinus, paraclival carotid arteries and the foramen lacerum.

The dura is thus exposed and the integrity of the basilar plexus, situated between the two layers of the dura of the upper clivus, should be respected to avoid copious bleeding. Bleeding from the basilar venous plexus is in fact often difficult to cauterize, but it may be managed with the use of hemostatic materials (Floseal Hemostatic Matrix®, Bayter Healthcare SA) and packing. The abducens nerve may be identified as traversing laterally the basilar plexus, and the paraclival ICA is also found.

For intradural lesions, a median longitudinal incision can be made initially on the outer layer of the dura. Then the internal layer is opened, with the visualization of the prepontine cistern and basilar artery (Figure 14).

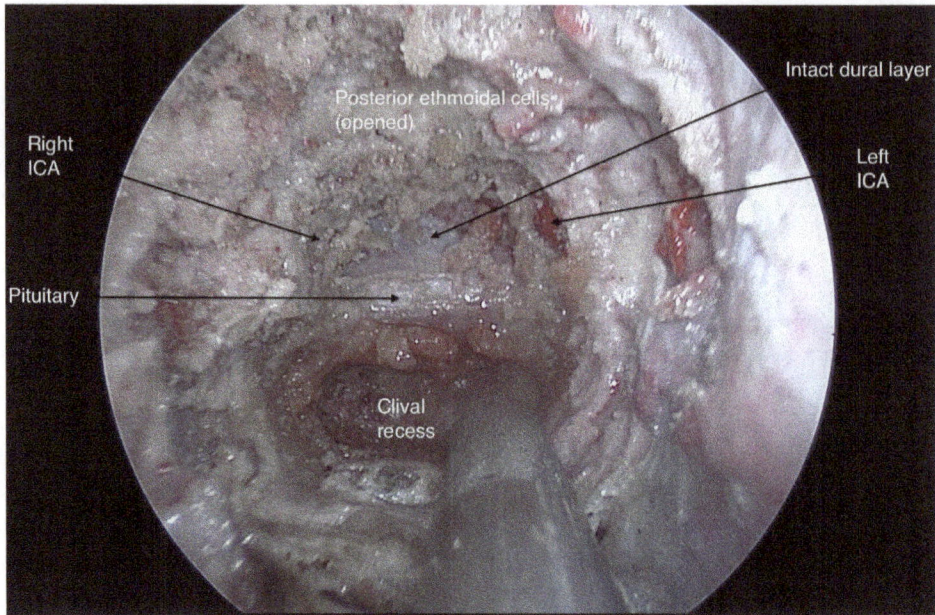

Figure 12. After a wide opening, the surgeon can choose the best sagittal corridor to reach the clival region of interest. The pituitary max be transposed to follow the supra-sellar corridor and gain access to the dorsum sellae or to the posterior clinoids or the clivus may be further drilled inferiorly. The lateral limits for the exposition are represented by the paraclival ICA. The vidian nerve should be identified and followed as it conducts directy to the foramen lacerum and may guide in defining the lateral limits of dissection.

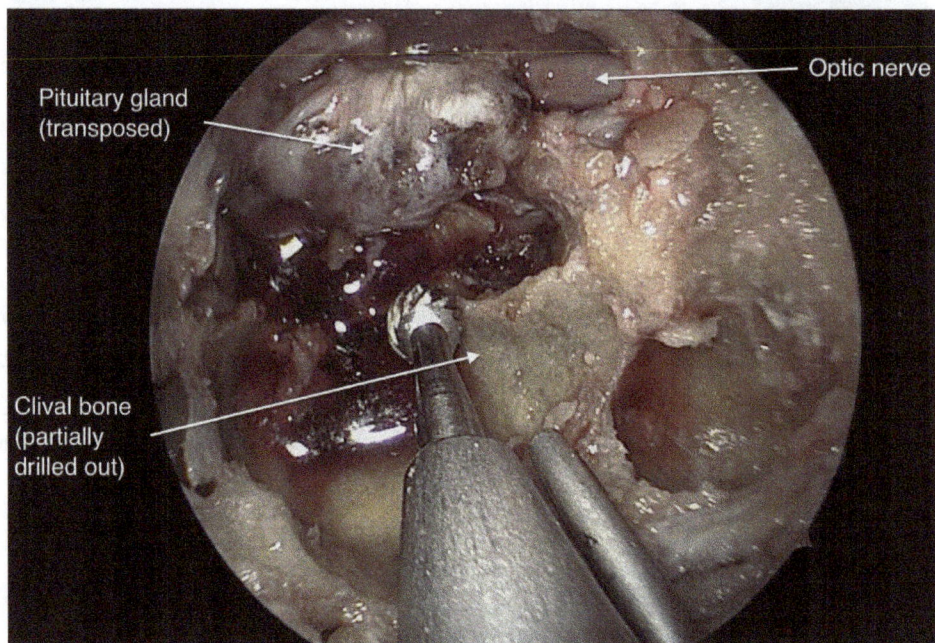

Figure 13. Drilling of the clival bone. The drilling is performed in a cranio-caudal fashion. It is important to respect dural integrity during this process.

The lesion is removed under endoscopic guidance in a piecemeal fashion with ultrasound dissectors. Intraoperative pathologic examination of tumor tissue is generally performed to decide on the extent of tumor resection on the basis of diagnosis.

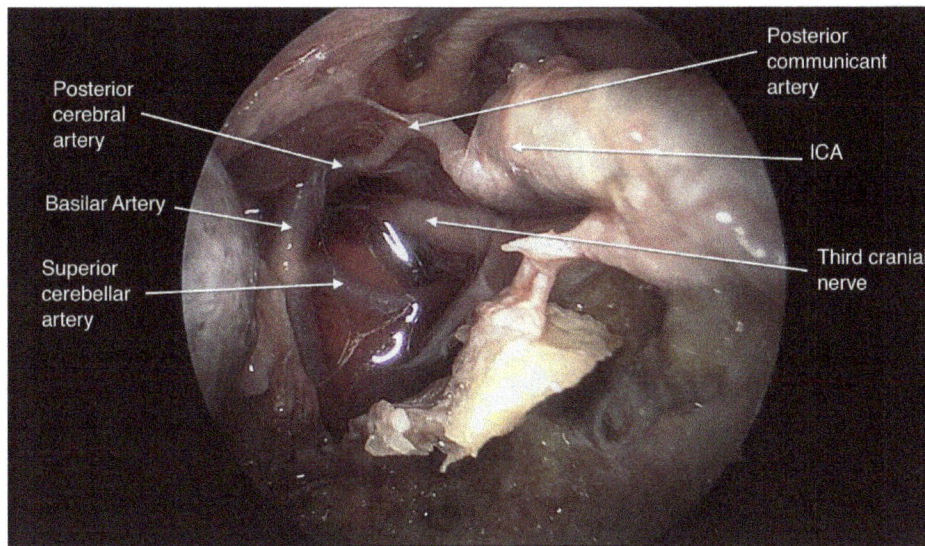

Figure 14. Exposition of the prepontine cistern in a cadaveric specimen. The two layers of the dura are opened and the posterior circulation is visualized.

The closure step is as important as the dissection and excision steps. A nasoseptal flap vascularized by the septal branches of the sphenopalatine artery may be prepared at the beginning of the procedure and displaced in the oropharynx, under the soft palate, to be protected during the surgery. It is important that the size of the pedicle of the flap stays sufficiently large to avoid necrosis of its borders. The use of the Hadad flap is now widespread, and it has allowed a significant reduction in the rate of postoperative CSF leaks after endoscopic techniques.

The reconstruction surface should be widened: flaps tend easily to shrink and we proposed the superposition of two nasoseptal flaps vascularized by branches of the posterior septal arteries in a lambdoid shape to ensure a correct closure. The middle turbinate resected at the beginning of the procedure may also be superimposed to increase the sealing in combination with biologic glue (Tisseel, Fibrin Sealant ®, Baxter AG).

3.3. Indications/management

Chordomas are slow-growing extra-axial tumors deriving from vestigial remnants of the notochord and the most common site at the sacrum and the clivus. A male predominance was described (3:1). They are considered low-grade malignancies but locally aggressive with a high recurrence rate. For this reason, gross total resection is fundamental but often difficult to achieve because of tumor extension and invasiveness and the proximity of important neurovascular structures. At clinical presentation, intracranial extension has normally occurred and complete resection is difficult in most cases (Figure 15).

When invading the basion, the most common presentation is represented by the XIIth cranial nerve palsy, while when the middle part of the clivus is interested (most common), chordomas may manifest as nasopharyngeal obstructive masses in cases of ventral extension or with VIth cranial nerve palsy in cases of dorsal extension. Chordomas arising at the upper third of the

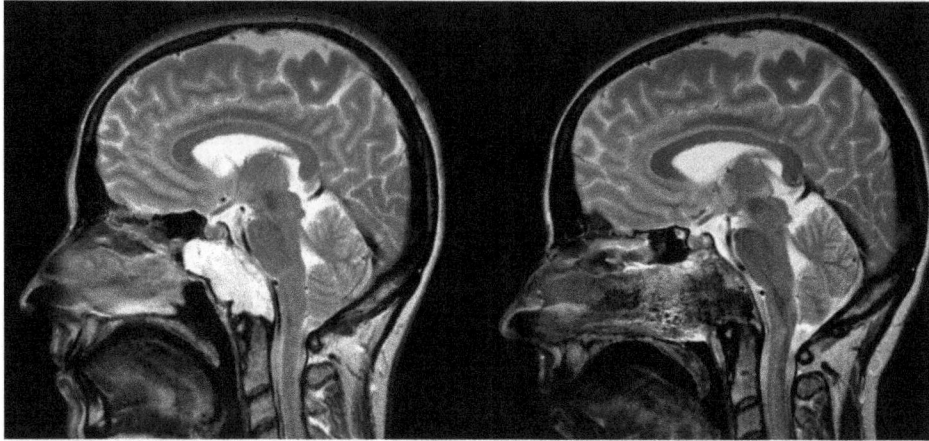

Figure 15. This young patient presented with neck pain. Preoperative sagittal T2-weighted cerebral MRI (left), showing a lesion involving the whole clivus. The sphenoidal and infrasphenoidal corridors were used to resect the lesion through EEEA. The postoperative MRI (right) shows a gross total resection of the lesion. The lesion was completely extradural. The patient was free of disease at 5-years follow-up.

clivus may present with hypopituitarism signs or bitemporal hemianopia due to chiasmal compression.

A lateral extension may also occur with consequent invasion of cavernous sinus in the upper part of the clivus or it may manifest with otologic symptoms like deafness, tinnitus and vertigo or facial paralysis because of involvement of the petrous bone.

Chondrosarcomas are malignant tumors derived from cartilaginous tissue arising from bone or soft tissues. They are less aggressive than other sarcomas but the natural history is characterized by multiple local recurrences after surgical excision. Distant metastases are rare. Both sexes are equally affected. About 75% of all cranial chondrosarcoma arise at the skull base, in particular in the middle cranial fossa. Imaging shows mottled calcifications within a soft tissue mass. Clinical manifestations are similar to those described for chordomas. Expansive lesions involving primarily the petrous apex may expand anteriorly and involve the clivus.

Meningiomas in particular may arise in close proximity to the porus acusticus or from a separate origin on the face of the petrous bone, and they may slowly extend to the clival region. They are five times more frequent in women, and the main clinical presentation is with vestibulocochlear symptoms. Secondarily, peripheral facial weakness or facial numbness are found accompanied by indirect signs of clival involvement in more advanced cases.

A complete local resection should be attempted along with resection or cauterization of dural attachment to minimize the risk of local recurrence.

The goal of every oncologic surgery should be gross total resection. However, to avoid complications and preserve neurovascular structures is the first compromise to accept when working in the clival region, and this is the first principle to guide the extent of resection.

Lesions showing wide intracavernous sinus extension, vascular encasement (ICA or vertebral artery) or brainstem involvement should be preoperatively planned as subtotal resection.

Furthermore, the extended endoscopic approach may be used as a valid alternative for debulking surgery or in palliative cases to limit the symptomatology of the patient or to allow a following complementary treatment, as radiotherapy or proton beam radiotherapy.

Traditionally clival lesions were treated through different trans-cranial approaches with a consequent important brain retraction, and a high risk of injury for the vessels and nerves crossed during the procedure [14-22].

The increased confidence in endoscopic techniques allowed a widespread application of the extended endoscopic approach to treat clival lesions. The first cadaveric study conducted in 2002 showed the feasibility of the procedure [23] and since then endoscopy has not ceased to find other applications. The main advantage is related to the avoidance of brain retraction and nerves crossing. Technological advancements allowed the development of a specialized instrumentation to work properly in the endonasal route, and many centers are pushing the application of endoscopic techniques far beyond the midline. Thanks to angled instruments, a dynamic 360° view may be obtained [24].

The results of the extended endoscopic approach for clival chordomas have been widely reported [7, 25-29]. In terms of gross total removal, it was equivalent or superior to classical open approaches [30, 31]. The extent of resection is the most important prognostic factors for survival in these cases, with a survival at 5 years of follow up dropping from 90% for GTR to 52% for partial resection [22]. The principal determinants for the surgical resection are the tumor volume and the lateral extension. The literature analysis shows how endoscopy represents an excellent approach for median lesions, with good results, especially for extra-dural lesions.

Following the increased experience with endoscopic techniques for extradural clival tumors, some centers started to use the trans-clival approach for the management of intradural tumors with good operative results [11, 13, 25, 31-33].

For lateral lesions or intradural lesions, however, the endoscopic approach is more complex, and it should be combined with traditional open approaches. After an excision as radical as possible, a complementary treatment through fractionated radiotherapy, stereotactic radio-surgery or proton beam radiotherapy represents the best management policy [34].

The tumor may thus be divided ideally into different compartments, which may be approached through a different surgical technique, endoscopic or transcranial, or treated with external irradiation. This conception allows minimizing the neurological morbidity and the complication rate because each technique is used safely. Furthermore, it is possible to realize a maximal resection with minimal access.

3.4. Complications

Both the extent of resection and the rate of complications are related to the experience of the first operator. The reconstructive step is as crucial as the excisional step, and it may be even more complicated in cases of large skull base defects. The first descriptive studies about the endoscopic skull base surgery reported an incidence of cerebrospinal fluid (CSF) leaks as high as 33.3% [27]. This complication may represent a medical emergency when not perceived in time because of the risk of infectious meningitis. CSF leak may be treated either with a surgical revision or conservatively with a lumbar drain. The main determinant factor is the surgeon's judgment about any intraoperative source of leakage. The CSF leak rate was severely reduced during the last years after the introduction of the vascularized nasospetal flap as described by Hadad [35], the gasket type seal and the multi-layered closure technique. The lumbar drain, which once was systematically used in the early postoperative period, may thus be avoided in most cases with a precocious mobilization of patients.

Infectious complications may be treated either with medical therapy or with surgical revision.

Vascular lesions may also occur, with early or delayed hemorrhagic complications (intracranial hematoma occurred in about 6% of cases according to Carrabba et al [36]). Though a careful dissection is realized, damage to the ICA may occur, often with catastrophic results. A preoperative occlusion test may help evaluate the consequences of an eventual ICA sacrifice. The consequences of an intraoperative ICA sacrifice may vary from the death of the patients to permanent neurological deficit to a simple Horner syndrome.

Cranial nerve palsies are significantly less frequent with the endoscopic approach when compared to the open approaches and transient in the majority of cases [36]. The majority of patients report an improvement in preoperative cranial nerve palsy due to surgical decompression. After surgery, patients mostly complain about transient minor symptoms as headache, blurred vision and nasal obstruction.

Patients having a postoperative syndrome of inappropriate antidiuretic hormone hypersecretion are also reported, as well as manifestations of hypopituitarism as a consequence of pituitary manipulation.

3.5. Limitations

Classical open approaches continue to be the gold standard for lesions extending lateral to the internal carotid artery, the vertebral arteries or lateral to the optic nerve, into the mastoid or inferior to the dens.

The excision of tumors extending into the cavernous sinus is actually possible with the endoscopic technique, but the postoperative cranial nerve palsy remains significant. A subtotal resection is performed in the majority of cases and the residual tumor may be treated with adjuvant stereotactic radiosurgery.

Furthermore, for intradural tumors a combined approach (extended endoscopic endonasal approach with transcranial microsurgery) is preferred.

4. Conclusion

The expanded endoscopic approach provides a good exposure to efficiently treat lesions of the clival region. This minimally invasive technique allows obtaining satisfying results in terms of oncological resection without skin incision and neurovascular retraction in a cohort of well-selected patients.

Author details

G. Cossu[1*], R.T. Daniel[1], M. George[2], F. Parker[3], N. Aghakhani[3], M. Levivier[1] and M. Messerer[1,3]

*Address all correspondence to: giulia.cossu@chuv.ch

1 Department of Neuroscience, Neurosurgical Unit, University Hospital of Lausanne, University of Lausanne, Faculty of Medicine and Biology, Lausanne, Switzerland

2 Department of E.N.T., University Hospital of Lausanne, University of Lausanne, Faculty of Medicine and Biology, Lausanne, Switzerland

3 Department of Neurosurgery, Kremlin Bicêtre Hospital, University of Paris Sud, Faculty of Medicine, Paris, France

The authors have no personal, financial or institutional interest.

References

[1] Stammberger H, Posawetz W. Functional endoscopic sinus surgery. Concept, indications and results of the Messerklinger technique. European Archives of Oto-Rhino-Laryngology : Official Journal of the European Federation of Oto-Rhino-Laryngological Societies. 1990;247(2):63-76.

[2] Messerklinger W. [Role of the lateral nasal wall in the pathogenesis, diagnosis and therapy of recurrent and chronic rhinosinusitis]. Laryngologie, Rhinologie, Otologie. 1987;66(6):293-9.

[3] Cappabianca P, Cavallo LM, De Divitiis E. Endoscopic endonasal transsphenoidal surgery. Neurosurgery. 2004;55(4):933-40; discussion 40-1.

[4] Carrau RL, Jho HD, Ko Y. Transnasal-transsphenoidal endoscopic surgery of the pituitary gland. The Laryngoscope. 1996;106(7):914-8.

[5] Kassam AB, Gardner P, Snyderman C, Mintz A, Carrau R. Expanded endonasal approach: fully endoscopic, completely transnasal approach to the middle third of the clivus, petrous bone, middle cranial fossa, and infratemporal fossa. Neurosurgical Focus. 2005;19(1):E6.

[6] Liu JK, Decker D, Schaefer SD, Moscatello AL, Orlandi RR, Weiss MH, et al. Zones of approach for craniofacial resection: minimizing facial incisions for resection of anterior cranial base and paranasal sinus tumors. Neurosurgery. 2003;53(5):1126-35; discussion 35-7.

[7]   Kassam AB, Prevedello DM, Thomas A, Gardner P, Mintz A, Snyderman C, et al. Endoscopic endonasal pituitary transposition for a transdorsum sellae approach to the interpeduncular cistern. Neurosurgery. 2008;62(3 Suppl 1):57-72; discussion 4.

[8]   Kassam AB, Vescan AD, Carrau RL, Prevedello DM, Gardner P, Mintz AH, et al. Expanded endonasal approach: vidian canal as a landmark to the petrous internal carotid artery. Journal of Neurosurgery. 2008;108(1):177-83.

[9]   Kassam A, Snyderman CH, Mintz A, Gardner P, Carrau RL. Expanded endonasal approach: the rostrocaudal axis. Part I. Crista galli to the sella turcica. Neurosurgical Focus. 2005;19(1):E3.

[10] Kassam A, Snyderman CH, Mintz A, Gardner P, Carrau RL. Expanded endonasal approach: the rostrocaudal axis. Part II. Posterior clinoids to the foramen magnum. Neurosurgical Focus. 2005;19(1):E4.

[11] Cappabianca P, Cavallo LM, Esposito F, De Divitiis O, Messina A, De Divitiis E. Extended endoscopic endonasal approach to the midline skull base: the evolving role of transsphenoidal surgery. Advances and Technical Standards in Neurosurgery. 2008;33:151-99.

[12] De Notaris M, Cavallo LM, Prats-Galino A, Esposito I, Benet A, Poblete J, et al. Endoscopic endonasal transclival approach and retrosigmoid approach to the clival and petroclival regions. Neurosurgery. 2009;65(6 Suppl):42-50; discussion 2.

[13] Schwartz TH, Fraser JF, Brown S, Tabaee A, Kacker A, Anand VK. Endoscopic cranial base surgery: classification of operative approaches. Neurosurgery. 2008;62(5): 991-1002; discussion 5.

[14] Al-Mefty O, Ayoubi S, Smith RR. The petrosal approach: indications, technique, and results. Acta Neurochirurgica Supplementum. 1991;53:166-70.

[15] Asaoka K, Terasaka S. Combined petrosal approach for resection of petroclival meningioma. Neurosurgical Focus. 2014;36(1 Suppl):1.

[16] Goel A, Desai K, Muzumdar D. Surgery on anterior foramen magnum meningiomas using a conventional posterior suboccipital approach: a report on an experience with 17 cases. Neurosurgery. 2001;49(1):102-6; discussion 6-7.

[17] Hakuba A, Liu S, Nishimura S. The orbitozygomatic infratemporal approach: a new surgical technique. Surgical Neurology. 1986;26(3):271-6.

[18] Javed T, Sekhar LN. Surgical management of clival meningiomas. Acta Neurochirurgica Supplementum. 1991;53:171-82.

[19] MacDonald JD, Antonelli P, Day AL. The anterior subtemporal, medial transpetrosal approach to the upper basilar artery and ponto-mesencephalic junction. Neurosurgery. 1998;43(1):84-9.

[20] Samii M, Knosp E. Approaches to the Clivus: Approaches to No Man's Land. Berlin: Springer-Verlag Berlin and Heidelberg GmbH & Co. K; 23 December 2011. p. 184.

[21] Seifert V, Raabe A, Zimmermann M. Conservative (labyrinth-preserving) transpetrosal approach to the clivus and petroclival region--indications, complications, results and lessons learned. Acta Neurochirurgica. 2003;145(8):631-42; discussion 642.

[22] Sen C, Triana AI, Berglind N, Godbold J, Shrivastava RK. Clival chordomas: clinical management, results, and complications in 71 patients. Journal of Neurosurgery. 2010;113(5):1059-71.

[23] Alfieri A, Jho HD, Tschabitscher M. Endoscopic endonasal approach to the ventral cranio-cervical junction: anatomical study. Acta Neurochirurgica. 2002;144(3):219-25; discussion 25.

[24] Cappabianca P, Alfieri A, De Divitiis E. Endoscopic endonasal transsphenoidal approach to the sella: towards functional endoscopic pituitary surgery (FEPS). Minimally Invasive Neurosurgery : MIN. 1998;41(2):66-73.

[25] Stippler M, Gardner PA, Snyderman CH, Carrau RL, Prevedello DM, Kassam AB. Endoscopic endonasal approach for clival chordomas. Neurosurgery. 2009;64(2): 268-77; discussion 77-8.

[26] Frank G, Sciarretta V, Calbucci F, Farneti G, Mazzatenta D, Pasquini E. The endoscopic transnasal transsphenoidal approach for the treatment of cranial base chordomas and chondrosarcomas. Neurosurgery. 2006;59(1 Suppl 1):ONS50-7; discussion ONS7.

[27] Dehdashti AR, Karabatsou K, Ganna A, Witterick I, Gentili F. Expanded endoscopic endonasal approach for treatment of clival chordomas: early results in 12 patients. Neurosurgery. 2008;63(2):299-307; discussion 9.

[28] Hong Jiang W, Ping Zhao S, Hai Xie Z, Zhang H, Zhang J, Yun Xiao J. Endoscopic resection of chordomas in different clival regions. Acta Oto-Laryngologica. 2009;129(1):71-83.

[29] Solares CA, Fakhri S, Batra PS, Lee J, Lanza DC. Transnasal endoscopic resection of lesions of the clivus: a preliminary report. The Laryngoscope. 2005;115(11):1917-22.

[30] Al-Mefty O, Borba LA. Skull base chordomas: a management challenge. Journal of Neurosurgery. 1997;86(2):182-9.

[31] Fraser JF, Nyquist GG, Moore N, Anand VK, Schwartz TH. Endoscopic endonasal minimal access approach to the clivus: case series and technical nuances. Neurosurgery. 2010;67(3 Suppl Operative):ons150-8; discussion ons8.

[32] Cavallo LM, Messina A, Gardner P, Esposito F, Kassam AB, Cappabianca P, et al. Extended endoscopic endonasal approach to the pterygopalatine fossa: anatomical study and clinical considerations. Neurosurgical Focus. 2005;19(1):E5.

[33] Cavallo LM, Messina A, Cappabianca P, Esposito F, De Divitiis E, Gardner P, et al. Endoscopic endonasal surgery of the midline skull base: anatomical study and clinical considerations. Neurosurgical Focus. 2005;19(1):E2.

[34] Daniel RT, Tuleasca C, Messerer M, Negretti L, George M, Pasche P, et al. Optimally invasive skull base surgery for large benign tumors. In: Berouma M, editor. Minimally Invasive Skull Base Surgery: Nova Science Publishers, Inc.; 2013.

[35] Hadad G, Bassagasteguy L, Carrau RL, Mataza JC, Kassam A, Snyderman CH, et al. A novel reconstructive technique after endoscopic expanded endonasal approaches: vascular pedicle nasoseptal flap. The Laryngoscope. 2006;116(10):1882-6.

[36] Carrabba G, Dehdashti AR, Gentili F. Surgery for clival lesions: open resection versus the expanded endoscopic endonasal approach. Neurosurgical Focus. 2008;25(6):E7.

9

Natural Orifice Translumenal Endoscopic Surgery of the GastroIntestinal Tract

Abdulzahra Hussain

Abstract

Research Focus - NOTES is a new technique that faces numerous challenges. Current technology, training and research activities are conducted to make it a safe and effective minimal access technique.

Research Methods Used - This chapter is based on the current evidence of published NOTES studies. Medline search is conducted through November to December 2014, including English literatures only. The search words are NOTES, natural orifice translumenal endoscopic surgery, hybrid NOTES and hybrid natural orifice translumenal endoscopic surgery; additional search words are specific for the titles like NOTES gastric, NOTES oesophageal, NOTES biliary, NOTES cholecystectomy, NOTES pancreatic, NOTES small bowel, NOTES colorectal and NOTES appendicectomy. Animal and human studies are selected after 2008. Small studies are excluded unless they report a novel approach or a new procedure.

Results/Findings of the Research - There is development in the technology by installing new platforms, instruments and closure devices to add more safety and security. There is also development in training and research activities across the continents; a number of NOTES procedures are performed safely on human beings including cholecystectomy, appendicectomy, peritoneoscopy, POEM and other procedures. Feasibility studies are conducted on animal and human cadaver models including numbers of complex procedures.

Main Conclusions and Recommendations - NOTES is evolving and gaining popularity. The growth rate however is slowed by challenges of the need for an ideal working platform and closure devices that are easy to use, cheap and time effective, in addition to the dedicated effective training.

Keywords: Upper GI NOTES, Lower GI NOTES, Oesophageal NOTES, Gastric NOTES, Duodenal NOTES, Liver NOTES, Pancreatic NOTES, Splenic NOTES

1. Introduction

Modern endoscopy began in 1805, when Phillip Bozzini first used a system to visualise the inside of the rectum and bladder through a mirror, a candle and a double-lumen ureteral catheter. The first source of inner light was invented by Bruck [1]. In 1878, Maximilian Carl-Friedrich Nitze introduced the first working cystoscope that contained a prismatic lens system and a channel through which you could insert a ureteral catheter, conducted in collaboration with Joseph Leiter [2]. Diagnostic methods of gastrointestinal tract have been evolving using flexible endoscopy. Dimitrij Oscarovic Ott (1855–1929) can undoubtedly be called the true pioneer of laparoscopy, especially of natural orifice translumenal endoscopic surgery (NOTES). In 1901 already he performed abdominal examinations via a transvaginal (Tv) access calling this procedure 'ventroscopy' [3]. In 1954 Hopkins made a crucial development by the idea of incorporating the light into scopes using the concept of multiple lenses separated by a room of air. Hopkins could never make the fibrescope, and it was a South African, Basil Hirschowitz, who made the first flexible fibreoptic gastroscope using Hopkins's idea [4]. Endoscopic retrograde cholangiopancreatography (ERCP) which was developed in 1968 and endoscopic ultrasound (EUS) in the 1980s are important milestones. With the development of sophisticated flexible scopes, it became feasible to conduct certain diagnostic and therapeutic GI procedures. Anthony Kalloo in 2000 reported the first peritoneoscopy on pigs [5]. Gastro-intestinal (GI) NOTES is a further development in the minimal access surgery (MAS). It has been received by surgical community with scepticism similar to what happened with the first laparoscopic cholecystectomy (LC) when Muhe introduced it for the first time to the German Surgical Society in 1985. In 2004 Rao and Reddy performed the first transgastric (Tg) appendicectomy [6]. In 2012, authors considered that rigid standard laparoscopy provided better organ visualisation, better lesion detection and better biopsy capability than the transgastric (Tg) and transrectal (Tr) NOTES approaches [7], and that is expected as NOTES still undergo refining and development which should push for more efforts to overcome these challenges. In spite of uncertainty, GI NOTES proved itself for a number of procedures that are applied in elective and emergency settings with significant contribution to improve the care and attained a high level of patient satisfaction and most importantly a great scale of safety and efficacy. The GI NOTES is gaining popularity but at slower rate compared to LC. It has been limited to the university institutions and big teaching tertiary centres across Europe, America and Asia. Nevertheless, large series are reported on human beings. Many centres are conducting feasibility studies on animals as well as cadavers and patients. Several obstacles are preventing the wide applications of NOTES. Of these is the need for advanced endoscopic and laparoscopic skills, infrastructure setting, funding and local health authority approval and health systems bureaucracy. Germany reports the highest number of human NOTES procedures in the Europe, while the USA is the leading state in the American continent.

1.1. Challenges to NOTES

1.1.1. Experience

The NOTES main tool is a flexible scope and unstable working platform. Preliminary endoscopic, and to less degree laparoscopic, experience is a pre-request for conducting NOTES procedures. An excellent endoscopic experience is crucial in conducting NOTES procedures [8]. A study from Germany showed endoscopic experience was the strongest influencing factor, whereas laparoscopic skills had limited impact on the performance of NOTES surgeons with previous endoscopic experience [9]. This can be explained by the ability of the endoscopist to adapt for movement and to perform procedure using unstable and flexible platform. Reputable institutions are organising training courses for NOTES, and a good example is Strasbourg in France. Training on animal models is providing opportunity of operating on living subjects and increasing the confidence of performing the procedure on patients [10]. An example of the training model is the endoscopic–laparoscopic interdisciplinary training entity (ELITE) used in Germany. One of the important issues in training is the willingness and interest of the junior surgeons to adapt NOTES in their institutions.

1.1.2. Governance, regulations and training

Extensive training is required for surgeons to overcome the vision–motion difficulty before they can perform NOTES safely and effectively [11]. Different bodies are sponsoring NOTES training in the USA, Europe, South America and Asia. NOSCAR and EAES are leading the research, training and development of NOTES. In 2005, the American Society of Gastrointestinal Endoscopy (ASGE) and the Society of American Gastrointestinal Endoscopic Surgeons (SAGES) formed the Natural Orifice Surgery Consortium for Assessment and Research (NOSCAR) and published the NOTES white paper [12, 13]. In Europe, the New European Surgical Academy (NESA) founded the NOS (Natural Orifice Surgery) working group, which is exploring another surgical route, the TransDouglas (Td) one. The NOS/SLO group is an interdisciplinary working group of the NESA. Its goal is to develop surgical procedures using the natural openings of the human body and "scarless" operations [14]. There are similar scientific bodies in South America like Brazilian group and also in Asia like Japanese, Chinese and Indian NOTES groups. The Virtual Translumenal Endoscopic Surgical Trainer (VTEST (TM)) is being developed as a platform to train for NOTES procedures and innovate NOTES tools and techniques [15]. Different tools are used in NOTES training courses. These include operating on animal models with an acceptable grade of satisfaction. One of such tool is the endoscopic–laparoscopic interdisciplinary training entity. A study has shown the constructing validity for the ELITE model which seems to be well suited for the training of NOTES as a new surgical technique [16].

1.1.3. Funding

The rising costs of healthcare are forcing all parties to consider both the medical risks/benefits and the economic efficiency of proposed tools and therapies [17]. Funding is required for research and for setting of the infrastructure to perform NOTES procedures on animals and patients. NOTES surgery needs extra cost for the instruments. The endoscopic closure devices, the working platforms and scope are very expensive compared to the classical laparoscopic instrumentations. Funding is a problem in the current era, and the leading teaching centres across America and Europe can afford it. The collaboration with businesses and industries has resulted in huge budget of funds to the NOTES research. For example, by 2009 Olympus has donated $1.25 million supporting NOTES activities in the USA [18]. Ethicon offered similar support and funding for NOSCAR research in the USA. The Center for Integration of Medicine and Innovative Technology's (CIMIT) investment in NOTES research will top $3 million overall, making CIMIT the largest financial sponsor of this technology worldwide [19].

1.1.4. Pressure of common acute and elective surgical take

Undertaking NOTES procedures in addition to the common surgical workload is adding a practical challenge. However, this can be resolved by dedicated time for specific NOTES activities. It is expected that NOTES will be a separate and distinguished speciality for the gastrointestinal surgeons.

1.1.5. Bureaucracy of health systems

It is not a surprise that the first reported NOTES procedure of appendicectomy was from the Hyderabad group in India which has less bureaucratic health system compared to Europe and the USA. The bureaucracy because of high grade of concerns about safety of any new technique or intervention. While this is a healthy issue, sometimes it defers innovations and frustrates surgeons who are trying to bring in reality and clinical practice new ideas and approaches. NOTES is not an exception to be rejected as a new method. In order to install NOTES technique, one would need extra efforts to pass through the hurdles that built up across modern health systems. In the UK we are much behind the fellow Europe states like Germany as far as NOTES is concerned. This may also be explained by less popularity of the technique in the UK. South London's Surrey University, Guildford, held the first ever NOTES training course in 2008. In the UK, there is no specific body to support NOTES research like NOSCAR in the USA or the NESA group of Europe.

1.1.6. Public opinion

As expected a study of 1006 patients demonstrated public's interest in these new techniques and thus gave further support to continued research and development in this area [20]. The Swanstrom group from the USA reported that majority of the patients surveyed (56%) would choose NOTES for their cholecystectomy [21]. It is not surprising that patients would choose an approach that provides excellent cosmetic and clinical outcomes with high safety profile [22]. Surgical societies are committed to work towards perfection, and NOTES is the ultimate approach for the management of a number of surgical conditions and provides extra benefits of minimal access techniques.

1.1.7. Septic complications

NOTES is not different from classical surgery of possible risk of infection. Intravenous antibiotics in addition to topical Betadine or chlorhexidine have effectively reduced microbial burden in both gastric and colonic mucosa in porcine model [23]. The common Tg and Tv routes are compared in animal models, and authors concluded that without gastric or vaginal lavage and antibiotic peritoneal irrigation, the Tg procedure has a higher infection rate than the Tv access. After antiseptic preparation, the bacterial load significantly decreased in the Tg group, which seems as safe as the sterile Tv approach [24]. However, in a study of 40 patients who underwent Roux-En-Y gastric bypass (RYGBP), contamination of the peritoneal cavity does occur with Tg endoscopic peritoneoscopy (TEP), but this does not lead to an increased risk of infectious complications [25]. Another study of 130 patients who underwent Tg NOTES showed that the risk of bacterial contamination secondary to peroral and Tg access is clinically insignificant [26]. Pure Tg endoscopic surgery results in less perioperative inflammatory response than laparoscopy in the early postoperative phase [27]. In a review of literature by the Darzi group, UK showed that recommendation requiring no preoperative preparation can be made for the Tg approach. Antiseptic irrigation is recommended for Tv (grade C) NOTES access, as is current practice [28].

1.1.8. Intraoperative NOTES complications

The management of intraoperative NOTES complications could be challenging. Adequate experience is therefore necessary to recognise and treat them to avoid morbidity and mortality and to minimise conversion to hybrid NOTES or open technique. Effective management of NOTES complications however is reported, for example, bleeding complications and splenic laceration [29]. For intestinal perforation, the case may be different. Authors found that small intestinal injuries are difficult to localise with currently available flexible endoscopes and accessories. Endoscopic clips, however, may be adequate for closure of small bowel lacerations if the site of injury is known [30]. A study has shown that urinary bladder injury occurring during NOTES can be successfully managed via a NOTES approach using currently available endoscopic accessories [31].

1.2. Principles of NOTES

1.2.1. Indications

NOTES approach is indicated in a variety of conditions across surgical specialities, not only gastrointestinal tract but also urology, gynaecology and thoracic field. NOTES indications could be an emergency or elective which is the majority. This chapter is concentrating on upper GI NOTES.

1.2.2. Access

1.2.2.1. Major sites for access

1.　Transgastric (Tg): The first human NOTES procedure was performed using Tg route. The experimental studies proved ultrasonography-guided access through the stomach to be feasible and safe without iatrogenic complications [32]. There are two challenges in the Tg route: the closure and the abdominal contamination and septic complications. The ideal

Tg access closure is expected to be easy, effective, cheap and less time consuming. Tg NOTES peritoneoscopy and the gastrotomy can be closed by deploying a 2-sided ECM occluder on animal model [33]. The results indicated that closure of gastrotomy by Eagle Claw VIII could withstand higher endoluminal pneumatic bursting pressure than endoclips [34]. Submucosal approach is a new and promising technique for the development of NOTES [35] (see Figure 1).

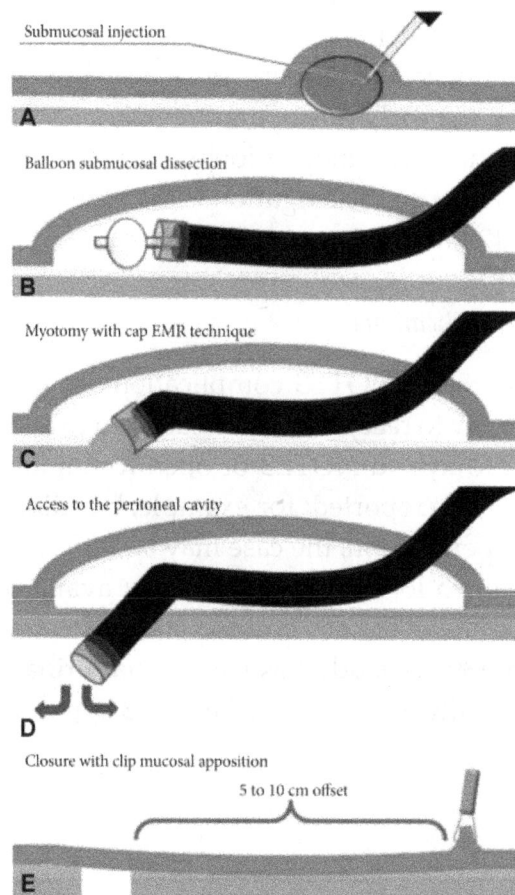

Figure 1. Submucosal tunnel technique is used (Lee SHI et al. 2012)

The Tg access closure is provided by different techniques including clips (over-the-scope clip), sutures, etc. [36, 37]. There are different closure methods in literature, but safety is shown in one of animal studies at least comparable to the classical laparoscopy procedure [38]. A novel gastric closure device, the loop-anchor purse-string (LAPS) closure system, had been described [39]. If hybrid technique is used, then laparoscopic stapler can be applied to the gastric access [40]. A multilayer extracellular matrix (ECM) occluder is assessed on animals, and it was safe and effective [41]. A loop and clip [KING closure], (see figure 2), [42] and QUEEN closure are other methods [43]. Self-approximating translumenal access technique (STAT) and implantation of a cellular matrix in the STAT tunnel are the two methods that have shown safety and efficacy on animal model [44]. There has been a method of testing support closure with T-tags and Padlock-G-clips over OVESCO OTS-clips and standard endoscopic clips [45].

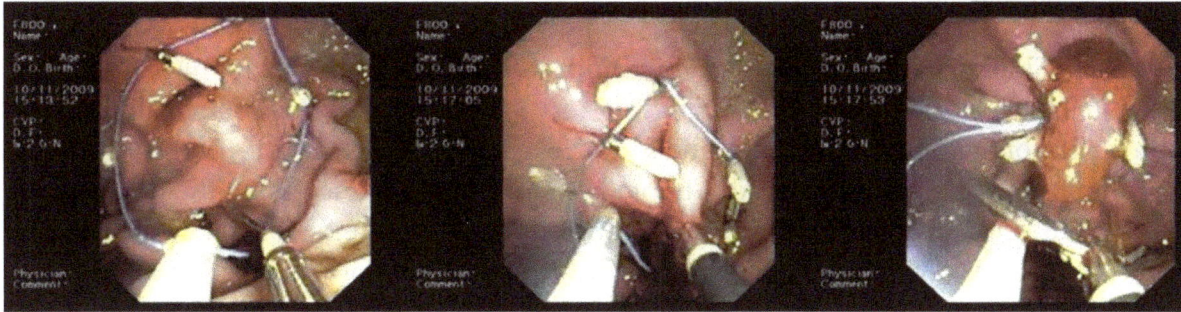

Figure 2. KING closure, loop and clip by Ryska O et al. 2012

2. Transvaginal (Tv): A recent meta-analysis confirmed high safety profile with this technique [46]. Infectious complications and the closure are the two important areas in this approach. A recent study of 102 Tv NOTES procedure reported only one case of infection following appendicectomy [47], which is comparable to the laparoscopic approach for similar pathology. Closure of the Tv access can be easier than Tg one [48]. Simple suturing under direct vision is the norm.

3. Transrectal (Tr): Animal studies have shown safety and efficacy [49]. The flexible endoscopic stapler is an effective device for the safe closure of a colon access, which in this feasibility study was equivalent to other well-established techniques [50]. Closure of Tr viscerotomy using end-to-end (EEA) circular stapler technique is feasible, easy to perform and histologically comparable to suture closure through a TEO platform. It may offer an attractive alternative for NOTES segmental colectomies and endoscopic resections [51]. The colostomy was closed by occlusion loop-and-clip (KING closure) technique [52]. To access the retroperitoneal space, significant challenges locating identifiable landmarks were faced mostly transrectally and improved in transgastric prone position [53].

4. Transvesical (Tve): Many animal studies have reported feasibility of NOTES procedures through the urinary bladder [54, 55]. Still there are no significant clinical applications on patients because of the challenging access closure and also because of the specimen delivery. J Bhullar et al. from Providence and medical centre, USA, used Vicryl loop for bladder access closure on a porcine model [56], (figure 3).

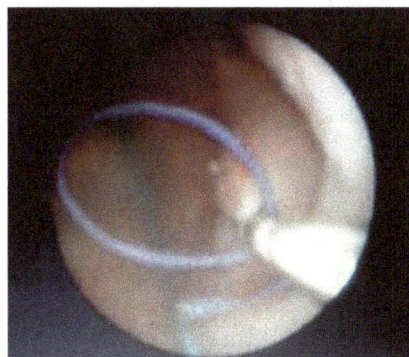

Figure 3. Vicryl loop closure of transvesical access (J Bhullar et al. 2012)

1.2.3. Instrumentation

Developing interfaces that are both intuitive and simple to use is crucial for NOTES dissemination [57]. The minimally invasive cardiac surgery (MICS) robot [58] is another step towards optimisation of the NOTES technique and to address the problems of optics, flexibility and the comfortable and adequate exposure. Abdominal navigation and accessing the pancreas was investigated on animals, and based on its success, pancreas resection was performed. A prototype multitasking platform "EndoSAMURAI" with the use of a biosimulation model and ex vivo porcine stomach was reported [59], (figure 5). There are new ancillary instruments like forceps, and training on using them is continuing [60]. The SPIDER platform is a sterile and disposable device that contains 4 working channels (2 flexible instrument delivery tubes positioned laterally and 2 rigid channels superiorly and inferiorly to accommodate an endoscope or any of the shelf rigid surgical instruments) [61]. This device has addressed some of the technical problems, and it is relatively expensive which limits its wide use. Authors concluded that the new manual handling system (MHS) is fully capable of achieving payload transport during a NOTES operation. The system is intuitive and easy to use. It dramatically decreases collateral trauma in the natural access point and can advantageously reduce the overall duration of a procedure [62]. The 3D display system is a great step in optics development. At least 34 systems are developed, for example, Aesculap's EinsteinVision (see Figure 4). This is in current use for laparoscopy and has the potential to improve the vision and anatomy at challenging NOTES procedures [63]. The Direct Drive Endoscopic System (DDES; Boston Scientific, Natick, MA) is a flexible laparoscopic multitasking platform that consists of a 55-cm steerable guide sheath that houses 3 lumens extending from a rail-based platform with interchangeable 4-mm instruments [64], (figure 6). Incisionless Operating Platform (IOP) is another flexible scope used for NOTES procedures including cholecystectomy [65].

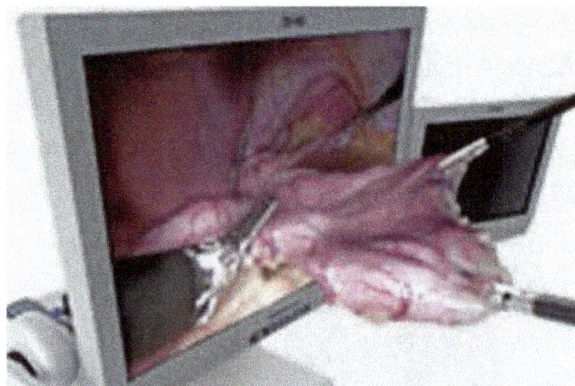

Figure 4. Aesculap's EinsteinVision® system

1.2.4. Anaesthesia

There are three main issues when using transoral access to perform upper GI NOTES procedures: The first one is to intubate via transnasal route to spare the oral space for NOTES flexible scope, the second issue is to position the patient according to the type of procedure, and the

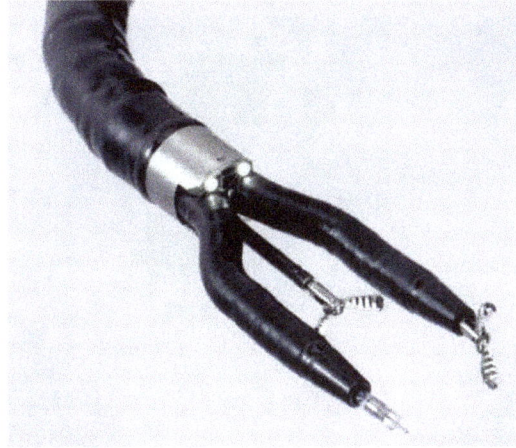

Figure 5. EndoSAMURAI platform, Yasuda K et al. 2014

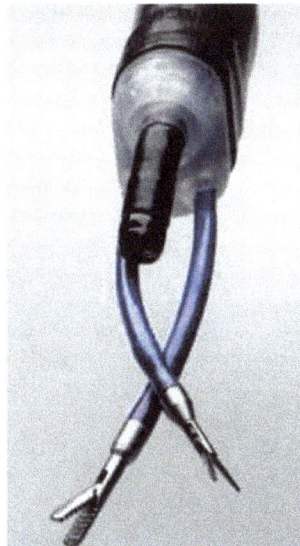

Figure 6. Direct Drive Endoscopic System (DDES), S Shaik et al. 2010

third point is to monitor ETCO2 [66], (figure 7). For other NOTES accesses, transnasal intubation is not necessary. Anaesthetic technique can be different from laparoscopic surgery. The effect of pneumoperitoneum may be not different; both techniques will have pneumoperitoneum if it is abdominal NOTES procedure. POEM procedure, for example, does not need pneumoperitoneum [67, 68]. Any patient that cannot tolerate pneumoperitoneum because of cardiopulmonary disease is not a candidate for NOTES procedure. Cardiorespiratory physiology is affected by laparoscopic procedure mainly because of pneumoperitoneum. However, the non-inferiority of NOTES compared to the laparoscopy is demonstrated from reported studies, although the evidence is limited by a number of researches [69]. When administering anaesthetic care to a patient undergoing NOTES, anaesthesiologists should closely monitor the patient's position as well as ETCO2 to minimise the incidence of mediastinal emphysema and pneumomediastinum and to ensure early detection of pneumoperitoneum-related respiratory and hemodynamic changes [70].

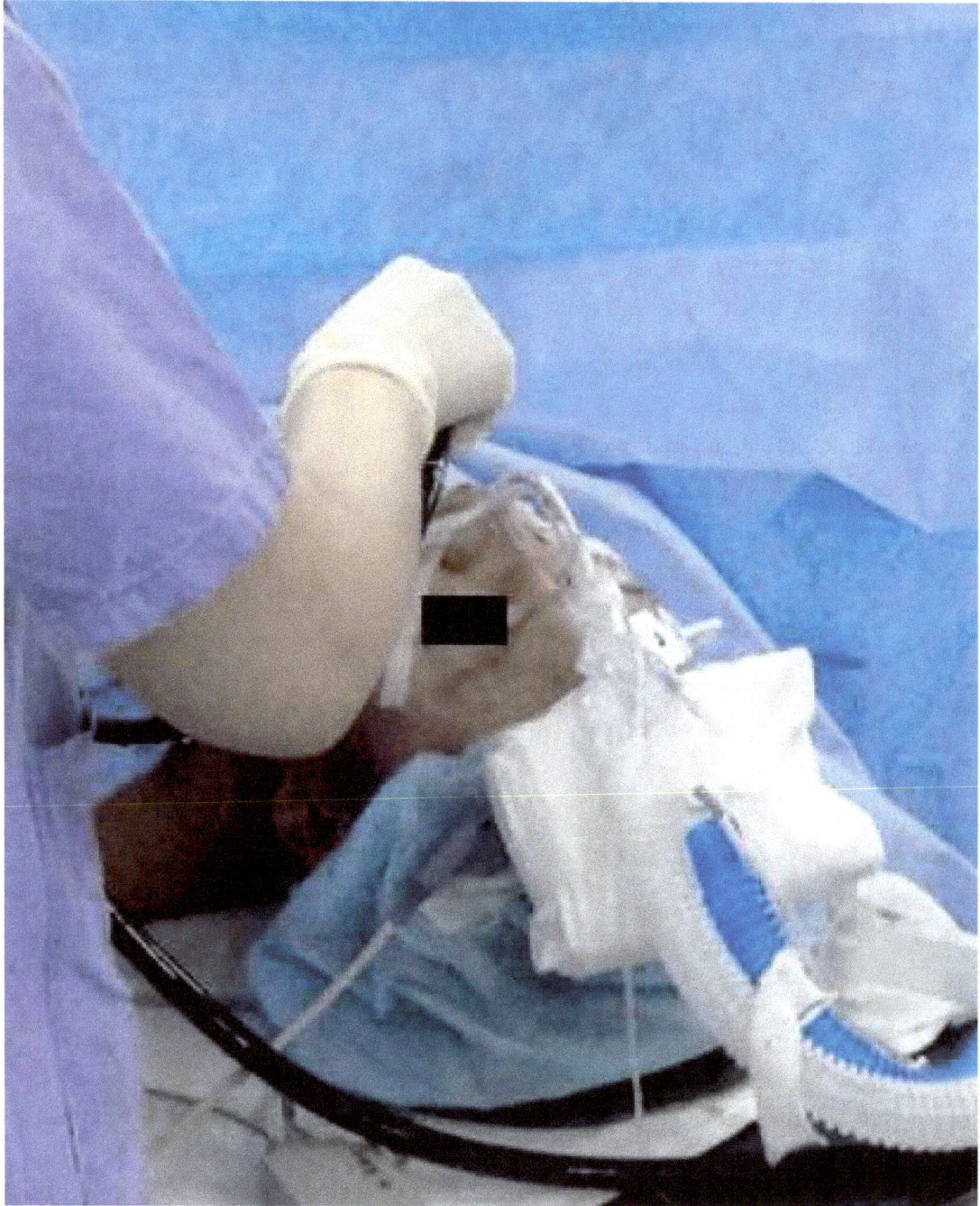

Figure 7. Transnasal intubation in upper GI NOTES. The patient was placed in the supine position and intubated via a nasal RAE™ tracheal tube. The endoscopic operator stood near the head of the patient and inserted the endoscope via the mouth (Ji Hyeon Lee et al. 2014)

1.2.5. Setting

NOTES units are part of surgical departments whether upper or lower GI, gynaecology and urology units. These units are usually located in well-established teaching hospitals. Theatre facilities are available for minimal access approach. Staffs are trained in NOTES, and they are familiar with the preparation and assistance.

1.2.6. Expertise

NOTES experience is crucial for the quality and safety of this intervention. The current guidelines advise to run through milestones of animal studies, cadaveric and live subject experimental and pilot projects. Once the learning curve is achieved after a number of procedures, NOTES can be performed under strict governance system. This has been achieved in a number of US and European states.

1.2.7. Complications

All minimal access surgery serious complications are those of organ injury due to suboptimal exposure that results from bad technique. It is anatomical and visual hallucination. This is to be avoided to provide the high grade of safety. Industries, related professionals and surgeons are striving to address all the issues that preclude safety.

2. Upper GI NOTES

2.1. Oesophagus NOTES

A number of oesophageal NOTES procedures are conducted safely on patients. Oesophageal discontinuity, which is a very complex procedure, is performed using a modification of NOTES [71]. The peroral endoscopic myotomy (POEM) for lower oesophageal conditions like achalasia has been performed on animals and patients with great success. NOSCAR has recently produced its white paper about the milestones of the POEM technique and the current opinion about the indications and quality and safety [72]. Distal oesophageal spasm that can progress to achalasia is another indication for POEM [73]. In 2002, Smith et al. found that the endoscopic stapling technique for the treatment of Zenker diverticulum results in a statistically significant shorter operative time, hospital stay and time to resume oral feedings compared with the standard open technique [74]. Transesophageal approach to posterior mediastinum has been reported on animal models [75]. Transoesophageal, anterior spinal NOTES reported lymph node resection, vagotomy, thoracic duct ligation, thymectomy, biopsy of the lung and pleura, epicardial coagulation, saline injection into the myocardium, pericardial fenestration and anterior thoracic spine procedures [76]. Exposure of the GOJ and placement of an anti-reflux prosthesis via a hybrid NOTES procedure were feasible, despite some complications [77]. Translumenal oesophago-oesophageal anastomosis was feasible on animal model [78]. Transoesophageal thoracic NOTES are a growing field. Diagnostic procedures have been well described. Closure of the oesophageal access is managed by different approaches including stenting [79].

2.2. Gastric NOTES

Gastric resection and specimen extraction through the upper GI route are reported by authors [80]. On animal models, a gastrojejunostomy was feasible with a 4-cm length using an anastomosing metal stent. After gastrotomy formation using a needle knife, a jejunotomy was then performed in the gastric cavity, which was followed by deployment of an anastomosing metal stent under fluoroscopic guidance [81]. Also on porcine model, combined NOTES and single trocar sleeve gastrectomy is feasible in a porcine model [82]. Through Tv NOTES gastrectomy for gastric submucosal tumours, with the assistance of two transabdominal ports, "oncologically acceptable" partial gastrectomy was successfully performed [83].

The hybrid NOTES technique is a combined method, including the advantages of both laparoscopic resection and endoscopic resection for gastric subepithelial tumours (SETs) [84]. After a 40-mm submucosal tunnel was created using an endoscopic submucosal dissection technique, in TGP, balloon dilation of a serosal puncture and intraperitoneal exploration were performed; in EFTR, a full-thickness incision and snaring resection were performed. Closure of the mucosal incision was performed by endoclips [85].

Hybrid sleeve gastrectomy (SG) and delivery of the specimen by transoral remnant extraction (TORE) are feasible and avoid port complications [86]. A study of 136 patients showed that Tv hybrid NOTES SG technique can be performed, but there is still a need for additional trocars through the abdominal wall [87]. Combined use of laparoscopy and NOTES enabled gastric pull-up without cervical and thoracic incisions [88]. NOTES omental repair of gastric perforation appears comparable to that of laparoscopy [89]. Hybrid NOTES resection of gastric gastrointestinal stromal tumour (GIST) was successfully reported on patients [90].

2.3. Duodenal NOTES

Currently, there is scarce of literatures on duodenal NOTES. This is because of rarity of duodenal pathologies that benefits from NOTES. Peritoneoscopy is actively used to assess upper GI tract including the duodenum [91]. This approach is feasible in selected series of patients [92].

2.4. Liver NOTES

Continued development of NOTES techniques may further alter the approaches to the biliary tract, liver and pancreas [93]. On animal models intraoperative NOTES-EUS is feasible to assess liver lesions [94]. Liver biopsy was performed successfully without any bleeding, and adequate samples were obtained in animal cases [95]. Using the Erbe Jet2 water-jet system, transanal and transvaginal wedge hepatic resection was successfully performed [96]. Tr liver resection and delivery of specimen were feasible and safe without problem of the rectal access [97]. Another study reported an animal liver wedge resection using MASTER robot [98]. Human cases of liver resection were reported as well. A combined laparoscopic Tv approach was used. Four 5-mm trocars were used. The liver parenchyma was divided using the harmonic scalpel, whereas the left hepatic vein was transected using the laparoscopic Tv vascular stapler. The specimen was placed in an Endobag and extracted transvaginally [99]. Complex liver surgery like hepatico-jejunostomy, major hepatic resection and transplantation is unlikely to be introduced at this stage due to the current limitations of the technique.

2.5. Pancreas NOTES

It is technically possible by EUS-guided NOTES procedures to achieve a systematic anterior and posterior access for NOTES transgastric peritoneoscopy and direct pancreatic endoscopic procedures [100]. Peripancreatic abscess can be managed by transgastric endoscopy and debridement with successful outcome, which provides great benefits of minimal access approach [101, 102]. NOTES cystogastrostomy for pancreatic pseudocyst management included endoscopic ultrasound (EUS)-guided puncture of the stomach just below the gastroesophageal (GOJ) junction to gain access to the pseudocyst, guidewire placement and then dilatation with a balloon to 18–20 mm. Endoscopic necrosectomy and debridement were performed, followed by transoral surgical anastomosis under endoscopic visualisation with the SurgAssist™ SLC 55 (Power Medical Interventions, Langhorne, PA) using 4.8-mm stapler [103]. A robotic platform to perform complex distal pancreatectomy on animal model was described [104].

2.6. Spleen NOTES

To dissect the upper end of the gastrosplenic ligament and the marginal region between the left diaphragm and upper pole of the spleen, a flexible single-channel endoscope was introduced into the peritoneal cavity simultaneously with the use of a rigid laparoscope. This is also providing the benefits of water-jet lens cleaning, effective suction and better visualisation in dissection of all splenic attachments and ligaments [105]. Hybrid splenectomy is performed on animal models without major complications indicating safety and feasibility [106]. Tv visualisation of the spleen and standard dissection of attachments were feasible, and splenectomy was completed using Tv stapling of the splenic hilum which is safely performed on patient [107].

2.7. Biliary NOTES

A comparison of the surgical errors during electrosurgery gallbladder dissection establishes that the NOTES procedure, while still new, is not inferior to the established laparoscopic cholecystectomy procedure [108]. NOTES cholecystectomy is the commonest upper GI procedure performed on patients. More than 3000 procedures are reported by now. Largest series of more than 2653 cases is from Germany [109]. Only 15% of NOTES cholecystectomy is performed in the USA. Two recent review studies showed increasing number of NOTES cholecystectomy [110, 111]. NOTES peritoneoscopy for accurate diagnosis and staging of intra-abdominal cancers is already in clinical use. Peritoneoscopy can accurately assess hepato-pancreatic-biliary malignancy and lymph node status [112].

2.8. Bariatric Surgery NOTES

Authors reported combined Tv and abdominal variant of SG on humans [113]. On animal models, hybrid NOTES SG is reported [114, 115]. The procedure was performed on humans using hybrid technique [116]. Roux-En-Y GBP was very challenging procedure and needed development of NOTES instruments to make it safe, feasible and time-effective operation.

Trials on human cadavers concluded feasibility, but long operative time mainly because of the lack of proper instrumentation resulting in insufficient tissue traction, countertraction and instrument manipulation complicated several steps during the procedure [117]. There are human series of hybrid NOTES RYGBP for obesity [118]. NOTES gastric band procedure was reported on a patient [119].(see table 1).

Authors	Year	Reference	Operation	Human subjects	Animal subjects
Spaun GO et al.	2010	[134]	Transcervical Heller's myotomy	Yes	Yes
Swanstrom et al.	2010	[135]	Oesophageal mobilisation	Yes	Yes
Welhelm et al.	2010	[77]	Anti-reflux surgery	No	Yes
Swanstrom et al.	2011	[136,137,72]	Endoscopic myotomy	Yes	No
Rieder et al.	2011	[138,74]	Zenker diverticulectomy	No	Yes
Ishimaru et al.	2011	[139]	Gastric pull through for oesophageal atresia	No	Yes
Turner et al.	2011	[140]	Closure of oesophageal access site	No	Yes
Turners et al.	2011	[141,79]	Stent closure of oesophageal access site	No	Yes
Rolanda et al.	2011	[142]	Peroral oesophageal segmentectomy	No	Yes
Cho et al.	2011	[143]	Resection of early gastric cancer	Yes	No
Abe et al.	2009	[144]	Gastric submucosal tumour resection	Yes	No
Nau et al.	2011	[118]	Staging pancreatic mass	Yes	No
			Hybrid gastric bypass	Yes	No
			Pure gastric bypass	Yes	No
Chiu et al.	2010	[145]	Tg gastrojejunostomy	No	Yes
Campos et al.	2010	[146]	Tg drainage of abdominal abscess	Yes	No
Cahill et al.	2009	[147]	Tv gastric lymph node mapping	No	Yes
Luo et al.	2012	[148]	Tg gastrojejunostomy	No	Yes
Ikeda et al.	2011	[149]	Gastric full-thickness resection	No	Yes
Lacey et al.	2009	[150,112,87]	Hybrid sleeve gastrectomy	Yes	No
Michalik et al.	2011	[117]	Hybrid gastric band	Yes	No
Branco et al.	2011	[151]	Transvesical peritoneoscopy, liver biopsy, appendix manipulation	Yes	No
Truong et al.	2012	[152]	Hybrid liver resection	Yes	No
Shi et al.	2011	[153]	Pure liver resection	No	Yes
Lehman et al.	2014	[122]	Cholecystectomy	Yes	No

Authors	Year	Reference	Operation	Human subjects	Animal subjects
			Peritoneum	Yes	No
			Gastric surgery	Yes	No
			Liver surgery	Yes	No
Bakker OJ et al.	2012	[101,102]	Tg pancreatic necrosectomy	Yes	No
Pallapothu et al.	2011	[103]	Cystogastrostomy	Yes	No
Targarona et al.	2009	[107]	Tv splenectomy	Yes	No

Table 1. Important upper GI NOTES procedures

3. Lower GI NOTES

3.1. Small bowel NOTES

Small intestinal anastomosis was performed in a porcine intestinal Tr NOTES model using two robotic arms and a camera inserted through the proctoscope and a rectal anterior wall incision [120]. NOTES gastroenterostomy with a biflanged lumen-apposing stent was reported recently by collaboration of French and US centres. The procedure was feasible and safe with only one minor complication [121]. This has the potential to treat variable distal gastric pathology by this type of NOTES anastomosis.

3.2. Appendicectomy

The first human NOTES procedure was Tg appendicectomy performed by Rao and Reddy in 2004 in India. Many cases were reported after that [122, 123]. German registry showed that more than 6% [182 cases] of human NOTES procedure was appendicectomy done by Tg and Tv routes. Not only slim patients but also morbidly obese patients benefited from NOTES appendicectomy [124]. A 5-mm trocar was inserted through the umbilicus and a 5-mm telescope was placed. A 12-mm trocar and a 5-mm grasper were inserted separately through the posterior fornix of the vagina under laparoscopic guidance. The appendix was divided with an endoscopic stapler through the Tv 12-mm trocar and removed from the same trocar [125].

3.3. Colonic NOTES

Pure NOTES resection and anastomosis of the large bowel were feasible, and the colorectal anastomosis was achieved using circular stapler [126]. Early clinical series of transanal TME with laparoscopic assistance (n = 72) were promising, with overall intraoperative and postoperative complication rates of 8.3% and 27.8%, respectively, similar to laparoscopic TME [127]. NOTES TME was feasible and safe in this series of patients with mid- or low rectal tumours [128]. Transanal full-thickness circumferential rectal and mesorectal dissections were performed, and a colorectal anastomosis was performed using a circular stapler with a single stapling technique. During the transanal approach, the gastrotomy was closed using four endoscopic clips [129]. On large series of human cadavers, transanal NOTES rectosigmoid resection with TME was feasible and demonstrates improvement in specimen length and operative time with experience. Transrectal retrograde rectosigmoid dissection was achieved in all attempts and showed numbers of lymph nodes similar to the laparoscopic group [130, 131]. A transrectal endoscopic device was used for optic assistance, colon dissection, ileum section and specimen retrieval. Transrectal MA-NOS total colectomy was assisted by three laparoscopic ports: A 12-mm port is used as the terminal ileostomy site [132]. Hybrid Tv resection of descending colon was feasible on animal model. Only one 5-mm transumbilical port was added for safety [133]. Long-segment Hirschsprung's disease was managed by NOTES. Authors reported the technique, which starts by a rectal mucosectomy 0.5 cm proximal to the dentate line and extending proximally to the level of the intraperitoneal rectum. Three cannulas were inserted through the muscular sleeve into the abdominal cavity. After colonic mobilisation, the ganglionic distal bowel segment was pulled through the anus and resected and the colo-anal anastomosis was created [134], (see table 2).

Authors	Year	Reference	Operation	Human subjects	Animal subjects
Demura et al.	2013	[119]	Small bowel anastomosis	No	Yes
Barthet M et al.	2015	[120]	Gastroenterostomy	Yes	No
Lehman et al.	2014	[122]	Appendicectomy	Yes	No
Bernhardt J et al.	2012	[125]	Sigmoid colectomy	No	Yes
Chouillard et al.	2014	[127]	TME	Yes	No
Park SJ et al.	2013	[128]	Rectosigmoid resection	No	Yes
Telem DA et al.	2013	[129]	TME [cadavers]	Yes	No
Lacy AM et al.	2012	[131]	Hybrid total colectomy	Yes	No
Alba mesa et al.	2012	[132]	Descending colon resection	No	Yes
Li N et al.	2013	[133]	Hirschsprung's segment resection	Yes	No

Table 2. Important lower GI NOTES procedures

4. Further research

NOTES is evolving and refinement of the technique is warranted for feasibility, safety, operative time effectiveness and practicality. Three hot areas are expected to be the focus for further research:

1.   Development of technology: this includes instruments, optics and working platforms.

2. Exploration of practicality of NOTES application in complex abdominal procedures and new fields like thoracic and retroperitoneal procedures.

3. Training: NOTES needs an advanced endoscopic and minimal access skills. Surgeons who already attended this level are those who are leading NOTES research in the respected academic institutions in the USA, Europe and Asia. What is needed is to organise an effective and specific dedicated training programme to produce NOTES trained surgeons. NOTES is expected to be an independent specialty that works to meet patient's expectation by making the most use of modern surgery and technology.

5. Conclusions

NOTES is gaining interest and popularity among surgeons. Many new procedures are reported as feasibility studies on animal models. Other procedures are starting to establish itself in clinical practice like NOTES cholecystectomy, appendicectomy and peritoneoscopy. Tv and Tg access routes are the commonest and closure technique is evolving to achieve a high degree of safety and effectiveness. Many new clinical procedures are introduced and currently are at experimental level. Development of the technology and instrumentation, effective training and support are expected to push NOTES further towards its long track of refinement and milestone journey towards an accepted and well-established standard technique.

Author details

Abdulzahra Hussain[1,2*]

Address all correspondence to: abdulzahra.hussain@nhs.net

1 Upper GI Surgeon at Airedale Hospital NHS Foundation Trust, Keighley, Bradford, UK

2 Honorary Senior Lecturer, King's College Medical School, London, UK

References

[1] Lau WY, Leow CK, Li AK. History of endoscopic and laparoscopic surgery. World J Surg. 1997;21(4):444-453.

[2] José FN. and Angel C.. NOTES, MANOS, SILS and other new laparoendoscopic techniques.World J Gastrointest Endosc. 2012; 4(6): 212-7.

[3] Hatzinger M1, Fesenko A, Sohn M. The first human laparoscopy and NOTES operation: Dimitrij Oscarovic Ott (1855-1929).Urol Int. 2014;92(4):387-91.

[4] http://www.baus.org.uk/Resources/BAUS/Documents/10-hopkins.pdf. Date of access 13/11/2014.

[5] Kalloo AN1, Singh VK, Jagannath SB, Niiyama H, Hill SL, Vaughn CA, Magee CA, Kantsevoy SV. Flexible transgastric peritoneoscopy: a novel approach to diagnostic and therapeutic interventions in the peritoneal cavity. Gastrointest Endosc. 2004 ; 60(1):114-7.

[6] Hussain A, Mahmood H. NOTES: current status and expectations. European Surgery.2008; 40(4);176-186.

[7] Von Renteln D1, Gutmann TE, Schmidt A, Vassiliou MC, Rudolph HU, Caca K. Standard diagnostic laparoscopy is superior to NOTES approaches: results of a blinded randomized controlled porcine study. Endoscopy. 2012;44(6):596-604.

[8] Auyang ED, Santos BF, Enter DH, Hungness ES, Soper NJ.Natural orifice translumenal endoscopic surgery (NOTES(®)): a technical review.Surg Endosc. 2011;25(10): 3135-48

[9] Gillen S1, Gröne J, Knödgen F, Wolf P, Meyer M, Friess H, Buhr HJ, Ritz JP, Feussner H, Lehmann KS. Educational and training aspects of new surgical techniques: experience with the endoscopic–laparoscopic interdisciplinary training entity (ELITE) model in training for a natural orifice translumenal endoscopic surgery (NOTES) approach to appendectomy. Surg Endosc. 2012;26(8):2376-82.

[10] Song S, Itawi EA, Saber AA. Natural orifice translumenal endoscopic surgery (NOTES). J Invest Surg. 2009;22(3):214-7.

[11] Cassera MA1, Zheng B, Spaun GO, Swanström LL. Optimizing surgical approach for natural orifice translumenal endoscopic procedures. Surg Innov. 2012;19(4):433-7.

[12] Rattner D, Kalloo AN, The SAGES/ASGE working group on natural orifice translumenal endoscopic surgery ASGE/SAGES working group on natural orifice translumenal endoscopic surgery. Surg Endosc. 2005;20(2):329–33.

[13] Rattner D. Introduction to NOTES white paper. Surg Endosc. 2006;20(2):185.

[14] http://www.nesacademy.org/projects.html. Date of access 03/12/2014.

[15] Dargar S1, Solley T, Nemani A, Brino C, Sankaranarayanan G, De S. The development of a haptic interface for the Virtual Translumenal Endoscopic Surgical Trainer (VTEST). Stud Health Technol Inform. 2013;184:106-8.

[16] Gillen S, Fiolka A, Kranzfelder M, Wolf P, Feith M, Schneider A, Meining A, Friess H, Feussner H.Training of a standardized natural orifice transluminal endoscopic surgery cholecystectomy using an ex vivo training unit. Endoscopy. 2011;43(10): 876-81.

[17] Schwaitzberg SD1, Hawes RH, Rattner DW, Kochman ML. Novel challenges of multi-society investigator-initiated studies: a paradigm shift for technique and technology evaluation. Surg Endosc. 2013;27(8):2673-7.

[18] http://www.endonurse.com/news/2009/07/olympus-donates-250-000-to-notes-research.aspx. Date of access 03/12/2014.

[19] http://www.cimit.org/programs-notes.html. Date of access 25/12/2014.

[20] Chow A1, Purkayastha S, Dosanjh D, Sarvanandan R, Ahmed I, Paraskeva P. Patient reported outcomes and their importance in the development of novel surgical techniques. Surg Innov. 2012;19(3):327-34.

[21] Swanstrom LL1, Volckmann E, Hungness E, Soper NJ. Patient attitudes and expectations regarding natural orifice translumenal endoscopic surgery. Surg Endosc. 2009;23(7):1519-25.

[22] Fei YF, Fei L, Salazar M, Renton DB, Hazey JW. Transvaginal surgery: do women want it. J Laparoendosc Adv Surg Tech A. 2014;24(10):676-83.

[23] Ryou M1, Hazan R, Rahme L, Thompson CC. An ex vivo bacteriologic study comparing antiseptic techniques for natural orifice translumenal endoscopic surgery (NOTES) via the gastrointestinal tract. Dig Dis Sci. 2012;57(8):2130-6.

[24] Yang QY1, Zhang GY, Wang L, Wang ZG, Li F, Li YQ, Ding XJ, Hu SY. Infection during transgastric and transvaginal natural orifice transluminal endoscopic surgery in a live porcine model. Chin Med J (Engl). 2011;124(4):556-61.

[25] Memark VC1, Anderson JB, Nau PN, Shah N, Needleman BJ, Mikami DJ, Melvin WS, Hazey JW. Transgastric endoscopic peritoneoscopy does not lead to increased risk of infectious complications. Surg Endosc. 2011;25(7):2186-91.

[26] Nau P1, Ellison EC, Muscarella P Jr, Mikami D, Narula VK, Needleman B, Melvin WS, Hazey JW. A review of 130 humans enrolled in transgastric NOTES protocols at a single institution. Surg Endosc. 2011;25(4):1004-11.

[27] Georgescu I1, Saftoiu A, Patrascu S, Silosi I, Georgescu E, Surlin V. Perioperative inflammatory response in natural orifice translumenal endoscopic surgery. Surg Endosc. 2013;27(7):2551-6.

[28] Sodergren MH1, Pucher P, Clark J, James DR, Sockett J, Matar N, Teare J, Yang GZ, Darzi A. Disinfection of the access orifice in NOTES: evaluation of the evidence base. Diagn Ther Endosc. 2011;(2011):245175. doi: 10.1155/2011/245175.

[29] Fyock CJ1, Kowalczyk LM, Gupte AR, Forsmark CE, Wagh MS. Complications during natural orifice translumenal endoscopic surgery: endoscopic management of splenic laceration and hemorrhage. J Laparoendosc Adv Surg Tech A. 2011;21(1):39-43.

[30] Fyock CJ1, Forsmark CE, Wagh MS. Endoscopic management of intraoperative small bowel laceration during natural orifice translumenal endoscopic surgery: a blinded porcine study. Surg Tech A. 2011;21(6):525-30.

[31] Fyock CJ1, Parekattil SJ, Atalah H, Su LM, Forsmark CE, Wagh MS. The NOTES approach to management of urinary bladder injury. JSLS. 2011;15(3):285-90.

[32] Donatsky AM. Assessing transgastric natural orifice transluminal endoscopic surgery prior to clinical implementation. Dan Med J. 2014;61(8):B4903.

[33] Sanz AF1, Hoppo T, Witteman BP, Brown BN, Gilbert TW, Badylak SF, Jobe BA, Nieponice A. In vivo assessment of a biological occluder for NOTES gastrotomy closure. Surg Laparosc Endosc Percutan Tech. 2014;24(4):322-6.

[34] Liu L1, Chiu PW, Teoh AY, Lam CC, Ng EK, Lau JY. Endoscopic suturing is superior to endoclips for closure of gastrotomy after natural orifices translumenal endoscopic surgery (NOTES): an ex vivo study. Surg Endosc. 2014 ;28(4):1342-7.

[35] Lee SH1, Cho WY, Cho JY. Submucosal endoscopy, a new era of pure natural orifice translumenal endoscopic surgery (NOTES).Clin Endosc. 2012;45(1):4-10.

[36] Sanz AF, Hoppo T, Witteman BP, Brown BN, Gilbert TW, Badylak SF, Jobe BA, Nieponice A. In vivo assessment of a biological occluder for NOTES gastrotomy closure. Surg Laparosc Endosc Percutan Tech. 2014;24(4):322-6.

[37] Sun G, Yang Y, Zhang X, Li W, Wang Y, Zhang L, Tang P, Kong J, Zhang R, Meng J, Wang X. Comparison of gastrotomy closure modalities for natural orifice transluminal surgery: a canine study. Gastrointest Endosc. 2013;77(5):774-83.

[38] Guarner-Argente C1, Beltrán M, Martínez-Pallí G, Navarro-Ripoll R, Martínez-Zamora MÀ, Córdova H, Comas J, De Miguel CR, Rodríguez-D'Jesús A, Almela M, Hernández-Cera C, Lacy AM, Fernández-Esparrach G. Infection during natural orifice transluminal endoscopic surgery peritoneoscopy: a randomized comparative study in a survival porcine model. J Minim Invasive Gynecol. 2011;18(6):741-6.

[39] Romanelli JR1, Desilets DJ, Chapman CN, Surti VC, Lovewell C, Earle DB. Loop-anchor purse-string closure of gastrotomy in NOTES(R) procedures: survival studies in a porcine model. Surg Innov. 2010;17(4):312-7.

[40] Dostalik J, Gunkova P, Gunka I, Mazur M, Mrazek T. Laparoscopic gastric resection with natural orifice specimen extraction for postulcer pyloric stenosis.Wideochir Inne Tech Malo Inwazyjne. 2014; 9(2): 282–285.

[41] Sanz AF1, Hoppo T, Witteman BP, Brown BN, Gilbert TW, Badylak SF, Jobe BA, Nieponice A. In vivo assessment of a biological occluder for NOTES gastrotomy closure. Surg Laparosc Endosc Percutan Tech. 2014;24(4):322-6.

[42] Ryska O, Martinek J, Filipkova T, Dolezel R, Juhasova J, Motlik J, Zavoral M, Ryska M. Single loop-and-clips technique (KING closure) for gastrotomy closure after

transgastric ovariectomy: a survival experiment. Wideochir Inne Tech Malo Inwazyjne. 2012 ;7(4):233-9.

[43] Hookey LC, Khokhotva V, Bielawska B, et al. The Queen's closure: a novel technique for closure of endoscopic gastrotomy for natural-orifice transluminal endoscopic surgery. Endoscopy. 2009;41(2):149–53.

[44] Gopal J1, Pauli EM, Haluck RS, Moyer MT, Mathew A. Intramural acellular porcine dermal matrix (APDM)-assisted gastrotomy closure for natural orifice transluminal endoscopic surgery (NOTES). Surg Endosc. 2012;26(8):2322-30.

[45] Azadani A1, Bergström M, Dot J, Abu-Suboh-Abadia M, Armengol-Miró JR, Park PO. A new in vivo method for testing closures of gastric NOTES incisions using leak of the closure or gastric yield as endpoints. J Laparoendosc Adv Surg Tech A. 2012 ; 22(1):46-50.

[46] Sodergren MH1, Markar S, Pucher PH, Badran IA, Jiao LR, Darzi A. Safety of transvaginal hybrid NOTES cholecystectomy: a systematic review and meta-analysis. Surg Endosc. 2014; (26) [Epub ahead of print].

[47] Wood SG1, Panait L, Duffy AJ, Bell RL, Roberts KE. Complications of transvaginal natural orifice transluminal endoscopic surgery: a series of 102 patients. Ann Surg. 2014;259(4):744-9.

[48] Zornig C1, Mofid H, Siemssen L, Wenck CH. Transvaginal access for NOTES. Chirurg. 2010;81(5):426-30.

[49] Kono Y1, Yasuda K, Hiroishi K, Akagi T, Kawaguchi K, Suzuki K, Yoshizumi F, Inomata M, Shiraishi N, Kitano S. Transrectal peritoneal access with the submucosal tunnel technique in NOTES: a porcine survival study. Surg Endosc. 2013;27(1):278-85.

[50] Sodergren M1, Clark J, Beardsley J, Bryant T, Horton K, Darzi A, Teare J. A novel flexible endoluminal stapling device for use in NOTES colotomy closure: a feasibility study using an ex vivo porcine model. Surg Endosc. 2011;25(10):3266-72.

[51] Diana M1, Leroy J, Wall J, De Ruijter V, Lindner V, Dhumane P, Mutter D, Marescaux J. Prospective experimental study of transrectal viscerotomy closure using transanal endoscopic suture vs. circular stapler: a step toward NOTES. Endoscopy. 2012 ;44(6):605-11.

[52] Ryska O1, Filípková T, Martínek J, Dolezel R, Juhás S, Juhásová J, Zavoral M, Ryska M. [Transrectal hybrid NOTES versus laparoscopic cholecystectomy--a randomized prospective study in a large laboratory animal] Rozhl Chir. 2011;90(12):695-700.

[53] Moran EA1, Bingener J, Murad F, Levy MJ, Gostout CJ. The challenges with NOTES retroperitoneal access in humans. Surg Endosc. 2011;25(4):1096-100.

[54] Bin X1, Bo Y, Dan S, Okhunov Z, Ghiraldi E, Huiqing W, Friedlander J, Liang X, Yinghao S, Kavoussi LR. A novel transvesical port for natural orifice translumenal endoscopic surgery. J Endourol. 2012;26(3):219-23.

[55] Jeong CW1, Oh JJ, Abdullajanov M, Yeon J, Lee HE, Jeong SJ, Hong SK, Byun SS, Lee SB, Kim HH, Lee SE. Pure transvesical NOTES uterine horn resection in swine as an appendectomy model. Surg Endosc. 2012;26(2):558-64.

[56] Bhullar JS, Subhas G, Gupta A, Jacobs MJ, Decker M, Silberberg B, Mittal VK. Transvesical NOTES: survival study in porcine model. JSLS. 2012;16(4):606-11.

[57] Kranzfelder M1, Schneider A2, Fiolka A2, Koller S2, Wilhelm D2, Reiser S2, Meining A2, Feussner H2. What do we really need? Visions of an ideal human-machine interface for NOTES mechatronic support systems from the view of surgeons, gastroenterologists, and medical engineers. Surg Innov. 2014;(23). pii: 1553350614550720. [Epub ahead of print].

[58] Thakkar S1, Awad M2, Gurram KC3, Tully S4, Wright C4, Sanan S4, Choset H4. A novel, new robotic platform for natural orifice distal pancreatectomy. Surg Innov. 2014(15). pii: 1553350614554232. [Epub ahead of print].

[59] Yasuda K, Kitano S, Ikeda K, Sumiyama K, Tajiri H. Assessment of a manipulator device for NOTES with basic surgical skill tests: a bench study. Surg Laparosc Endosc Percutan Tech. 2014;24(5):e191-5.

[60] Addis M1, Aguirre M, Frecker M, Haluck R, Matthew A, Pauli E, Gopal J. Development of tasks and evaluation of a prototype forceps for NOTES. JSLS. 2012;16(1): 95-104.

[61] Villamizar N1, Pryor AD. SPIDER and flexible laparoscopy: the next frontier in abdominal surgery. Surg Technol Int. 2010 ;20:53-8.

[62] Midday J1, Nelson CA, Oleynikov D. Improvements in robotic natural orifice surgery with a novel material handling system. Surg Endosc. 2013;27(9):3474-7.

[63] http://www.bbraun.com. Date of access 21/12/2014.

[64] Sohail N Shaikh and Christopher C Thompson. Natural orifice translumenal surgery: Flexible platform review.World J Gastrointest Surg. 2010;27; 2(6): 210-6.

[65] Swanström L, Swain P, Denk P. Development and validation of a new generation of flexible endoscope for NOTES. Surg Innov. 2009;(16):104-10.

[66] Ji Hyeon Lee, Chan Jong Chung, Seung Cheo Lee, Ho Jin Shin. Anesthetic management of transoral natural orifice transluminal endoscopic surgery: two cases report. Korean J Anesthesiol. 2014;67(2):148-52.

[67] Schaefer M. Natural orifice transluminal endoscopic surgery (NOTES): implications for anesthesia. F1000 Med Rep. 2009;1:80. doi: 10.3410/M1-80.

[68] Phalanusitthepha C, Inoue H, Ikeda H, Sato H, Sato C, Hokierti C. Peroral endoscopic myotomy for esophageal achalasia. Ann Transl Med. 2014;2(3):31.

[69] Grabowski JE, Talamini MA. Physiological effects of pneumoperitoneum. J Gastrointest Surg. 2009;13(5):1009-16.

[70] Pucher P1, Sodergren MH, Alkhusheh M, Clark J, Jethwa P, Teare J, Yang GZ, Darzi A. The effects of natural orifice translumenal endoscopic surgery (NOTES) on cardiorespiratory physiology: a systematic review. Surg Innov. 2013;20(2):183-9.

[71] Chang ET1, Ruhl DS, Kenny PR, Sniezek JC. Endoscopic management of esophageal discontinuity. Head Neck. 2014;(1). doi: 10.1002/hed.23883 [Epub ahead of print].

[72] Modayil R, Savides T, Scott DJ, Swanstrom LL, Vassiliou MC. Per-oral endoscopic myotomy white paper summary. NOSCAR POEM White Paper Committee, Stavropoulos SN, Desilets DJ, Fuchs KH, Gostout CJ, Haber G, Inoue H, Kochman ML, Gastrointest Endosc. 2014;80(1):1-15.

[73] Achem SR1, Gerson LB. Distal esophageal spasm: an update. Curr Gastroenterol Rep. 2013;15(9):325.

[74] Smith SR1, Genden EM, Urken ML. Endoscopic stapling technique for the treatment of Zenker diverticulum vs standard open-neck technique: a direct comparison and charge analysis. Arch Otolaryngol Head Neck Surg. 2002;128(2):141-4.

[75] Woodward TA, Jamil LH, Wallace MB. Natural orifice trans-luminal endoscopic surgery in the esophagus. Gastrointestinal Endoscopy Clinics of North America. 2010;20(1):123-138.

[76] Magno p, Khashab MA, Mas M, Giday SA, Buscaglia JA, Shin EJ, Dray X, and Kalloo AN. Natural orifice translumenal endoscopic surgery for anterior spinal procedures. Minim Invasive Surg. 2012;2012: 365814. doi: 10.1155/2012/365814.

[77] Wilhelm D1, Meining A, Schneider A, Von Delius S, Preissel A, Sager J, Fiolka A, Friess H, Feussner H. NOTES for the cardia: antireflux therapy via transluminal access. Endoscopy. 2010;42(12):1085-91.

[78] Ishimaru T1, Iwanaka T, Hatanaka A, Kawashima H, Terawaki K. Translumenal esophageal anastomosis for natural orifice translumenal endoscopic surgery: an ex vivo feasibility study. J Laparoendosc Adv Surg Tech A. 2012;22(7):724-9.

[79] Brian G Turner, Denise W Gee. Natural orifice transesophageal thoracoscopic surgery: A review of the current state. World J Gastrointest Endosc. 2010; 2(1):3-9.

[80] Dostalik J1, Gunkova P2, Gunka I3, Mazur M2, Mrazek T1. Laparoscopic gastric resection with natural orifice specimen extraction for postulcer pyloric stenosis. Wideochir Inne Tech Malo Inwazyjne. 2014;9(2):282-5.

[81] Yi SW1, Chung MJ, Jo JH, Lee KJ, Park JY, Bang S, Park SW, Song SY. Gastrojejunostomy by pure natural orifice transluminal endoscopic surgery using a newly de-

signed anastomosing metal stent in a porcine model. Surg Endosc. 2014;28(5): 1439-46.

[82] Elazary R1, Schlager A2, Khalaileh A2, Mintz Y2. Laparoscopic sleeve gastrectomy with transgastric visualization: another step toward totally NOTES procedures. Surg Innov. 2014;21(5):464-8.

[83] Nakajima K1, Takahashi T1, Yamasaki M1, Kurokawa Y1, Miyazaki Y1, Miyata H1, Takiguchi S1, Mori M1, Doki Y1. [Transvaginal natural orifice translumenal endoscopic surgery partial gastrectomy: initial clinical experience] Nihon Geka Gakkai Zasshi. 2013;114(6):303-7.

[84] Heo J1, Jeon SW. Hybrid natural orifice transluminal endoscopic surgery in gastric subepithelial tumors. World J Gastrointest Endosc. 2013;16;5(9):428-32.

[85] Lee SH1, Kim SJ, Lee TH, Chung IK, Park SH, Kim EO, Lee HJ, Cho HD. Human applications of submucosal endoscopy under conscious sedation for pure natural orifice transluminal endoscopic surgery. Surg Endosc. 2013;27(8):3016-20.

[86] Dotai T1, Coker AM, Antozzi L, Acosta G, Michelotti M, Bildzukewicz N, Sandler BJ, Jacobsen GR, Talamini MA, Horgan S. Transgastric large-organ extraction: the initial human experience. Surg Endosc. 2013;27(2):394-9.

[87] Buesing M1, Utech M, Halter J, Riege R, Saada G, Knapp A. [Sleeve gastrectomy in the treatment of morbid obesity. Study results and first experiences with the transvaginal hybrid NOTES technique] Chirurg. 2011;82(8):675-83.

[88] Ishimaru T1, Iwanaka T, Kawashima H, Terawaki K, Kodaka T, Suzuki K, Takahashi M. A pilot study of laparoscopic gastric pull-up by using the natural orifice translumenal endoscopic surgery technique: a novel procedure for treating long-gap esophageal atresia (type a). J Laparoendosc Adv Surg Tech A. 2011;21(9):851-7.

[89] Moran EA1, Gostout CJ, McConico AL, Michalek J, Huebner M, Bingener J. Assessing the invasiveness of NOTES perforated viscus repair: a comparative study of NOTES and laparoscopy. Surg Endosc. 2012;26(1):103-9.

[90] Mori H1, Kobara H, Kobayashi M, Muramatsu A, Nomura T, Hagiike M, Izuishi K, Suzuki Y, Masaki T. Establishment of pure NOTES procedure using a conventional flexible endoscope: review of six cases of gastric gastrointestinal stromal tumors. Endoscopy. 2011;43(7):631-4.

[91] Alford C, Hanson R. Evaluation of a transvaginal laparoscopic natural orifice transluminal endoscopic surgery approach to the abdomen of mares. Vet Surg. 2010;39(7): 873-8.

[92] Hyder Q1, Zahid MA, Ahmad W, Rashid R, Hadi SF, Qazi S, Haider HK. Diagnostic transgastric flexible peritoneoscopy: is pure natural orifice transluminal endoscopic surgery a fantasy? Singapore Med J. 2008;49(12):e375-81.

[93]   Potter K1, Swanstrom L. Natural orifice surgery (NOTES) and biliary disease, is there a role? J Hepatobiliary Pancreat Surg. 2009;16(3): 261-5.

[94]   Fyock CJ, Kirtane TS, Forsmark CE, Wagh MS. Intraoperative NOTES endosonography and identification of mock hepatic lesions. Surg Laparosc Endosc Percutan Tech. 2012;22(1):e1-4.

[95]   Tagaya N1, Kubota K. NOTES: approach to the liver and spleen. J Hepatobiliary Pancreat Surg. 2009;16(3):283-7.

[96]   Shi H1, Jiang SJ, Li B, Fu DK, Xin P, Wang YG. Natural orifice transluminal endoscopic wedge hepatic resection with a water-jet hybrid knife in a non-survival porcine model. World J Gastroenterol. 2011;17(7):926-31.

[97]   Ohdaira T1, Endo K, Abe N, Yasuda Y. Transintestinal hepatectomy performed by hybrid NOTES using a customized X-TRACT Tissue Morcellator with an electrifiable round cutter. J Hepatobiliary Pancreat Surg. 2009;16(3):274-82.

[98]   Phee SJ1, Ho KY, Lomanto D, Low SC, Huynh VA, Kencana AP, Yang K, Sun ZL, Chung SC. Natural orifice transgastric endoscopic wedge hepatic resection in an experimental model using an intuitively controlled master and slave transluminal endoscopic robot (MASTER). Surg Endosc. 2010;24(9):2293-8.

[99]   Truong T1, Arnaoutakis D, Awad ZT. Laparoscopic hybrid NOTES liver resection for metastatic colorectal cancer. Surg Laparosc Endosc Percutan Tech. 2012;22(1):e5-7.

[100] Saftoiu A1, Bhutani MS, Vilmann P, Surlin V, Uthamanthil RK, Lee JH, Bektas M, Singh H, Ionut D, Gheonea, Pactrascu S, Gupta V, Katz MH, Fleming JB. Feasibility study of EUS-NOTES as a novel approach for pancreatic cancer staging and therapy: an international collaborative study. Hepatogastroenterology. 2013;60(121):180-6.

[101] Wang XW, Fan CQ, Wang L, Guo H, Xie X, Zhao GC, Zhao XY. Transoralgastric gastroscopic debridement for peripancreatic abscess: a special case report. Hepatogastroenterology. 2011;58(110-111):1801-4.

[102] Endoscopic transgastric vs surgical necrosectomy for infected necrotizing pancreatitis: a randomized trial. Bakker OJ, Van Santvoort HC, Van Brunschot S, Geskus RB, Besselink MG, Bollen TL, Van Eijck CH, Fockens P, Hazebroek EJ, Nijmeijer RM, Poley JW, Van Ramshorst B, Vleggaar FP, Boermeester MA, Gooszen HG, Weusten BL, Timmer R; Dutch Pancreatitis Study Group.JAMA. 2012;07(10):1053-61.

[103] Pallapothu R1, Earle DB, Desilets DJ, Romanelli JR. NOTES(®) stapled cystgastrostomy: a novel approach for surgical management of pancreatic pseudocysts. Surg Endosc. 2011;25(3):883-9.

[104] Thakkar S, Awad M, Gurram KC, Tully S, Wright C, Sanan S, Choset H. A novel, new robotic platform for natural orifice distal pancreatectomy. Surg Innov. 2014;(15). pii: 1553350614554232 [Epub ahead of print].

[105] Tomikawa M1, Akahoshi T, Kinjo N, Uehara H, Hashimoto N, Nagao Y, Kamori M, Kumashiro R, Maehara Y, Hashizume M. Rigid and flexible endoscopic rendezvous in spatium peritonealis may be an effective tactic for laparoscopic megasplenectomy: significant implications for pure natural orifice translumenal endoscopic surgery. Surg Endosc. 2012; 26(12): 3573-9.

[106] Tagaya N1, Kubota K. NOTES: approach to the liver and spleen. J Hepatobiliary Pancreat Surg. 2009;16(3):283-7.

[107] Targarona EM, Gomez C, Rovira R, Pernas JC, Balague C, Guarner-Argente C, Sainz S, Trias M. NOTES-assisted transvaginal splenectomy: the next step in the minimally invasive approach to the spleen. Surg Innov. 2009;16(3):218-22.

[108] Nemani A1, Sankaranarayanan G, Olasky JS, Adra S, Roberts KE, Panait L, Schwaitzberg SD, Jones DB, De S. A comparison of NOTES transvaginal and laparoscopic cholecystectomy procedures based upon task analysis. Surg Endosc. 2014;28(8): 2443-51.

[109] Lehmann KS1, Zornig C, Arlt G, Butters M, Bulian DR, Manger R, Burghardt J, Runkel N, Pürschel A, Köninger J, Buhr HJ. [Natural orifice transluminal endoscopic surgery in Germany : Data from the German NOTES registry.] Chirurg. 2014; (5) [Epub ahead of print].

[110] A Hussain. Upper GI natural orifice translumenal endoscopic surgery: what is new? European Surgery. 2014; 46(1): 3-11.

[111] Sodergren MH1, Markar S, Pucher PH, Badran IA, Jiao LR, Darzi A. Safety of transvaginal hybrid NOTES cholecystectomy: a systematic review and meta-analysis. Surg Endosc. 2014;26 [Epub ahead of print].

[112] Yasuda K1, Kitano S. Lymph node navigation for pancreatic and biliary malignancy by NOTES. J Hepatobiliary Pancreat Sci. 2010;17(5):617-21.

[113] Chouillard EK1, Al Khoury M, Bader G, Heitz D, Elrassi Z, Fauconnier A. Intercontinental Society of Natural Orifice, Endoscopic, Laparoscopic Surgery (i-NOELS), Poissy, France. Combined vaginal and abdominal approach to sleeve gastrectomy for morbid obesity in women: a preliminary experience. Surg Obes Relat Dis. 2011;7(5): 581-6.

[114] Elazary R, Schlager A, Khalaileh A, Mintz Y. Laparoscopic sleeve gastrectomy with transgastric visualization: another step toward totally NOTES procedures. Surg Innov. 2014;21(5):464-8.

[115] Mintz Y, Horgan S, Savu MK, Cullen J, Chock A, Ramamoorthy S, Easter DW, Talamini MA. Hybrid natural orifice translumenal surgery (NOTES) sleeve gastrectomy: a feasibility study using an animal model. Surg Endosc. 2008;22(8):1798-802.

[116] Fischer LJ, Jacobsen G, Wong B, Thompson K, Bosia J, Talamini M, Horgan S. NOTES laparoscopic-assisted transvaginal sleeve gastrectomy in humans--description of preliminary experience in the United States. Surg Obes Relat Dis. 2009;5(5):633-6.

[117] Hagen ME1, Wagner OJ, Swain P, Pugin F, Buchs N, Caddedu M, Jamidar P, Fasel J, Morel P. Hybrid natural orifice transluminal endoscopic surgery (NOTES) for Roux-en-Y gastric bypass: an experimental surgical study in human cadavers. Endoscopy. 2008;40(11):918-24.

[118] Nau P, Anderson J, Yuh B, Muscarella P Jr, Christopher Ellison E, Happel L, Narula VK, Melvin WS, Hazey JW. Diagnostic transgastric endoscopic peritoneoscopy: extension of the initial human trial for staging of pancreatic head masses. Surg Endosc. 2010 ;24:1440-6.

[119] Michalik M, Orlowski M, Bobowicz M, Frask A, Trybull A. The first report on hybrid NOTES adjustable gastric banding in human. Obes Surg. 2011;21:524-7.

[120] Demura Y, Ishikawa N, Hirano Y, Inaki N, Matsunoki A, Watanabe G. Transrectal robotic natural orifice translumenal endoscopic surgery (NOTES) applied to intestinal anastomosis in a porcine intestine model. Surg Endosc. 2013; 27(12): 4693-701.

[121] Barthet M, Binmoeller KF, Vanbiervliet G, Gonzalez JM, Baron TH, Berdah S. Natural orifice transluminal endoscopic surgery gastroenterostomy with a biflanged lumen-apposing stent: first clinical experience (with videos). Gastrointest Endosc. 2015 ; 81(1):215-8.

[122] Tian Y, Wu SD, Chen YH, Wang DB. Transvaginal laparoscopic appendectomy simultaneously with vaginal hysterectomy: initial experience of 10 cases. Med Sci Monit. 2014;10(20):1897-901.

[123] Lehmann KS1, Zornig C, Arlt G, Butters M, Bulian DR, Manger R, Burghardt J, Runkel N, Pürschel A, Köninger J, Buhr HJ. [Natural orifice transluminal endoscopic surgery in Germany: Data from the German NOTES registry.] Chirurg. 2014 Jul 5 [Epub ahead of print].

[124] Yagci MA1, Kayaalp C1, Ates M1. Transvaginal appendectomy in morbidly obese patient. Case Rep Surg. 2014;2014:368640. doi: 10.1155/2014/368640.

[125] Knuth J, Heiss MM, Bulian DR. Transvaginal hybrid-NOTES appendectomy in routine clinical use: prospective analysis of 13 cases and description of the procedure. Surg Endosc. 2014;28(9):2661-5.

[126] Bernhardt J, Köhler P, Rieber F, Diederich M, Schneider-Koriath S, Steffen H, Ludwig K, Lamadé W. Pure NOTES sigmoid resection in an animal survival model. Endoscopy. 2012;44(3):265-9.

[127] Emhoff IA1, Lee GC, Sylla P. Transanal colorectal resection using natural orifice translumenal endoscopic surgery (NOTES). Dig Endosc. 2014 Jan;26(1):29-42.

[128] Chouillard E, Chahine E, Khoury G, Vinson-Bonnet B, Gumbs A, Azoulay D, Abdalla E. Notes total mesorectal excision (TME) for patients with rectal neoplasia: a preliminary experience.Surg Endosc 2014;28; (11):3150-7.

[129] Park SJ, Lee KY, Choi SI, Kang BM, Huh C, Choi DH, Lee CK. Pure NOTES rectosigmoid resection: transgastric endoscopic IMA dissection and transanal rectal mobilization in animal models. J Laparoendosc Adv Surg Tech A. 2013;23(7):592-5.

[130] Telem DA, Han KS, Kim MC, Ajari I, Sohn DK, Woods K, Kapur V, Sbeih MA, Perretta S, Rattner DW, Sylla P. Transanal rectosigmoid resection via natural orifice translumenal endoscopic surgery (NOTES) with total mesorectal excision in a large human cadaver series. Surg Endosc. 2013;27(1):74-80.

[131] Rieder E1, Spaun GO, Khajanchee YS, Martinec DV, Arnold BN, Smith Sehdev AE, Swanstrom LL, Whiteford MH. A natural orifice transrectal approach for oncologic resection of the rectosigmoid: an experimental study and comparison with conventional laparoscopy. Surg Endosc. 2011;25(10):3357-63.

[132] Lacy AM, Saavedra-Perez D, Bravo R, Adelsdorfer C, Aceituno M, Balust J. Minilaparoscopy-assisted natural orifice total colectomy: technical report of a minilaparoscopy-assisted transrectal resection. Surg Endosc. 2012;26(7):2080-5.

[133] Alba Mesa F, Amaya Cortijo A, Romero Fernandez JM, Komorowski AL, Sanchez Hurtado MA, Sanchez Margallo FM. Totally transvaginal resection of the descending colon in an experimental model. Surg Endosc. 2012;26(3):877-81.

[134] Li N, Zhang W, Yu D, Sun X, Wei M, Weng Y, Feng J. NOTES for surgical treatment of long-segment hirschsprung's disease: report of three cases. J Laparoendosc Adv Surg Tech A. 2013;23(12):1020-3.

[135] Spaun GO, Dunst CM, Arnold BN, Martinec DV, Cassera MA, Swanström LL.Transcervical heller myotomy using flexible endoscopy. J Gastrointest Surg. 2010;14:1902-9.

[136] Swanstrom LL, Dunst CM, Spaun GO. Future applications of flexible endoscopy in esophageal surgery. Gastrointest Surg. 2010;14 Supple 1:S127-32.

[137] Swanstorm LL, Rieder E, Duns CM. A stepwise approach and early clinical experience in peroral endoscopic myotomy for the treatment of achalasia and esophageal motility disorders. J Am Coll Surg. 2011;213:751-6.

[138] Rieder E, Martine DV, Duns CM, Sandstorm LL. Flexible endoscopic Zenkers diverticulotomy with a novel bipolar forceps: a pilot study and comparison with needle-knife dissection. Surg Endosc. 2011;25:3273-8.

[139] Ishimaru T, Iwanaka T, Kawashima H, Terawaki K, Kodaka T, Suzuki K, Takahashi M. A pilot study of laparoscopic gastric pull-up by using the natural orifice translumenal endoscopic surgery technique: a novel procedure for treating long-gap esophageal atresia (type a). J Laparoendosc Adv Surg Tech A. 2011;21:851-7.

[140] Turner BG, Kim MC, Gee DW, Dursun A, Mino-Kenudson M, Huang ES, Sylla P, Rattner DW, Brugge WR. A prospective, randomized trial of esophageal submucosal tunnel closure with a stent versus no closure to secure a transesophageal natural orifice transluminal endoscopic surgery access site. Gastrointest Endosc. 2011;73:785-90.

[141] Turner BG, Cosigner S, Kim MC, Mino-Kenudson M, Ducharme RW, Surti VC. Stent placement provides safe esophageal closure in thoracic NOTES (TM) procedures. Surg Endosc. 2011; 25:913-8.

[142] Rolanda C, Silva D, Bronco C, Madeira I, Macedo G, Correia-Pinto J. Peroral esophageal segmentectomy and anastomosis with single transthoracic trocar: a step forward in thoracic NOTES. Endoscopy. 2011;43:14-20.

[143] Cho WY, Kim YJ, Cho JY, Bok GH, Jin SY, Lee TH, Kim HG, Kim JO, Lee JS. Hybrid natural orifice transluminal endoscopic surgery: endoscopic full-thickness resection of early gastric cancer and laparoscopic regional lymph node dissection - 14 human cases. Endoscopy. 2011;43:134-9.

[144] Abe N, Takeuchi H, Yanagida O, Masaki T, Mori T, Sugiyama M, Atomi Y. Endoscopic full-thickness resection with laparoscopic assistance as hybrid NOTES for gastric submucosal tumor. Surg Endosc. 2009;23:1908-13.

[145] Chiu PW, Wai Ng EK, Teoh AY, Lam CC, Lau JY, Sung JJ. Transgastric endoluminal gastrojejunostomy: technical development from bench to animal study (with video). Gastrointest Endosc. 2010;71:390-3.

[146] Campos JM, Evangelista LF, Neto MP, Pagnossin G, Fernandes A, Ferraz AA, Ferraz EM. Translumenal endoscopic drainage of abdominal abscess due to early migration of adjustable gastric band. Obes Surg. 2010;20:247-50.

[147] Cahill RA, Asakuma M, Perretta S, Dallemagne B, Marescaux J. Gastric lymphatic mapping for sentinel node biopsy by natural orifice transluminal endoscopic surgery (NOTES). Surg Endosc. 2009;23 :1110-6.

[148] Luo H, Pan Y, Min L, Zhao L, Li J, Leung J, Xue L, Yin Z, Liu X, Liu Z, Sun A, Li C, Wu K, Guo X, Fan D. Transgastric endoscopic gastroenterostomy using a partially covered occluder: a canine feasibility study. Endoscopy. 2012;44:493-8.

[149] Ikeda K, Sumiyama K, Tajiri H, Yasuda K, Kitano S. Evaluation of a new multitasking platform for endoscopic full-thickness resection. Gastrointest Endosc. 2011;73:117-22.

[150] Lacy AM, Delgado S, Rojas OA, Ibarzabal A, Fernandez-Esparrach G, Taura P. Hybrid vaginal MA-NOS sleeve gastrectomy: technical note on the procedure in a patient. Surg Endosc. 2009;23:1130-7.

[151] Branco F, Pini G, Osório L, Cavadas V, Versos R, Gomes M, Authoring R, Correia-Pinto J, Lima E. Transvesical peritoneoscopy with rigid scope: feasibility study in human male cadaver. Surg Endosc. 2011;25:2015-9.

[152] Truong T, Arnaoutakis D, Awad ZT. Laparoscopic hybrid NOTES liver resection for metastatic colorectal cancer. Surg Laparosc Endosc Percutan Tech. 2012;22:e5-7.

[153] Shi H, Jiang SJ, Li B, Fu DK, Xin P, Wang YG. Natural orifice transluminal endoscopic wedge hepatic resection with a water-jet hybrid knife in a non-survival porcine model. World J Gastroenterol. 2011;17:926-31.

10

Guidelines for Reprocessing Non-Lumened, Heat-Sensitive ENT Endoscopes

Matteo Cavaliere and Maurizio Iemma

Abstract

Endoscopes have become an indispensable instrument in the ENT department, but their use has introduced potential health risks such as the infection transmission.

Numerous guidelines have been issued for both digestive and respiratory endoscopes, while to date specific references to ENT endoscopes do not exist. The diagnostic ENT endoscope does not generally have an operative channel, it is shorter, thinner and has a much more frequent usage. As a consequence the guidelines for digestive or respiratory endoscopes are not always functional for the ENT department.

This paper proposes:1. to standardize the correct way to carry out the disinfection procedure of heat-sensitive non-lumened ENT endoscopes, 2. to guarantee the disinfection within a limited time frame, appropriate for an ENT out-patients department.

In the initial phase the critical areas encountered in ENT endoscopy were determined. This was followed by a research of the literature in order to identify existing guidelines for the reprocessing of endoscopes with a view to establishing a common disinfection procedure of non-lumened ENT endoscopes. Finally, the new methods of disinfection, developed specifically for the reprocessing of ENT endoscopes were examined and discussed.

Keywords: Heat-sensitive ENT endoscopes, Cleaning, Disinfection

1. Introduction

The introduction of the endoscopes into clinical practice has certainly improved the diagnosis and treatment of numerous pathologies, but has also brought the risk of transmission of infections.

In the Literature, [1] the incidence of infection appears to be 1 per every 1,800,000 endoscopic procedures performed (0.000056%).

Considering the high number of endoscopic procedures performed daily worldwide, the endoscopy-related infections are those most often associated with the medical device.

In nearly all of the infections transmitted, the problem is a defect in the cleaning and disinfection procedures, [2, 3, 4] in particular during

- the pre-washing step (12%),

- the washing/disinfection step (73%),

- drying and storage (12%).

Flexible endoscopes are heat-sensitive and therefore cannot be sterilised in an autoclave, but must be disinfected. [5]

In otorhinolaryngology, unlike digestive and respiratory endoscopy, to date, no specific guidelines yet exist. ENT diagnostic endoscopes do not have the operating channel, their size is smaller and their use is more frequent, including in outpatient situations.

Then, the guidelines used in digestive and respiratory endoscopy are not always functional in the ENT department, since they do not consider the dynamism and intensity of the work carried out there.

2. Objectives

This document proposes to

1. standardise the correct method of disinfection procedures for heat-sensitive, non-channelled ENT endoscopes,

2. reduce the risk of transmitting infections,

3. increase operator safety,

4. guarantee disinfection in fast times.

3. Methods

In the initial phase, we identified the main critical procedures within ENT endoscopy departments. Next, we researched the literature to find all the guidelines on reprocessing endoscopes.

Lastly, we discussed the new disinfection methods designed specifically for the reprocessing of ENT endoscopes.

In order to form a basis for the guidelines for the reprocessing of flexible ENT endoscopes, the working group decided to conduct a survey among the Italian ENT departments with the objective to gather information regarding the methodologies actually employed for the disinfection of heat-sensitive, non-lumened endoscopes. Two hundred and seventy two questionnaires were sent out to the ENT departments. The questionnaire was divided into six sections: the first dealt with general information, sections 2 to 5 considered the four principle reprocessing methods of flexible ENT endoscopes (automated, manual immersion, wipes and sheaths). The last section considered the storage of the endoscopes.

The information requested referred to the way the endoscope was reprocessed by each participant and an evaluation of the method in relation to the needs of the department.

4. Survey findings

The following general considerations emerged from the study:

- The average number of endoscopic visits per day was around 10 and the majority of the doctors referred to difficulties in performing more examinations due to the limited number of instruments and the time necessary for reprocessing.

- Reference to guidelines is made in just above 30% of cases, they are not always the same and generally refer to gastroendoscopes/bronchoscopes (Figure 1).

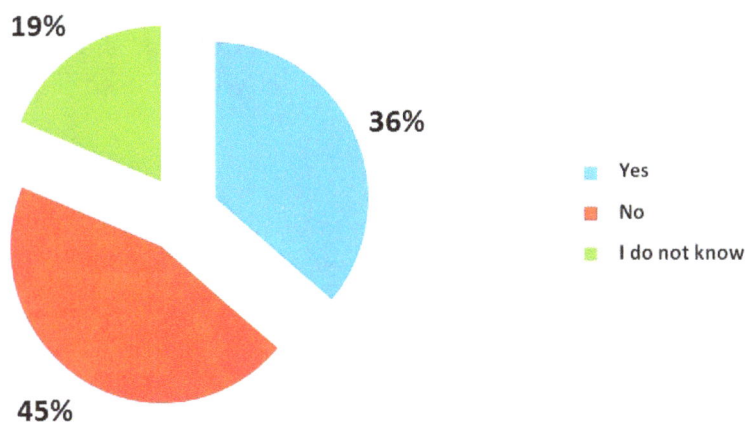

Figure 1

- *Manual immersion is the principle method (about 70% of cases)* for the disinfection of ENT endoscopes (Figure 2), followed by the sheath, which in 50% of cases is used in conjunction with other methods. The automated endoscope reprocessor (AER) is present in about 20% of the departments, but in over 60% of cases is used in conjunction with other systems, evidence maybe of the difficulties of habitual usage.

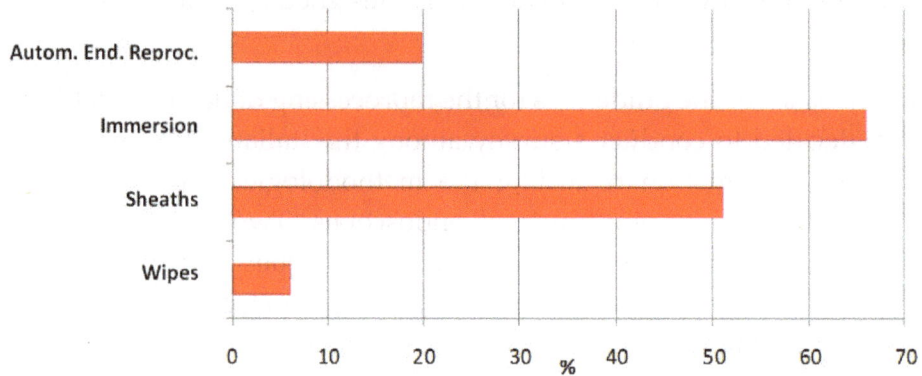

Figure 2

a.   Immersion

- Immersion is the most utilized method, both as a sole method and as a method used in conjunction with others. A basin or tray is mostly utilized for the immersion of the instrument.

- The leak test is performed in about 80% of cases.

- The enzymatic detergent is mostly used in the pre-cleaning step (about 50% of cases), while simple soap and water in about 20%. The time taken for pre-cleaning is normally less than 5 minutes, but can exceed 15.

- At least in 42% of cases the same detergent is re-used. It must be remembered that the detergent does not have any biocidal activity and so it is plausible that microbes can survive in the solution. As a consequence, a new solution should be used on each occasion.

- A wide variety of disinfectants are used for the disinfection step, mainly peracetic acid based, but also glutaraldehyde and orthophthalaldehyde are used (Figure 3).

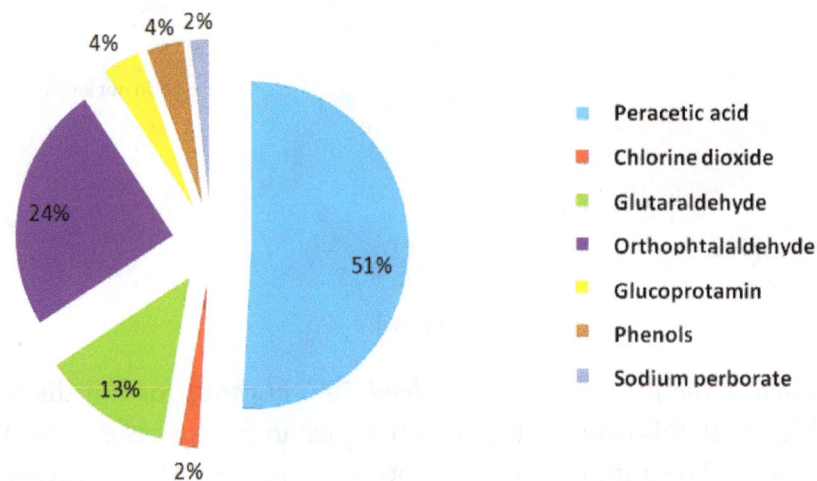

Figure 3

- From an analysis of the disinfectants used, it was noted that not all the products have been tested according to current European norms (EN 14885) and that different contact times have been indicated for the same product. *It is therefore important to underline that even if the disinfectants have the same molecular base, the formulations may be different and consequently the way in which they are used can be different.*

- The majority of disinfectants are multi-use which makes it difficult to implement a traceability system.

- For 75% of cases, the rinse step is performed by using tap water and is completed in less than 5 minutes.

- *The use of a traceability system is practically impossible with a re-usable disinfectant, but 95% of the respondents would appreciate a registration system.*

- In the evaluation of the method employed, *the respondents highlighted the problems of traceability and personal protective equipment.*

- The sheath is used in more than 30% of cases after disinfection, mainly for patients with a perceived risk of infection.

- Microbiological controls of the instrument are performed in less than 20% of cases.

b. Sheaths

- About 30% of ENT departments use exclusively the sheath. *It is mainly used in conjunction with other reprocessing methods, primarily for cases where the instrument must be used on patients with a recognized risk of infection.*

- Respondents expressed a critical evaluation regarding:

    1. the less than optimal adherence of the sheath,

    2. possible damage to the instrument, particularly during removal (50% of respondents),

    3. possible tearing of the sheath (17% of cases),

    4. reduced image quality (70% of respondents),

    5. patient discomfort, particularly children.

- The main reason for using the sheath is for better instrument turnaround (Figure 4), which can mean less expenditure for instruments. Avoiding cross-contamination and chemical products and practical usage are other important motivations.

- The overall evaluation is positive, but some *perplexity remains, particularly regarding traceability and the cost/benefit relationship* (from the sample the average cost of the sheath is around €10, but it can cost up to €25).

- The literature regarding the use of the sheath is limited, but where it exists, it is clearly indicated that the instrument needs to be cleaned and disinfected with ethanol after the sheath is removed in order to be equivalent with high-level disinfection. From the replies this occurs in only 2% of cases.

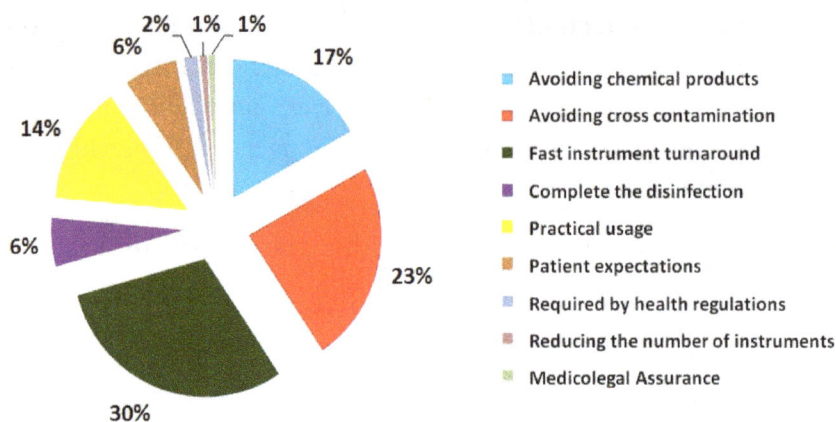

Figure 4

- Microbiological controls are performed in 17% of cases and leak tests in 82%.

c.   Automated endoscope reprocessors (AERs)

- In most cases, they are used in conjunction with sheaths (more than 50% of cases).

- In more than 33% of cases, the AER is not located in the department but in a central sterilization centre, affecting instrument rotation times.

- Cycle times vary between 20 and 30 minutes, which when added to the time for transporting endoscopes (when the endoscope is reprocessed outside the department) means that *the rotation time is about 1 hour in 70% of cases.*

- Pre-cleaning is mainly performed with an enzymatic detergent (75% of cases), but soap and water or only water are also used.

- The automatic reprocessors use mainly chemical disinfectants, notably single-use peracetic acid.

- The AERs can contain up to four instruments per cycle and in 75% of cases, both flexible and rigid scopes at the same time.

- Rinsing is normally performed while the instrument is automatically dried in only 50% of cases.

- The majority of AERs provide a confirmation print out for validation purposes, but the print outs are not always filed in a special record book.

- Microbiological controls are performed in 50% of cases, normally on a monthly basis and leak tests are nearly always performed.

d.   Wipes

- They are used by less than 10% of respondents probably due to their recent introduction.

- The leak test is performed less often compared to other systems (60% of cases).

- The overall evaluation is favourable, both regarding the practicality and the traceability.

- For patients with a known risk of infection, normally the sheath is also used.

e.   Storage

There are diversified methods of storing the instrument between one visit and another (Figure 5).

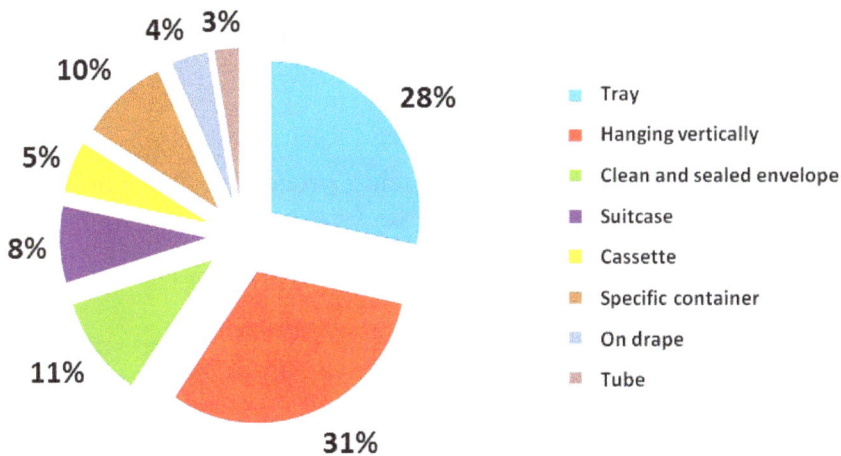

Figure 5

It is worth noting that about 10% of respondents store the instrument in its case, which actually represents one of the main sources of contamination.

From the answers, it can be seen that over 50% of respondents believe the instrument can be contaminated during storage, but, despite this risk, the disinfection cycle is performed in only 33% of cases on instruments being taken out of storage.

5. Principle problems related to endoscope reprocessing

Schematically, the problems most frequently encountered with endoscope reprocessing are associated with [6]:

- environment,

- organization of endoscopic activity,

- personnel.

Problems associated with the environment:

1.   the room or the disinfection area is not equipped with an extractor hood despite the use of certain disinfectants where it is specified,

2.   the presence of a sharp smell due to the disinfectant solution,

3. insufficient space in relation to the volume of activity,

4. no distinct separation between dirty and clean work surfaces,

5. environmental cleaning can be of poor quality.

Problems associated with the organization of endoscopic activity:

1. excessive volumes of activity in relation to staff allocation and equipments available.

2. unplanned endoscopic examinations affect the organization of the programmed work.

Problems associated to personnel:

1. Insufficient number of nurses,

2. the personnel are not aware of the reprocessing procedures or, when they are available, they are not known or shared,

3. respect of safety precautions by the operators is not optimal,

4. specific training of the personnel involved is not always performed.

6. Principles of hygiene in the endoscopic procedures [7, 8]

Abiding to the basic principles of hygiene represents the foundation for the control of risks of infection associated with endoscopic procedures.

These basic principles must be applied to

- equipment and medical devices,

- environmental surfaces,

- health operator behaviour.

The equipment and medical devices *are the principle vehicles for cross-infections in that they are continually contaminated by microbes originating from assistance to patients.*

They must be carefully cleaned and subjected to a process of high-level disinfection (or sterilization in the case of devices which can be placed in the autoclave) according to the indications of the manufacturer.

The environmental surfaces *are likewise a vehicle* for cross-infections in that they are continuously contaminated not only by environmental microbes but also by those originating from assistance to patients. The objective of the cleaning and disinfection of the surfaces is to ensure a low-level bacterial count and interrupt the risk of transmission of pathogens. *Sanitization should be performed with water and detergent.*

Disinfection should be performed preferably with chlorine-based disinfectants to ensure the destruction of the more resistant microbes.

The area where the disinfection of the endoscope takes place should be distinct from where the endoscopic examination is performed. A separate and specific room is "highly preferable"; but in the reality of the ENT department, unlike others such as gastroenterology, it is possible that the reprocessing of the endoscope is carried out in the same room as the patient's examination. It is necessary therefore *to highlight the need to ensure a clear division between contaminated areas (where the used instruments are placed) and clean areas (from where the reprocessed instruments are picked up)* so that the used instruments are completely separate from the reprocessed ones, avoiding risks of cross-contamination.

The *wash basins* should be of adequate dimension to allow the complete immersion of the instruments, without causing damage, preferably in steel (ceramic basins can be the cause of damage due to knocks to the terminal part of the instrument).

The necessity or not to install an extractor hood should be evaluated in function of the room and the equipment installed. It is absolutely necessary and essential if chemical products are used in open containers. Automatic systems which incorporate a device for the handling of vapours do not necessarily require the hood.

Where the room is not naturally ventilated, an *air ventilation system* needs to be installed (supply and extraction) in order to reduce to a minimum the exposition of everybody to the potentially harmful vapours (e.g. glutaraldehyde). In Italy, the limit of 10 air changes per hour is considered acceptable.

Operator behaviour *is critical for the prevention of cross-infections. Fundamentally, the principle that all patients are potential carriers of infections should be considered.*

Standard precautions

- should be applied by all health operators for all patients who receive assistance, irrespective of the diagnosis or the presumed state of infection,

- have the objective protecting health personnel and patients,

- should be based on the following healthcare practices:

  1. washing of hands and use of gloves,

  2. use of face masks, eye protection, smocks.

Written procedures should be present in all working environments with clear indications of each stage of the process.

Personnel must be taught to apply the "standard precautions" published periodically by the C.D.C. (Control Diseases Center of Atlanta) for infection control and should know:

- the procedure for cleaning and disinfecting each device,

- the conduct to follow in case of an alarm or malfunctioning of equipment,

- the biological and chemical risks which can be incurred during the disinfection procedure and how they should be encountered.

The responsibility of the disinfection procedure for endoscopes is attributed both to the nursing staff and to the doctor using the instrument. [5]:

- *the nurse and healthcare operator* are responsible for performing decontamination, pre-cleaning and disinfection of the equipment,

- *the head nurse of the operating unit* is responsible for verifying that the procedure is carried out correctly,

- *the doctor* using the instrument must visibly check that the instrument has been reprocessed before performing the examination,

- *the head consultant of the operating unit* is responsible for overseeing organizational aspects.

Endoscopes are very delicate instruments and therefore should be handled only by trained operators authorized to use and disinfect them.

The ENT operating unit together with the infection control unit should organize courses to train how to use and disinfect the endoscopes correctly and should keep an up to date list of all authorized personnel.

7. Risk of infection in endoscopy

The sources of infection are represented by infected or colonized patients [9] and by environment [10], in particular, the water used to rinse the endoscopes. Where possible, rinsing in sterile water is recommended. Differently, rinsing in high-quality drinking water is also acceptable using a bacteria-retentive filtering system (0.2 μ).

An observational study [11] conducted at 26 hospitals in the United States revealed that the endoscopes and bronchoscopes can be improperly disinfected due to inappropriate disinfectant solution, lack of control of the disinfectant's concentration, failure to clean all the parts of the endoscope and failure to measure manual disinfection times.

The *degree of risk* is classified as

- low when there is contact with healthy skin,

- intermediate when there is contact with the mucous membranes or superficially damaged skin,

- high for penetration into tissue or sterile cavities or into the vascular system.

The degree of risk determines the reprocessing level of the instrument used: *the risk of infection of the ENT endoscopes* (entering into contact with mucous membranes or damaged skin) *is intermediate and the high-level disinfection is then required.* [12, 7, 8]

High-level disinfection presumes the inactivation of all the bacteria, mycobacteria, fungi and viruses, but not necessarily of all bacterial spores. In ENT this is sufficient to have a guarantee regarding the transmission of pathogenic microorganisms for both the doctor and the patient.

7.1. High-level disinfection of endoscopes: traditional and emerging methods [13– 14]

We have categorized disinfection systems into two types:

1. *Traditional:*

   - *Immersion:* the operator manually performs all the steps of the disinfection,

   - *Automatic:* the disinfection is handled automatically without manual intervention,

2. *Emerging,* methods designed specifically for the ENT department:

3. *Complete reprocessing using wipes,*

4. *Immersion systems electronically controlled by a microprocessor:* part of the process is handled by the operator and part occurs automatically,

5. *Sterile protective sheaths*: constitute a protective barrier of the endoscope and not a system of disinfection.

The steps to reprocess endoscopes common to all traditional disinfection systems are described in Table 1. We must first emphasize the following points:

1. *reprocess the endoscope immediately after use* to prevent the formation of encrustations and consequent damage to the instrument.

2. *the entire endoscope must be cleaned and disinfected:* to be avoided are the wall tubes fitted in cui only the insertion tube of the instrument is placed, preventing contact between the control head and the disinfectant.

After analysing the reference literature, the authors suggest the following recommendations divided according to the type of disinfection system (Table 2).

In the following, we provide in detail the main considerations and evaluations for each system presented.

8. Traditional systems

1. Manual disinfection system by immersion

The manual procedure is relatively inexpensive but has the following disadvantages:

- errors or forgetfulness,

- lack of traceability,

- risk of contact between operators and contaminated material,

- damage to the instruments,

- disinfection times of at least 20 minutes.

2. Automatic disinfection systems

While until very recently only automatic systems for gastroscopies and bronchoscopies were available, today several companies realized washer-endoscopes for non-channelled ENT endoscopes.

The automatic systems can

- automatically cleanse, disinfect and dry,

- perform only the disinfection step.

These systems are composed of

- a tub for the disinfectant and one for the cleaning solution,

- a basin with a cover for the positioning of the endoscope. Washer-disinfector-endoscopes normally can reprocess several endoscopes simultaneously,

- a panel for setting the washing cycle (in general, the time and the temperature of the washing and disinfection sequences).

The disinfectant is transferred from the tub to the basin containing the endoscope and remains here for the time indicated on the technical sheet. This is followed by rinsing and the endoscope is ready for re-use.

In order to reduce the risk of contaminations, the washer-disinfector-endoscopes are usually equipped with thermal auto-disinfection systems.

It is advisable to position washer-disinfector in well-ventilated areas separated from those in which occurs the endoscopic examination.

When buying a washer-disinfector-endoscope, one should pay attention to the following aspects:

- automatic loading of cleanser and disinfectant,

- capacity to reprocess more than one endoscope simultaneously,

- programmability,

- the possibility of performing a complete cycle of cleansing, disinfection and rinsing,

- cycle time,

- the type of disinfectants for which the system is certified and their cost per cycle,

- the possibility of performing auto-disinfection/auto-sterilization,

- the presence of visual and sound alarms,

- required space,

- registration of procedures performed, an aspect strongly advised today because of medical–legal lawsuits. In general, the data that is recorded and/or printed are

  ○ identification number of the instrument;

- o details of the operator;

- o operating parameters relating to procedures;

- date and time of the procedure.

The automatic procedures therefore

- standardizes the process, reducing the possibility of errors,

- allows the immersion of the entire endoscope,

- makes it possible to "track" the procedures by printing a receipt after every disinfection cycle,

- reduces the risk of contact between operators or environment and contaminated instruments,

- reduces the risk of damage to endoscopes.

The main disadvantages are

- the cost of equipment and maintenance expenses; *some companies have product-specific washer-disinfector-endoscopes for ENT, smaller and less expensive* (Figure 6),

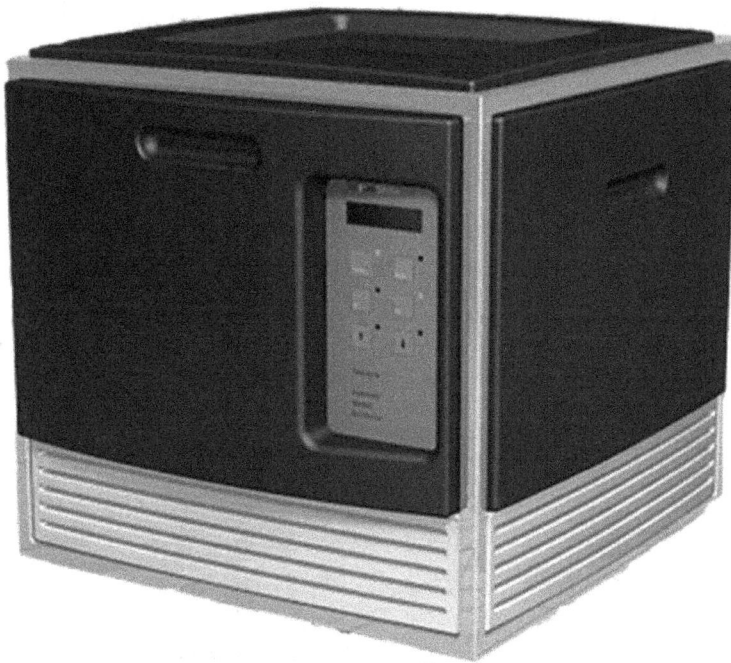

Figure 6

- the possibility of recontamination of the endoscopes by the same washer-disinfector,

- time required for the disinfection process (in general at least 20 minutes).

9. Emerging systems

9.1. Manual disinfection system with wipes

The disinfection system by means of wipes is a manual sporicidal disinfection treatment of semi-critical, non-channelled and heat-sensitive endoscopes.

The active ingredient used is chlorine dioxide (ClO_2), patented under the name "Tristel".

The Tristel Wipe System consists of a wipe for the pre-disinfection cleaning step, a wipe for the disinfection process and one for the post-disinfection rinsing step. The mechanical wiping action increases the efficacy of the cleaning and disinfection. The wipes are single-use and thus permit tracking of the procedures.

Treatment time is only 2–3 minutes allowing a notable reduction in disinfection times compared with other disinfectants in immersion methods. The Tristel Wipe System was in fact designed for the rapid turnaround of the ENT endoscope.

In addition, the wipes are non-toxic and non-irritating, thus allowing manual wiping technique not possible with the other traditional high-level disinfectants.

This simple system, however, is manual and can lead to different results between the various operators: accurate training is necessary to ensure that all operators are capable of optimal performance.

9.2. Immersion disinfection system electronically controlled by a micro-processor

This is a high-level disinfection system of the endoscopes by immersion controlled electronically. *The time necessary for disinfection is 5 minutes*, but the overall treatment time depends on the cleaning and rinsing method used, respectively, before and at the end of disinfection.

The system (Figure 7) consists of a base unit with a cover in which the instrument is placed, after cleaning, and to which is added the high-level disinfectant, ClO_2-based [15, 16].

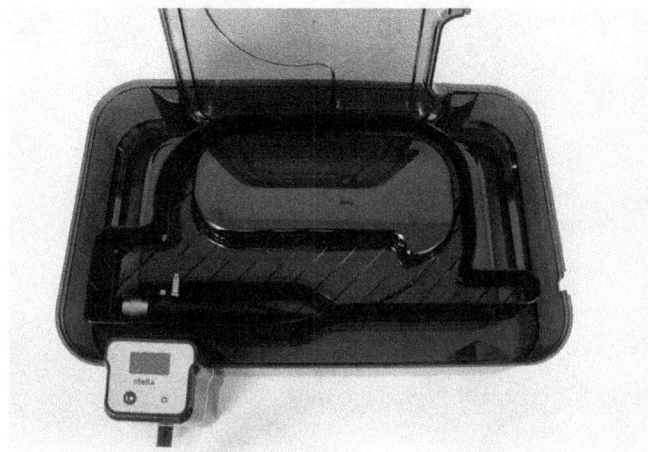

Figure 7

At the end of the disinfection cycle, the disinfectant is automatically emptied out in the sink and the instrument is rinsed manually.

At the end of the treatment, the base unit can be used as an aseptic container for short-term storage and/or for transport of the endoscope. The base unit and the cover are made of polycarbonate resin and can tolerate up to 30 autoclave cycles.

The micro-processor records every disinfection cycle and the recorded data can be downloaded on to the PC and archived, making it possible *to track the entire process*.

Placing the instrument in the empty unit and removing it only when the disinfectant is emptied out *avoids any skin contact with the disinfectant.*

Furthermore, the system is easily transportable because no connection to the electrical network is necessary; the only installation requirement is its positioning close to a sink in order to empty out the used disinfectant.

The immersion system with electronic control, by means of the micro-processor, ensures adequate contact time with the disinfectant and potentially damaging chemical overexposure, in addition to the ability to track the entire procedure.

9.3. Sterile protective sheaths

This is an endoscope encasing system that can represent an alternative to the high-level disinfection of endoscopes (Figure 8).

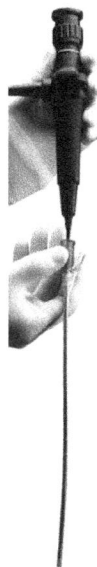

Figure 8

Various studies [17, 18] have demonstrated *the necessity to clean the entire endoscope with an enzymatic cleanser, followed by a disinfectant with 70% ethanol*, immediately after the removal of the sheath, in order to guarantee the equivalent of a high-level disinfection. In fact, it was seen that small viruses are capable of penetrating the sheath.

From our investigation conducted at ENT departments in Italy in 2010, we have seen that the practice of cleaning and disinfecting is done in only 2% of cases after removal of the encasing.

The advantage of this system is *the speed*.

The *disadvantages* are represented by:

- an increase of the diameter of the endoscope with the subsequent discomfort for the patient,

- the possibility of contamination of the control head unprotected,

- the risk of breakage of the sheath during the exam [19],

- the possibility of damage to the endoscope when removing the sheath,

- vision is not optimal,

- costs: endoscopes of various brands moreover require specific sheaths and their cost ranges from 8 to 25 euros.

To remember:

- The choice of disinfection systems should be made in agreement between the head of the operating unit, the hospital pharmacy, the hospital infection control committee and the indications of the endoscope manufacturer.

- Endoscopes which cannot be fully immersed should be substituted.

- Instruments should be reprocessed immediately after use because if allowed to dry for a long period, the residues can become encrusted and even damage the instrument.

- If the endoscope is immersed for too long a period, the outer casing and the seals can be damaged.

- The endoscopic examination should be avoided for patients with suspected Creutzfeldt-Jakob disease (prions are resistant to all forms of conventional sterilization). When the endoscope is considered really necessary, a dedicated endoscope should be used, maybe single-use, or else an instrument which is reaching the end of its life cycle. After use, the endoscope must be put in quarantine until definitive confirmation of the pathology.

10. Disinfection of endoscopes contaminated by HVB, HVC, HIV or mycobacterium [20, 21]

At the time of writing, there have been no reports of the transmission of viruses by means of bronchoscopes, while cases of the transmission of HBV and HBC by means of gastroendoscopes inadequately reprocessed have been reported.

The majority of viruses, including HVB, HVC and HIV, are quickly neutralized with disinfection solutions. The major risks of virus transmission reside in the unsuccessful removal of biological residues during the manual pre-clean, which allows the virus to avoid contact with the disinfectant.

Mycobacterium are responsible for an elevated percentage of contamination incidents referred to in the literature. All cases of tuberculosis have been attributed to the failed observance of infection control procedures.

Although some authors have sustained the need for longer disinfection times for endoscopes after use in patients affected by mycobacterium, this strategy is not required if infection control guidelines are carefully followed. Numerous studies have, for example, demonstrated that immersion for 20 minutes in a basic 2% solution of glutaraldehyde at 20°C, after an adequate pre-clean, significantly reduces the bacterial count of *M. Tuberculosis*.

11. Disinfection of endoscopes contaminated by prions [22– 23]

Prions are responsible for transmissible spongiform encephalopathy (TSE), capable of provoking degenerative diseases to the central nervous system in animals and man.

The most frequent disease from prions is Creutzfeldt Jakob Disease (CJD); other forms include variant Creutzfeldt Jakob Disease (vCJD), Gertsmann Straussler Scheinker syndrome (GSS), Fatal Familial (FFI), insomnia and Kuru.

Prions are resistant to common disinfectant substances. The tissues at high risk of infection include the brain, the dura mater, the spinal cord and the eyes, while tissues at low risk include cerebrospinal fluid, liver, lymph nodes, kidneys, lungs and spleen.

There have been no indications of cases of CJD attributable to devices contaminated with blood. Recognized cases of CJD as iatrogenic have been attributed to contaminated medical devices such as cerebral electrodes, cerebral neurosurgical instruments, dura mater grafts, corneal grafts, gonadotropins and human growth hormones.

From an analysis of the literature, it can be deduced that *endoscopes (apart from those used in neurosurgery) are devices which do not normally come into contact with tissues at risk of TSE* and consequently, even when used during diagnostic procedures on high-risk patients, standard reprocessing protocols are adequate.

The primary and principle preventive measure, however, in the case of high-risk patients, is *to limit endoscopic examinations exclusively to when necessary. If the examination is effectively necessary, it is advisable to designate one endoscope for such patients also for the future.*

In the case of an endoscopic examination which envisages contact with high and low risk tissues in a probably or certainly infected patient, the WHO guidelines indicate special treatments (sodium hydroxide, sodium hypochlorite, phenol, sterilization in autoclave) which are not compatible with endoscopes.

Seeing that the most common disinfectants used for endoscopes are not efficacious and considering the high cost of the instrument, some authors suggest covering the endoscope with a plastic sheath as a partial protection which can be eliminated after use as a special waste.

The ENT endoscopic procedures can, however, be managed without any special precautions due to the fact that the tissues with which there is contact are not considered infectious. For these patients, the standard protocols of pre-cleaning and high-level disinfection are adequate.

12. Biological controls

The monitoring infections resulting from endoscopic procedures cannot be an indicator of the efficacy of disinfection since infections are rarely linked to the execution of the endoscopic exam performed.

Moreover, the culture methods currently in use have not been rigorously validated, with the danger of underestimating or overestimating results, consequently causing potential harm to patients and health facilities. [24]

In the absence of adequate scientific evidence, the APIC (Association for Professionals in Infection Control and Epidemiology) and the CDC (Centres for Disease Control and Prevention) do not recommend routine microbiological tests and advise them *only in cases of epidemics*.

13. Tracking systems [5]

In every endoscopy unit, it is desirable to have a registration system in which the following information would need to be recorded for each procedure:

- examination number,
- patient generality,
- doctors and nurses generality,
- type of procedures,
- time,
- endoscope identification number,
- type of disinfection carried out.

The nursing coordinator of the unit should maintain

- documentation relating to installation, testing and maintenance of the washer-disinfector-endoscope machines (up to 5 years following the end of service),
- user's manuals for all the equipment,

- registration of biological controls carried out on the washer-disinfector-endoscope machines and on the endoscopes (at least 5 years),

- a copy of the print-out issued by the washer-disinfector-endoscopes, certifying the disinfection cycle (at least 5 years).

14. Disinfectants for the reprocessing of heat-sensitive, non-lumened ENT endoscopes

The survey findings indicated that peracetic acid and orthophthalaldehyde are the high-level disinfectants most commonly used for endoscopes. Chlorine dioxide is a disinfectant which is being increasingly used over the past few years.

Often, it is possible to find different disinfection solutions used for the same type of endoscope in the same hospital, and the use of a disinfectant as opposed to another is dependent on the operating unit.

Before examining the principle disinfectants, it is necessary to consider the following points regarding choice and usage [25, 26]:

1. Disinfectants must be registered at the Health Ministry and the technical bulletin should clearly indicate

- how to use,

- concentrations,

- contact times,

- temperature,

- pH.

2. Choose the disinfectant which is compatible with the endoscope in accordance with the indications of the instrument manufacturer.

3. The choice of solutions should be made in agreement with the pharmacy, health management and the heads of the operating units involved.

4. The disinfectants in use must be managed and stored in such a way as to avoid contamination (for example, containers handled with dirty hands and gloves, partial closure of packaging, etc).

5. When the disinfectant is re-usable, it is necessary

- to test the minimum effective concentration (MEC) at the beginning of the day. Results should be documented and the solution discarded when inferior to MEC,

- discard the disinfection solution at the end of the indicated usage period irrespective of the MEC. In cases where the disinfectant is added to AERs, the determination of the expiry date should be based on the original preparation date.

Monographs of the most commonly used disinfectant solutions are reported below *according to the information supplied by the manufacturers and the data from scientific literature.*

14.1. Glutaraldehyde (e.g. Cidex, Asep, Glutaster basica, Sporex) [27, 28]

Active ingredient

Glutaraldehyde or glutaric aldehyde in aqueous solution has a colourless or verging on yellow clear appearance and a pungent odour. The most common usage is a 2% *alkaline* solution.

Characteristics

Glutarladehyde is mainly commercialized in an acid form which is stabile for long periods when stored in cool conditions and in tightly closed container (up to 5 years).

Before use, glutaraldehyde must be "activated" by adding a buffer and surfactant in order to obtain a pH of 7.5–8.5. The activator (e.g. bicarbonate) is supplied separately and is used to obtain a working solution *stable for 14 days.* This period of validity refers to the activated solution in its original bottle, while the period of reusability should be considered in function of the concentration level, generally not less than 1.5% (the concentration diminishes in time and in function of the number of disinfections).

Mode of action

Glutaraldehyde is also defined as glutaric dialdehyde because it is endowed with two aldehydic groups (CHO), positioned at the extremes of the molecule, which are the real source of biocidal action; they are directly involved in the alkylation of sulphide, carboxylic, amino and hydroxyl groups of the proteins of the microorganism, causing an irreversible alteration of the protein synthesis and the nucleic acids.

Glutaraldehyde is not deactivated significantly by organic material even though its presence renders the disinfection less effective due to the fixative capability of glutaraldehyde, which creates a protective covering that prevents the destruction of the microbial cells. It is recognized in fact that glutaraldehyde is not efficacious against biofilm.

Spectrum of activity

The spectrum of activity of glutaraldehyde is almost complete but the contact times vary notably according to conditions, e.g. a 2% solution in laboratory has been demonstrated to be active in

- 1–2 minutes against bacteria in vegetative form (e.g. *Staphylococcus aureus*, including the penicillin, *Pseudomonas aeruginosa, Escherichia coli*),

- 5–10 minutes against viruses (e.g. *Poliovirus* Type 1, *Coxsackie* B1, ECHO 6, *Rotavirus*, HAV, HBV, HCV, HTLV-III/LAV),

- 10 minutes against yeasts, fungi and moulds (e.g. *Trichophyton interdigitalis, Microsporum gypseum, Candida albicans, Aspergillus niger*),

- 20 minutes against *Mycobacterium tuberculosis* whereas the activity is slower against other types of mycobacterium (at least 60 minutes) due to the lipidic component in the cellular wall which makes them almost impermeable. The contact time can be reduced by using a 3–4% solution and/or increasing the temperature to 25°C,

- 3 hours against spores. Concentrations less than 2% do not offer guarantees of being sporicidal, even with an increase in the contact time.

Material compatibility

Glutaraldehyde is not corrosive to metals and does not present particular problems for rubber, plastic, glass and optical fibres. It is necessary, however, to take precautions:

- objects in carbon steel should not remain in contact with the solution for more than 24 hours.

- it is necessary to avoid contact between different metals during immersion (danger of causing an electrolytic reaction, capable of corroding instruments).

Toxicity/precautions

Glutaraldehyde is a toxic, irritant and sensitizing substance and can cause, in the case of inadequate rinsing, rhinoconjunctivitis, asthma, diarrhoea and abdominal cramp.

The main risk of glutaraldehyde toxicity is run by the staff who have to handle it, because:

- frequent contact with the skin can cause dermatitis and a persistent yellow or brown colouring of the skin,

- contact with the eyes can cause reddening of the conjunctiva or grievous damage to the cornea.

- irritation to the conjunctiva with burning, lachrymation and reddening,

- damage to the respiratory system with bronchitis, dyspnoea, bronchial asthma,

- damage to the central nervous system with headache, depression,

- ingestion can cause from moderate to marked irritation to the mouth, throat, oesophagus and stomach, pains in the chest and abdomen, nausea, vomiting, diarrhoea, dizziness, drowsiness, shock.

The product did not result to be carcinogenic, for inhalation, on laboratory animals after continued exposure.

The literature reports TLV/TVA[1]values from 0.2 to 0.05 ppm.

For these reasons *the use of glutaraldehyde must*

---

1 Threshold limit value-time weighted average: average concentration of a chemical agent weighted on an exposure level of 8 hours and for 40 hours per week, to which operators may be exposed without adverse effects for their health being apparent.

1.   *Envisage the use of adequate personal protective equipment:*

   • protective eyewear,

   • authorized ventilators with filters for organic vapours, only in the presence of elevated vapours,

   • protective smock,

   • butyl or nitrile gloves or a double pair of latex gloves.

2.   *Envisage use in a ventilated environment, in closed containers and in the presence of adequate extraction systems.*

3.   Envisage staff training for correct usage and relative information regarding toxicity.

In the case of exposure, the first aid measures depend on the affected site:

• Contact with eyes: wash with plenty of water for at least 10 minutes. Remove contact lenses if possible to do easily. Visit the optician.

• Skin contact: remove contaminated clothes and wash with soap and water the affected parts of the skin. Consult a doctor if irritation persists.

• Ingestion: the product can cause ulceration and inflammation of the upper digestive system; it is preferable, therefore, not to cause vomiting but to resort to a cautious gastric lavage.

• Inhalation: transfer the person to a ventilated area. Artificial respiration may be necessary.

The use of glutaraldehyde as a high-level disinfectant is in constant decline, not particularly for reasons of efficacy, but rather for reasons linked to staff health and safety issues. It is worth noting that this chemical solution can no longer be used in British hospitals.

Disposal

The starting concentration of glutaraldehyde (2%) is possibly harmful. The concentration level, however, diminishes progressively due to re-use, evaporation and progressive dilutions.

According to Italian legislation, which has adopted European norms, disposal of the exhausted solution to sink is permitted, considering the high levels of dilution by water used daily for patient care. The sink must, however, be in a well-ventilated environment and disposal should be followed by running water to accelerate the discharge. Attention must be taken disposing large quantities directly into the sewers due to possible damage to the purification system through the inhibition of bacterial activity.

Indications for use

2% glutaraldehyde is indicated for the high-level disinfection of endoscopes and semi-critical medical devices with a contact time of not less than 20 minutes at a temperature of 20°C or more.

A contact time of 1 hour is advisable for bronchoscopes due to the slower mycobacterial activity. A satisfactory sporicidal activity is achieved after 3 hours.

After studying glutaraldehyde residues in plastic and rubber, after immersion in 2% glutaral-dehyde, it was concluded that a 2 minute rinse is sufficient to significantly reduce the quantity of the active ingredient absorbed in the exposed material, with the exception of natural rubbers for which a prolonged soak and rinse is recommended.

14.2. Orthophthalaldehyde (e.g. Cidex OPA, Opaster) [29– 30]

Active ingredient

An aromatic dialdehyde in commerce for a few years also in Italy, generally used at a concentration of 0.55% in an aqueous solution, with a lowly accentuated odour and blue colour. It is stable at 15–30°C for 2 years.

Characteristics

Unlike glutaraldehyde, orthophthalaldehyde (OPA) is ready to use and does not require activation. Once opened, the unused solution can be stored in the original bottle for up to 2 months while the solution poured into the disinfection tray can be used for no more than 14 days, providing that the concentration level is superior to the MEC (at least 0.3%) indicated by special test stripes. After 14 days the product must be disposed, even if the concentration is still superior to the MEC.

Mode of action

In the case of bacteria, OPA provokes the formation of crossed bonds between the cytoplasmic membrane lipoproteins with a subsequent cementation effect on the external layer of the cell and limitation of the exchanges. The periplasmic enzymes are also deactivated with consequent rapid death of the cell.

In the case of fungi and yeasts, the main interaction site is the chitin, principle component of the cellular wall, as well as the superficial enzymes present in the cellular membrane. As with glutaraldehyde, OPA is not effective against biofilm.

Spectrum of activity

OPA is capable of performing a rapid disinfection action in just 5 minutes at room temperature (20°C) on the majority of tested microorganisms, with the exception of spores for which higher concentrations and contact times (1% for 10–12 hours or 0.55% for 24 hours) are required.

Specifically, in laboratory, it is effective in:

- 5 minutes against bacteria in vegetative form (e.g. *Staphylococcus aureus, Pseudomonas aeruginosa, Salmonella choleraesuis, Enterococcus, Escherichia coli*).

- 5 minutes against viruses (*Adenovirus, Coxsackie virus, Citomegalovirus, Herpes simplex, HIV-1*, Human *Coronavirus, Influenza* Type A, *Poliovirus, Rhinovirus*),

- 5 minutes against yeasts, fungi and moulds (*Candida albicans, Aspergillus niger* and Trichophyton mentagrophytes),

- 5 minutes against *Mycobacterium bovis, M. avium, M. terrae, M. smegmatis,*

- 10 hours against the spores *Clostridium difficile* and *Bacillus subtilis*.

Material compatibility

OPA has proved to be compatible with a wide range of materials commonly used in the production of re-usable medical devices (metal, plastic, elastomers and adhesives) and, in many cases, it was found to be less aggressive than glutaraldehyde. Endoscopic instruments have undergone tests and are considered to be compatible with the solution. For prolonged contact times (greater than 15 minutes), the substrates with which it comes into contact can be subjected to permanent discolouring.

Toxicity/precautions

OPA is a molecule less volatile than glutaraldehyde and its toxicity, considering the same target organs, is of minor relevance.

Exposure to OPA has different effects according to the type of contact:

- Ingestion can cause irritation to the pharynx, esophagus and stomach with nausea, vomiting and diarrhoea.

- Skin contact can cause temporary blotches and slight irritations mainly after prolonged exposure. Such symptoms usually disappear when exposure is terminated.

- Eye contact can cause marks, excessive lachrymation and conjunctivitis.

- Inhalation: OPA is not considered volatile and is not thought to carry risks for inhalation during normal use. Exposure to spray or particulate can provoke, however, bland irritation to respiratory tracts with coughing and sneezing.

This product does not result to be mutagenic, embryotoxic or terotogenic in humans. Its components are not considered carcinogenic.

Occupational exposure limits have not, however, been established.

As with glutaraldehyde, the use of OPA also must

1. *Envisage the use of adequate personal protective equipment:*

    - protective eyewear,

    - authorized ventilators with filters for organic vapours, only in the presence elevated vapour concentrations,

    - protective smock,

    - butyl or nitrile gloves or a double pair of latex gloves.

2. *Envisage use in a ventilated environment and in closed containers* (if these requisites are satisfied, extraction systems are not necessary).

3. Envisage staff training for correct usage and relative information regarding toxicity.

In case of exposure, the same first aid measures for glutaraldehyde are valid:

- Eye contact: wash with plenty of water for at least 10 minutes. Remove contact lenses if possible to do easily. Visit the optician.

- Skin contact: remove contaminated clothes and wash the affected parts with soap and water. Consult a doctor if irritation persists.

- Ingestion: the product can cause ulceration and inflammation of the upper digestive system if ingested; it is preferable, therefore, not to cause vomiting but to resort to a cautious gastric lavage.

- Inhalation: transfer the person to a ventilated area. Artificial respiration may be necessary.

Disposal

According to Italian legislation, as with glutaraldehyde, disposal of the exhausted solution to sink is permitted, taking into account the high levels of dilution by water used daily for patient care. The sink must, however, be in a well-ventilated environment and disposal should be followed by running water to accelerate the discharge. The disposal of large quantities directly into the sewers can, however, cause damage to the purification system through the inhibition of bacterial activity.

Indications for use

0.55% OPA is indicated for the high-level disinfection of endoscopes and semi-critical medical devices with a contact time of at least 5 minutes at a temperature of 25°C in an AER and 12 minutes at 20°C in a manual immersion system.

Rinsing for at least 1 minute with copious water is sufficient to remove all traces of the disinfectant.

14.3. Peracetic acid (e.g. Nu Cidex, Steris, Persafe, Gigasept, Adaspor, Oxydrox, Perax liquid, Steradrox, Anioxide, SP3) [31, 32]

Active ingredient

Peracetic acid solutions are colourless or slightly yellow aqueous solutions, with a pungent odour and pH of around 6, containing a mixture of hydrogen peroxide and acetic acid.

The peracetic acid solutions commonly used in the medical field are:

- diluted working solution from concentrates,

- working solutions prepared by automatic systems which control all variables (dilution, temperature, contact times and pH),

- prepared to a defined concentration (0.35%).

Characteristics

Peracetic acid is an unstable compound and therefore it is necessary to store the concentrated solutions in bottles, preferably in a cool environment. *The working solutions should be prepared and are valid from 1 hour to 12 days depending on the type of dilution, on the pre-cleaning procedure and on the minimum recommended concentration.*

Mode of action

It has not been defined definitively; the activity seems to be linked to the strong oxidizing power both at the cellular membrane level of the microorganism (interruption of the chemiosmotic function) and inside the microbial cell (irreversible damage to the essential enzymatic system).

Being an oxidant, peracetic acid cleans and de-scales eventual deposits of the material.

Spectrum of activity

Peracetic acid is characterized by a rapid disinfection activity. A 0.35% solution in laboratory was seen to be effective in 10 minutes at room temperature against the following microorganisms:

- Bacteria in vegetative form (e.g. *Staphylococcus aureus, Pseudomonas aeruginosa, Enterococcus, Escherichia coli*).

- Viruses such as HCV, HIV, HBV, *Coronarovirus.*

- Yeasts, fungi and moulds (*Candida albicans, Aspergillus niger*).

- Mycobacterium such as *Mycobacterium tuberculosis, M. avium, M. terrae, M. smegmatis.*

- Spores of *Clostridium sporogenes, Bacillus subtilis, Bacillus cereus.*

Material compatibility

The activated solution demonstrates good compatibility with materials commonly present in medical devices, particularly endoscopes and AERs. It can cause discolouring of the insertion tube.

Toxicity/precautions

The concentrated solutions (>0.35%) and the peracetic acid vapours in contact with the skin and the mucous membranes can cause irritation, sometimes even severe; for this reason, it is necessary to rinse carefully all disinfected medical devices and wear appropriate personal protective equipment during handling:

- mask for acid vapours in case of emergency,

- protective gloves (neoprene or heavy rubber),

- protective eyewear,

- complete protective clothing.

The 0.15% commercial solutions are neither corrosive nor irritants (only slightly for the eyes).

The literature indicates TLV/TVA[2] values of 10 ppm.

In case of exposure, the following are required:

- Eye contact: wash with plenty of water for at least 10 minutes. Remove contact lens if possible to do easily. Visit the optician.

- Skin contact: remove contaminated clothes and wash with soap and water the affected parts of the skin. Consult a doctor if irritation persists.

- Ingestion: the product can cause ulceration and inflammation of the upper digestive system if ingested; it is preferable, therefore, not to cause vomiting but to resort to a cautious gastric lavage.

- Inhalation: transfer the person to a ventilated area. Artificial respiration may be necessary.

Disposal

Peracetic acid is not harmful and does not pollute the environment because it breaks down into acetic acid, water and oxygen.

Indications for use

Cartridges containing 35% peracetic acid inserted into a specific AER obtain, in controlled conditions, a 0.2% solution and operate at around 55°C with a contact time of 12 minutes. This does not seem to be a particularly suitable system for flexible endoscope reprocessing due to the cost of each cycle.

The stabilized and buffered 0.35% solution has, according to studies, the same indications, being effective in 5 minutes against bacteria, fungi, virus and mycobacterium and 10 minutes against spores. It should be prepared as a working solution and is stable for 24 hours. It can be used for up to 20 cycles or up to a concentration of not less than 2500 ppm.

Even though the solution contains anti-corrosion inhibitors, it is not recommended for use in AERs which contain aluminium or copper. Tests have demonstrated variations in the plating of rigid endoscopes which contain such metals.

The technical bulletin for the 0.15% stabilized solution indicates a contact time of 10–15 minutes for high-level disinfection and 30 minutes for sporicidal action. This solution must also be activated and disposed of every 24 hours.

As confirmed by the study carried out among the ENT departments, there are a variety of products marketed under the name of peracetic acid. The usage and the contact times vary according to the product and consequently it is necessary, to carefully follow the instructions supplied by the manufacturer, as well as verifying the compatibility of the product with the instruments which need to be disinfected.

14.4. Chlorine dioxide (e.g. ClO$_2$ Tristel) [26, 35, 36]

Active ingredient

A molecule composed of one atom of chlorine and two atoms of oxygen (ClO$_2$). The biocidal power of ClO$_2$ has long been recognized for use in different industrial applications and for the

---

2 Threshold limit value-time weighted average: average concentration of a chemical agent weighted on an exposure level of 8 hours and for 40 hours per week, to which operators may be exposed without adverse effects for their health being apparent.

disinfection of drinking water. The particular characteristic of this disinfectant is its broad spectrum of activity in rapid contact times at low levels of concentration. Its oxidizing capacity is the equivalent of 2.5 times that of chlorine. It can be used in manual systems, electronically controlled manual systems and also automatic systems.

Characteristics

ClO_2 is an unstable gas, it cannot be transported and therefore *must be generated at the moment of use*. The patented Tristel method envisages generation by means of mixing a sodium chlorite solution with a mixture of organic acids, prevalently citric acid. The almost instantaneous reaction between the two precursors produces chlorous acid, which in turn dissociates to release a ClO_2 gas in solution for immediate use at a level of concentration suitable for the sporicidal disinfection of semi-critical medical devices. The concentration of ClO_2 (read by spectrophotometry immediately at the end of the activation time) in the wipes system is 175–225 ppm (approximately 0.02%) while the diluted liquid format for immersion is 50–60 ppm (0.005–0.006%).

Mode of action

ClO_2 reacts almost instantaneously with of all types of microorganisms, creating an electron transfer to form a breach in the surface from which all vital constituents pour out of the microorganism with consequent destruction by lysis. The particular means of microbial destruction prevents bacteria, fungi and viruses developing resistance to the molecule and creating mutant strains.

Spectrum of activity

The ClO_2 activity in its different formulations has been tested microbiologically in laboratories according to the European norms EN 14885 to demonstrate its effectiveness.

It is effective *in 30 seconds in the ready–to-use format and in 5 minutes in the diluted liquid format for immersion on the following microorganisms*:

- Spores (e.g. *Bacillus subtilis* and *Clostridium difficile*),

- Mycobacterium (e.g. *M. tuberculosis, M. avium* e *M. terrae*),

- Viruses (e.g. HBV, HCV, HIV, *Poliovirus* Type 1, *Adenovirus, Orthopoxvirus*),

- Fungi (e.g. *Candida albicans, Aspergillus niger*),

- Bacteria (e.g. *Staphylococcus aureus, Pseudomonas aeruginosa, Enterococcus*).

Material compatibility

Instrument integrity is guaranteed when used with single-use ClO_2, providing the instructions are followed: *no damage has ever been noted from using the wipes system, neither after extensive laboratory testing nor after a decade of use in the field.*

Toxicity/precautions

The safety for people using ClO_2 has been confirmed by toxicological studies performed on both humans and animals. The results demonstrated that at the concentrations used there are no reactions or contraindications. It is however recommended to use gloves during handling.

Disposal

The solution of ClO_2 decomposes into a simple saline solution and consequently has no negative impact on the environment and does not entail additional disposal costs.

Indications for use

ClO_2 is indicated for the high-level disinfection of endoscopes and semi-critical medical devices. The formulation used in the wipes system is ready to use with a contact time of 30 seconds, while the diluted liquid formulation has a contact time of 5 minutes.

There is only one dilution with water at room temperature and pH adjustment is unnecessary.

14.5. Glucoprotamin (e.g. Sekusept Plus, Sekumatic) [36]

Active ingredient

Glucoprotamin is a substance with a wide spectrum of activity obtained from the reaction of glutamic acid and coco alkyl propylene diamine. Both precursors are natural compositions and therefore highly biodegradable.

Characteristics

A clear aqueous solution, yellow in colour, not volatile, which must be diluted in water from 1–4% without the necessity of additional activators. It is usable in both manual and automatic systems.

The solution is valid for 14 days.

Mode of action

Glucoprotamin operates by disrupting the cell membrane, by inhibiting the activity of the principle enzymes and denaturing the cell proteins.

Spectrum of activity

Glucoprotamin has a wide spectrum of activity against bacteria (including mycobacterium), yeast and fungi, enveloped viruses and partially effective against non-enveloped viruses. It acts specifically on the following microorganisms:

- Bacteria (tested on *Pseudomonas aeruginosa, Escherichia coli, Staphylococcus aureus, Micrococcus luteus, Enterococcus hirae, Gemella morbillorum, Corynebacterium* spp.),

- Mycobacterium (tested on *M. tuberculosis, M. avium* and *M. terrae*),

- Viruses (tested on HIV, HBV, HCV),

- Yeasts (tested on *Candia albicans*).

The contact time for bacteria is 5 minutes and 15 minutes for yeasts.

Material compatibility

The product has been tested and approved for use on Olympus and Storz endoscopes, Rusch anesthesia materials and Martin instruments.

Toxicity/precautions

Health risks: eye irritation.

The literature indicates TLV/TVA[3] values of 500 ppm.

Respiratory tract protection: none, in normal usage conditions.

Hand protection: wear protective gloves in nitrilic or butylic rubber.

Eye protection: wear protective eyewear.

Skin protection: none, in normal usage conditions.

In case of exposure, the following first-aid measures should be adopted:

- Eye contact: wash with plenty of water for at least 10 minutes. Remove contact lens if possible to do easily. Visit the optician.

- Skin contact: remove contaminated clothes and wash with soap and water the affected parts of the skin. Consult a doctor if the irritation persists.

- Ingestion: the product can cause ulceration and inflammation of the upper digestive system if ingested; it is preferable, therefore, not to cause vomiting but to resort to a cautious gastric lavage.

- Inhalation: transfer the person to a ventilated area. Artificial respiration may be necessary.

Disposal

The discharge of the product into the water network is damaging to microflora, microfauna and aquatic organisms for a brief period.

According to Italian legislation, disposal of the exhausted solution to sink is permitted, considering the high levels of dilution by water used daily for patient care. The sink must, however, be in a well-ventilated environment and disposal should be followed by running water to accelerate the discharge.

Indications for use

Glucoprotamin is indicated for the high-level disinfection and simultaneous detersion of flexible endoscopes, anaesthesia materials and semi-critical medical devices.

---

3 Threshold limit value-time weighted average: average concentration of a chemical agent weighted on an exposure level of 8 hours and for 40 hours per week, to which operators may be exposed without adverse effects for their health being apparent.

Glucoprotamin has been taken into consideration because its usage in some ENT departments was found in the survey findings. Evaluation studies of its microbial efficacy currently available indicate a wider spectrum of activity than intermediate disinfectants, but its efficacy against spores, a fundamental requisite for a high-level disinfectant, is not documented. Further research is necessary in order to confirm its use for the reprocessing of endoscopes.

15. Conclusions

15.1. General norms

1. Every patient should be considered a potential source of infection and consequently, each examination and all reprocessing procedures must be performed with the same accuracy.

2. The responsibility of the disinfection process is attributed to the nursing staff and the doctor using the instrument.

3. The choice of disinfection systems should be made in agreement between the head of the operating unit, the hospital pharmacy and the hospital infection control committee.

4. Staff should wear personal protective equipment during the endoscopic procedure and in the various phases of reprocessing of the instrument.

5. Contaminated and clean areas should be distinctly divided.

6. Disinfection should be performed by adequately trained staff, whose competence is periodically checked.

7. Periodic microbiological controls are not advisable as an indicator of the disinfection process. In case of suspected contamination, endoscope, tap water and instruments used in the disinfection process should be microbiologically tested.

8. When there is a suspected or ascertained case of infection, consult the hospital infection control committee.

15.2. Reprocessing steps

1. After the endoscopic exam, a leak test and a visual check of the integrity of the instrument should be performed before reprocessing.

2. Endoscopes which cannot be completely immersed should be substituted.

3. Before using the pre-clean or disinfection solution, consult the technical bulletin and the safety data sheet: concentration levels, temperature, contact time should be respected in order to achieve an effective disinfection.

4. The thorough cleaning of the instrument (immediately after use) with a detergent solution in order to remove soil and organic material is fundamental for a successful disinfection.

5. The disinfectant should be registered with the Health Ministry and the registration includes the indication of how to use, the concentrations, contact time, temperature and pH.

6. In the case of the disinfectant being reusable, it is necessary to:

    • Test the MEC of the disinfectant at the beginning of each working day. The results should be documented and the solution should be disposed if the concentration is below the minimum required.

    • Dispose of the disinfection liquid at the end of the period indicated for use without taking into account the MEC.

7. Rinse the endoscope according to indications and dry before storing. The humidity increases the risk of infections.

8. Keep a register of the endoscope usage and of the management and disinfection of eventual AERs.

15.3. Disinfection systems

The ideal disinfection system should allow

• standardization of the process, to reduce the possibility of error,

• rapid turnaround of endoscopes,

• reduction of risks of operator contamination,

• reduction of risks of damage to endoscopes.

Advantages and disadvantages of the various disinfection systems are indicated so that everyone can choose the one most adaptable to their local situation (human and economic resources, available space, volume of activity, number of endoscopes).

1. Manual immersion systems do not require big investments but have the following disadvantages:

• risks of errors or forgetfulness,

• inadequate "traceability",

• risk of operator contamination,

• risk of environmental contamination,

• damage to endoscopes,

• disinfection times of at least 20 minutes.

2. AERs:

• standardized process which avoids errors or forgetfulness,

- allows "traceability" of the process,

- reduces possible operator contact with contaminated instruments,

- reduces the possibility of environmental contamination,

- reduces risk of damage to endoscopes.

Possible disadvantages:

- equipment and maintenance costs,

- adequate space for installation of equipment (often at a distance from the endoscopic room with consequent loss of time due to transport and the increased risk of damage to the instrument during transport),

- time required for the disinfection process (normally at least 20 minutes). Added to transport times, the endoscope may not be available before 1 hour.

Some manufacturers produce AERs specifically for ENT endoscopes, smaller than those used for gastroenterology, easier to locate and at lower cost.

3. The wipes system using ClO_2

- allows a rapid rotation of the instrument (less than 5 minutes),

- allows traceability because the wipes are single use.

Although easy to use, the system is manual and therefore requires careful and continuous staff training to ensure that the procedure is performed correctly.

4. Manual immersion system with microprocessor:

- guarantees the contact time and avoids over exposure to chemistry which can potentially damage the instrument,

- allows traceability,

- has lower purchase and maintenance costs compared to AERs.

The pre-clean step and the rinse step are both manual and therefore require care.

5. Sterile protective sheaths:

allow a rapid rotation of the instrument, but the correct usage envisages cleaning and disinfection after sheath removal.

Disadvantages include

- possible discomfort for the patient,

- optical part of the endoscope not protected against contamination,

- possible rupture of the sheath during patient visit,

- possible damage to the endoscope when removing the sheath,

- hampered visuals,

- cost.

The choice of the disinfection system is made in consultation with the Director of the Unit, the Pharmacy Service and the Infection Control Task.

The nursing staff as well as the doctor using the endoscope are responsible for the disinfection process and must be adequately trained.

Author details

Matteo Cavaliere* and Maurizio Iemma

*Address all correspondence to: matorl@inwind.it

Department of Otorhinolaryngology, University Hospital "San Giovanni di Dio e Ruggi d'Aragona", Salerno, Italy

References

[1] American Society for Gastrointestinal Endoscopy (ASGE). Technology Assessment Committee Position Paper. Transmission of infection by gastrointestinal endoscopy. Gastrointest Endoscopy 1993;36:885–8.

[2] Birnie GC, Quigley A, Clements GB, et al. Endoscopic transmission of hepatitis B virus. Gut 1983;24:171–4.

[3] Bronowicki JP, Venard V, Botte C. Patient-to-patient transmission of hepatitis C virus during colonoscopy. N Engl J Med 1997;337:237–40.

[4] Morris J, Duckworth GJ, Ridgway GL. Gastrointestinal endoscopy decontamination failure and the risk of transmission of blood-borne viruses: a review. J Hosp Infect 2006;63:1–13.

[5] Agenzia Sanitaria Regionale dell'Emilia-Romagna. Reprocessing degli endoscopi. Indicazioni operative. Dossier 133, Bologna; 2006.

[6] Heeg P. Reprocessing endoscopes: national recommendations with a special emphasis on cleaning. The German perspective. J Hosp Infect 2004;56:S23–6.

[7] CDC. Guideline for Disinfection and Sterilization in Healthcare Facilities. University of North Carolina, Chapell Hill; 2008.

[8] CDC. Guideline for Isolation Precautions: Preventing Transmission of Infectious Agents in Healthcare Settings. University of North Carolina, Chapel Hill; 2004.

[9]   CCLIN Sud-Ouest-Centre de coordination de lutte contre les infections nosoco-
      miales. Prevéntion du risque infectieux en imagerie médicale non interventionnelle.
      Bordeaux 2004.

[10] Culver DA, Gordon SM, Mehta AC. Infection control in the bronchoscopy suite. Am J
      Respir Crit Care Med 2003;167:1050–6.

[11] Rutala WA, Weber DJ. Reprocessing endoscopes: United States perspective. J Hosp
      Infect 2004;56(2):27–39.

[12] Spaulding EH. Chemical disinfection of material and surgical materials. In: Block SS
      (ed.) Disinfection, Sterilization and Preservation. Philadelphia: Lea & Febiger; 1968,
      pp. 617–641.

[13] APIC Guidelines Committees. APIC Guideline for infection prevention and control
      in flexible endoscopy. Am J Infect Control 2000;28:138–55.

[14] Beilenhoff U, Neumann CS, Biering H, et al. ESGE/ ESGENA guideline for process
      validation and routine testing for reprocessing endoscopes in washer disinfectors, ac-
      cording to European Standard EN ISO 15883 parts 1,4 and 5. Endoscopy 2007;39:85–
      94.

[15] Isomoto H, Urata M, Kawazoe K, et al. Endoscope disinfection using chlorine dioxide
      in an automated washer-disinfector. J Hosp Infect 2006;63:298–305.

[16] Coates D. An evaluation of the use of chlorine dioxide (Tristel One-Shot) in an auto-
      mated washer/disinfector (Medivator) fitted with chlorine dioxide generator for de-
      contamination of flexible endoscopes. J Hosp Infect 2001;48:55–65.

[17] Alvarado CJ, Anderson AG, Maki DG. Microbiological assessment of disposable ster-
      ile endoscopic sheaths to replace high-level disinfection in reprocessing: a prospec-
      tive clinical trial with nasopharyngoscopes. Am J Inf Control 2009;37:408–13.

[18] Baker KH, Chaput MP, Clavet CR, et al. Evaluation of endoscope sheaths as viral
      barriers. Laryngoscope 1999;109:636–9.

[19] Awad Z, Pothier DD. A potential danger of flexible endoscopy sheaths: a detached
      tip and how to retrieve it. J Laryngol Otol 2009;123:243–4.

[20] Martin Y.H., Floss H., Zuhlsdorf B. The importance of cleaning for the overall results
      of processing endoscopes. J Hosp Infect 2004;56:S16–22.

[21] Schembre DB. Infectious complications associated with gastrointestinal endoscopy.
      Gastrointest Endosc Clin N Am 2000;10:215–31.

[22] Ippolito G, Petrosillo N, Suzzi R. Rischio di trasmissione iatrogena e nosocomiale
      dell'agente della malattia di Creutzfeldt-Jakob e misure di prevenzione. GIIO
      1997;4(2):66-71

[23] OMS World Health Organization. Infection control guidelines for transmissible spongiform encephalopathies. 2000.

[24] Beilenhoff U, Neumann CS, Rey JF, et al. ESGE-ESGENA guideline for quality assurance in reprocessing: Microbiological surveillance testing in endoscopy. Endoscopy 2007;39:175–81.

[25] ECRI. Healthcare Product Comparison System. Duodenoscopes; Gastroscopes; Choledoscopes 2004;2:1–10.

[26] Society of Gastroenterology Nurses and Associates. Guidelines for the use of high-level disinfectants and sterilants for reprocessing of flexible gastrointestinal endoscopes. Gastroenterol Nurs 2004;27(4):198–206.

[27] Agolini G, Raitano A, Vitali M. Glutaraldeide, una saga tutta italiana. View & Review, 1999;7:7–15.

[28] Scott E., Gorman S. Glutaraldeyde. In: Block SS (ed.). Disinfection, Sterilization and Preservation. Philadelphia, Lippincott Williams & Wilkins, 2001.

[29] McDonnel G, Pretzer D. New and developing chemical antimicrobials. In: Rutala WA, Weber DJ and the Healthcare Infection Control Practices Advisory Committee. (eds.). Draft Guideline for Disinfection and Sterilization in Healthcare Facilities. CDC, 2002.

[30] Rutala WA, Weber DJ. Disinfection of endoscopes: review of new chemical sterilants used for high-level disinfection. Infect Control Hosp Epidemiol 1999;20(1):69–76.

[31] Curti C. Una gestione razionale dei principi attivi usati per la disinfezione/sterilizzazione ospedaliera; schede monografiche: Acido peracetico. In: Raitano A, Curti C, Agolini G. (eds.) Igiene e disinfezione clinica nelle strutture ospedaliere. Principi e tecniche applicate per gli anni 2000. Edizioni Kappadue, 2002.

[32] Malchesky PS. Medical application of peracetic acid. In: Block SS. (ed.). Disinfection, Sterilization and Preservation. Philadelphia, Lippincott Williams & Wilkins, 2001.

Permissions

The contributors of this book come from diverse backgrounds, making this book a truly international effort. This book will bring forth new frontiers with its revolutionizing research information and detailed analysis of the nascent developments around the world.

We would like to thank all the contributing authors for lending their expertise to make the book truly unique. They have played a crucial role in the development of this book. Without their invaluable contributions this book wouldn't have been possible. They have made vital efforts to compile up to date information on the varied aspects of this subject to make this book a valuable addition to the collection of many professionals and students.

This book was conceptualized with the vision of imparting up-to-date information and advanced data in this field. To ensure the same, a matchless editorial board was set up. Every individual on the board went through rigorous rounds of assessment to prove their worth. After which they invested a large part of their time researching and compiling the most relevant data for our readers.

The editorial board has been involved in producing this book since its inception. They have spent rigorous hours researching and exploring the diverse topics which have resulted in the successful publishing of this book. They have passed on their knowledge of decades through this book. To expedite this challenging task, the publisher supported the team at every step. A small team of assistant editors was also appointed to further simplify the editing procedure and attain best results for the readers.

Apart from the editorial board, the designing team has also invested a significant amount of their time in understanding the subject and creating the most relevant covers. They scrutinized every image to scout for the most suitable representation of the subject and create an appropriate cover for the book.

The publishing team has been an ardent support to the editorial, designing and production team. Their endless efforts to recruit the best for this project, has resulted in the accomplishment of this book. They are a veteran in the field of academics and their pool of knowledge is as vast as their experience in printing. Their expertise and guidance has proved useful at every step. Their uncompromising quality standards have made this book an exceptional effort. Their encouragement from time to time has been an inspiration for everyone.

The publisher and the editorial board hope that this book will prove to be a valuable piece of knowledge for researchers, students, practitioners and scholars across the globe.

List of Contributors

Kenro Kawada, Tatsuyuki Kawano, Toshihiro Matsui, Masafumi Okuda, Taichi Ogo, Yuuichiro Kume, Yutaka Nakajima, Katsumasa Saito, Naoto Fujiwara, Tairo Ryotokuji, Yutaka Miyawaki, Yutaka Tokairin, Yasuaki Nakajima and Kagami Nagai
Department of Esophageal and General Surgery, Tokyo Medical and Dental University, Tokyo, Japan

Taro Sugimoto
Department of Otorhinolaryngology, Tokyo Medical and Dental University, Tokyo, Japan

Takashi Ito
Department of Human Pathology, Tokyo Medical and Dental University, Tokyo, Japan

J. G. Calleary, T. Lee, B. Burgess, R. Hejj and P. Naidu
Department of Urology, Pennine Acute Hospitals, North Manchester General Hospital, Crumpsall, Manchester, UK

Taku Sakamoto, Masayoshi Yamada, Takeshi Nakajima, Takahisa Matsuda and Yutaka Saito
Endoscopy Division, National Cancer Center Hospital, Tokyo, Japan

Lela Migirov and Michael Wolf
Department of Otolaryngology- Head and Neck Surgery, Sheba Medical Center, affiliated to the Sackler School of Medicine, Tel Aviv University, Israel

Phillip L. Chaffin, Jonathan M. Grischkan, Prashant S. Malhotra and Kris R. Jatana
Department of Otolaryngology-Head and Neck Surgery, Nationwide Children's Hospital and Wexner Medical Center at Ohio State University, Columbus, Ohio, USA

Somchai Amornyotin
Department of Anesthesiology and Siriraj GI Endoscopy Center, Faculty of Medicine Siriraj Hospital, Mahidol University, Bangkok, Thailand

Boonsam Roongpuvapaht, Kangsadarn Tanjararak and Ake Hansasuta
Department of Otolaryngology Head and Neck Surgery, Ramathibodi Hospital, Faculty of Medicine, Mahidol University, Thailand

G. Cossu, R. T. Daniel and M. Levivier
Department of Neuroscience, Neurosurgical Unit, University Hospital of Lausanne, University of Lausanne, Faculty of Medicine and Biology, Lausanne, Switzerland

M. Messerer
Department of Neuroscience, Neurosurgical Unit, University Hospital of Lausanne, University of Lausanne, Faculty of Medicine and Biology, Lausanne, Switzerland
Department of Neurosurgery, Kremlin Bicêtre Hospital, University of Paris Sud, Faculty of Medicine, Paris, France

M. George
Department of E.N.T., University Hospital of Lausanne, University of Lausanne, Faculty of Medicine and Biology, Lausanne, Switzerland

F. Parker and N. Aghakhani
Department of Neurosurgery, Kremlin Bicêtre Hospital, University of Paris Sud, Faculty of Medicine, Paris, France

Abdulzahra Hussain
Upper GI Surgeon at Airedale Hospital NHS Foundation Trust, Keighley, Bradford, UK
Honorary Senior Lecturer, King's College Medical School, London, UK

Matteo Cavaliere and Maurizio Iemma
Department of Otorhinolaryngology, University Hospital "San Giovanni di Dio e Ruggid'Aragona", Salerno, Italy

Index